Drug Misuse and Motherhood

The growing use of illicit drugs among women has become a major concern for health professionals and social services. The reluctance of drug-using women to seek help from drug agencies and to disclose their use of drugs to antenatal, midwifery and social services is now officially recognised by government agencies. However, devising an appropriate strategy that will overcome these fears will not be easy without a better understanding of their causes and effects.

Drug Misuse and Motherhood gives drug-using mothers a voice. Based on longitudinal research and in-depth interviews it provides new insights and much-needed information in five key areas:

- family life
- pregnancy
- motherhood
- service delivery and development
- implications for policy.

The user-perspective of this book is balanced by the professional viewpoint on the same issues. It offers a unique source of data for researchers and fresh inspiration for practitioners working in the field.

Hilary Klee, **Marcia Jackson** and **Suzan Lewis** are all at Manchester Metropolitan University.

Drug Misuse and Motherhood

Hilary Klee, Marcia Jackson and Suzan Lewis

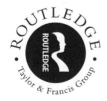

London and New York

First published 2002
by Routledge
11 New Fetter Lane, London EC4P 4EE

Simultaneously published in the USA and Canada
by Routledge
29 West 35th Street, New York, NY 10001

Routledge is an imprint of the Taylor & Francis Group
© 2002 Routledge

Typeset in Times by Florence Production Ltd, Stoodleigh, Devon
Printed and bound in Great Britain by MPG Books Ltd, Bodmin,
Cornwall

British Library Cataloguing in Publication Data
A catalogue record for this book is available from the British
Library

Library of Congress Cataloging in Publication Data
Drug misuse and motherhood / Hilary Klee,
    Marcia Jackson, and Suzan Lewis.
        p. cm.
    Includes bibliographical references and index.
    1. Women–Great Britain–Drug use. 2. Pregnant women–Great
    Britain–Drug use. 3. Mothers–Great Britain–Drug use. 4. Drug
    abuse–Great Britain–Prevention. I. Klee, Hilary. II. Jackson,
    Marcia, 1965– . III. Lewis, Suzan.

HV5824.W6 D79 2002
362.29'085'20941–dc21

ISBN 0–415–27194–0 (hbk)
ISBN 0–415–27195–9 (pbk)

Contents

List of figures   xi
Authors and contributors   xiii
Preface   xvii
Acknowledgements   xix
The research base   xxi

PART I
**The changing context: women, drugs and family
   life**   I

1 **Women, family and drugs**   3
   HILARY KLEE

   Mothers who use drugs 3
   Stigmatisation: counterproductive consequences 5
   Self-medication by women 6
   Parenting: changing family patterns 7
   The children 8
   *Perpetuating a cycle of substance misuse – the need for service
      intervention 10*
   References 11

2 **Women's use of drugs: gender specific factors**   15
   SAMANTHA WRIGHT

   The importance of gender specificity 15
   Gender differences: drug use 16
   Gender differences: the social context of drug use 19
   *Gender differences: access to and experience of drug treatment
      services 20*
   Summary 26
   References 27

3   **Concepts of motherhood**   32
     SUZAN LEWIS

     Motherhood as natural, instinctive and fulfilling 32
     Concepts of the 'good mother' 34
     Motherhood as work 36
     Motherhood as a social construction 37
     Ambivalent mothers and social pressures 38
     The idealisation and blaming of mothers 39
     Summary 41
     References 42

PART II
Approaching motherhood: the pregnancy   **45**

4   **Preparing for motherhood**   47
     HILARY KLEE AND SUZAN LEWIS

     Adapting 47
     Drug-using women – a disadvantaged group 48
     Coping 55
     The support needs of pregnant women 56
     Approaching the professionals 57
     Models of motherhood 60
     Conclusions 61
     References 62

5   **Antenatal care: expectations and experiences**   63
     HILARY KLEE

     Failure to attend 63
     The need for reassurance 68
     The need for information 71
     Evaluation of antenatal services 73
     Professional collaboration 75
     Summary and conclusions 76
     References 77

6   **Drugs and pregnancy**   78
     HILARY KLEE

     Drug use: the early months 79
     Methadone: attempts to reduce and abstain 82

Independent action 86
Quality of information: the health professionals' perspectives 88
Conclusions 90
References 91

7 Informal support: partners and mums   **93**
HILARY KLEE

Introduction 93
Partners 94
Mothers 99
Conclusions 102
References 103

8 Practitioner views of pregnant drug users   **105**
MARCIA JACKSON AND HILARY KLEE

The uptake of services 105
Practitioners' views of drug users' parenting capacity 108
Alternative professional perspectives 109
Moves towards professional collaboration 115
Drugs knowledge, education and training 119
Conclusions 122
References 122

PART III
Motherhood   **125**

9 Hospital confinement   **127**
HILARY KLEE

Admission to hospital 127
Infant health 133
Admission to Special Care Baby Unit (SCBU) 136
Treating Neonatal Abstinence Syndrome 140
Staying on in hospital 141
Summary and conclusions 143
References 144

10 Drugs and parenting   **145**
HILARY KLEE

Early demands 145
The positive aspects of motherhood 149

Coping 150
Risk factors and parents' prevention strategies 152
Conclusions 161
References 163

11   Relapse: missing the window of opportunity   **165**
HILARY KLEE

Coping with demands 165
*The relative importance of support and continuing drug use by
    the partner 168*
A role for grandmothers 170
Friends 171
Seeking professional support 172
Summary and conclusions 175
References 175

12   Mothering and drugs: four case studies   **177**
MARCIA JACKSON

Case 1: Mandy 177
Case 2: Diane 183
Case 3: Linda 186
Case 4: Brenda 190
Summary 193

13   Child protection: social workers' views   **195**
JULIAN BUCHANAN AND LEE YOUNG

The ideology of child protection: from 'care' to 'control' 196
*The restructuring of the welfare state and its impact on social
    work 200*
Child protection: social workers' views 202
Conclusion 207
Recommendations 208
References 209

PART IV
Service delivery and development   **211**

14   Neonatal Abstinence Syndrome   **213**
STEPHEN WALKINSHAW, BENJAMIN SHAW AND CATHERINE SINEY

Prediction of neonatal opiate withdrawal 214

Identification and recognition of Neonatal Abstinence
  Syndrome 216
Summary 221
References 221

**15 The role of drug services for pregnant drug users: the
    Liverpool approach**   **224**
SUSAN RUBEN AND FRANCES FITZGERALD

Aims and objectives of the Pregnancy Support Group 225
Agreed protocol for the Pregnancy Support Group 225
The pregnancy clinic 226
Initial assessment by the drug services 228
The care plan 230
*Sharing antenatal care: the role of the specialist health
  visitor 235*
Sharing postnatal care 236
Summary 237
References 238

**16 The drug liaison midwife: developing a model of maternity
    services for drug-using women from conception to creation**   **239**
FAYE MACRORY

The background to the project 239
Building the framework 242
The role of the drug liaison midwife 244
Antenatally: through birth and beyond 246
Conclusion 248
References 248

**17 Providing care for pregnant women who use drugs:
    the Glasgow Women's Reproductive Health Service**   **250**
MARY HEPBURN

The Glasgow Women's Reproductive Health Service 250
Effects of drug use on pregnancy 252
*Management of problem drug use in pregnancy:
  general principles 253*
Obstetric management 256
Social management 258
Summary 259
References 260

PART V
Implications for policy   261

18 Overcoming the barriers   263
HILARY KLEE

Negative discrimination: being judged 264
Exposure of drug use 265
Professional inconsistency on drug management 266
Professional credibility and patient confidence 266
Fear of social work intervention 268
Working together: professional consistency 272
Summary and conclusions 274
References 275

19 Dilemmas of child welfare and drug dependence   276
HILARY KLEE

Reconciling the irreconcilable 276
Reducing the risk 277
Social work dilemmas 278
The advantages of family therapy 280
Relevance to the UK 281
Conclusion: avoiding family break-up 283
References 283

**20 Drugs policy and practice development in the
United Kingdom**   285
HILARY KLEE

International service guidelines and recommendations 286
The United Kingdom 288
Services for drug-using parents: the UK guidelines for
    inter-agency working 289
Models of care: the drug liaison midwife 291
Models of care: multi-agency collaboration 292
Models of care: advocacy 294
The case conference 294
The future of services for drug-using pregnant women 295
References 296

Notes   298
Index   299

Figures

14.1   Liverpool neonatal drug withdrawal chart   219
14.2   Liverpool guidelines for management of drug
        withdrawal   220

Authors and contributors

Julian Buchanan is a Senior Lecturer at the North East Wales Institute of Higher Education. He worked as a drug specialist in the 1980s where he pioneered a risk reduction approach to drug-using offenders. He was also involved in establishing one of the largest interagency community drug teams in the UK. He has researched and written widely on the subject of drug use.

Frances Fitzgerald has been a Health Visitor since 1990. Prior to moving to work as a Specialist Health Visitor at the Liverpool Drug Dependency Clinic, she worked as a Child Protection Facilitator in addition to her role as Health Visitor. She has particular responsibility for pregnant and newly delivered drug-misusing mothers, and acts as an on-site resource for drug services in relation to child protection issues. She also works with, and supports, other Health Visitors in Liverpool who have drug-misusing mothers on their case loads.

Mary Hepburn trained first as a GP, then as an obstetrician and gynae-cologist. She established, and is a consultant in charge of, the Glasgow Reproductive Health Service for women with social problems, including drug use. She is currently senior lecturer at Glasgow University jointly in the Departments of Obstetrics/Gynaecology and Social Policy/Social Work, and Honorary Consultant Obstetrician and Gynaecologist at the Glasgow Royal Maternity Hospital. Her clinical interests concern the effects of deprivation on health, and the design and delivery of appropriate services for those with special needs.

Marcia Jackson studied psychology at Manchester Metropolitan University. She subsequently worked as a drugs counsellor in North Manchester and was also a volunteer for a street-based project, offering information and practical advice to prostitutes working in the city centre. She returned to Manchester Metropolitan University some years later to conduct this research into the needs of drug users during pregnancy and early motherhood. Marcia is currently a full-time mother to her two young daughters.

Hilary Klee is Research Professor in Psychology and Director of the Centre for Social Research on Health and Substance Abuse (SRHSA) at the Manchester Metropolitan University, UK. Her research has covered a wide range of drug misuse and health concerns, for example: polydrug use and the misuse of prescribed pharmaceuticals; HIV-related risk behaviour; peer-group leaders and prevention; pregnancy, motherhood and drugs; drug-using parents; and drug use among the young homeless. Her special interests lie in the areas of amphetamine misuse, and women's use of drugs.

Suzan Lewis is Professor in Psychology at Manchester Metropolitan University and one of the Directors of the multi-site Work–Life Research Centre. Her main research interests are family and work, and gender issues. Her previous publications include: *The Work–Family Challenge. Rethinking Employment*, Sage (1996); *Dual Earner Families. International Perspectives*, Sage (1992) and *Career Couples*, Unwin Hyman (1989). She is co-editor of the international journal *Community, Work and Family*.

Faye Macrory was responsible for the development of the post of Drug Liaison Midwife in Manchester which aimed to improve the accessibility and appropriateness of maternity services for drug-using women and their families. An interagency collaborative support system was established across city-wide services to enhance the quality of care for this client group. She also works with a non-statutory street agency that serves the needs of sex workers, giving antenatal care when required. Her role in the treatment support of pregnant drug users also includes providing training both locally and nationally about the many complex issues associated with drug use. She is well known for her work to improve services for drug-using pregnant women. She was awarded an MBE in 1997 for her dedication in this area.

Susan Ruben is Consultant Psychiatrist at the Liverpool Drug Dependency Clinic. She has been a Consultant in Liverpool since 1998 and has been active in developing a range of services for drug misusers within Liverpool. Her particular interest has included setting up a Multi-Agency Pregnancy Support Group which takes a holistic approach to substance misuse. She is a member of the Government's Advisory Council on the Misuse of Drugs. In view of her interest in motherhood it seems appropriate to mention that she was also named *Liverpool Echo*'s 'Mum of the Year' in 1994.

Benjamin Shaw is a Consultant Neonatologist at the Liverpool Women's Hospital. His major interests are neonatal respiratory disorders and neonatal withdrawal. With Cath Siney he is responsible for developing guidelines for the management of drug withdrawal in neonates and an assessment chart associated with those guidelines for use by ward staff. He is a member of the Pregnancy Support Group which is part of the Specialist Drug Service for pregnant drug users in Liverpool.

Catherine Siney was the first Drug Liaison Midwife in the country, starting the service in Liverpool in 1990. The service links Liverpool Maternity and Gynaecology Services with agencies providing care and/or treatment throughout the city and its surrounding areas for people who have drug problems. She lectures regularly at universities and for health authorities in the UK and abroad. She has published papers and articles in medical, nursing and midwifery journals and has contributed chapters to a number of books. She has also contributed to and edited two books, *The Pregnant Drug Addict* (1995) and *Pregnancy and Drug Misuse* (1999).

Stephen Walkinshaw is Consultant in Maternal and Foetal Medicine in Liverpool. He co-ordinates the services provided for high risk pregnancies within Central Liverpool and has responsibility for the care of women requiring preterm delivery transferred from other hospitals in Mersey Region. His research focuses on pragmatic, randomised clinical trials.

Samantha Wright worked for the Centre for Social Research on Health and Substance Abuse (SRHSA) between 1995 and 1999 researching a variety of projects in the drugs field including the effectiveness of treatment for amphetamine users, drug-using parents, the education and employment histories of drug team clients, and steroid use among bodybuilders. She has a strong interest in women's drug use, and in the dynamics of family life among drug users.

Lee Young is Lecturer and Course Director of the MA in Social Work course at the University of Liverpool. He worked in the area of children and families social work for many years. His last five years in practice were as a specialist social worker at the Liverpool Drug Dependency Unit, where he was instrumental in setting up a multi-agency support group for pregnant drug users – a model now reproduced in a number of other areas. He has researched and published in the area of policy and practice in relation to drug services and drug use more generally.

Preface

The idea for this book emerged during research on pregnant drug users that had been conducted over several years with only small-scale funding and with little expectation of sustaining it in the long term. We are grateful to the Department of Health for their support that enabled us to complete the study and to extend and complement the data with research on parenting.

The misuse of drugs by women is a growing interest among health professionals and policy makers in the UK and in other developed nations. International seminars and conferences on the topic have been sponsored by the World Health Organisation, the Council of Europe Pompidou Group and the United Nations. Many others have been organised at national level. The inadequacy of drug treatment services has been noted consistently, and the absence of information about women's needs, including those of pregnant women, has become a matter of concern. The needs of women have now assumed an increasingly important part of the range of topics for further research and attention by service providers and policy makers. There is a particular interest in pregnant drug users and drug-using mothers as drug use by women of child-bearing age increases and is not matched by a corresponding rise in those known to treatment and maternity services. All data suggest that they fear the exposure of their use of drugs to the authorities and avoid contact.

The early literature on maternal drug use, mostly published in the US, focused on foetal damage and this issue induced increasingly punitive reactions in some states with the adoption of mandatory drug testing and treatment. In the UK the problem has been raised only rarely in the media and is mainly associated with child deaths through the accidental consumption of methadone prescribed for a parent. However, attitudes towards drug-using mothers have hardened further, partly through their involvement in the transmission of HIV infection to their children, which has intensified their fears and social isolation.

Drug users challenge the ideal image of the caring mother. Women are seen as providers and guardians of their family's health. In particular, they are responsible for children's health, and substance abuse is regarded as incompatible with that role. The phenomenon is universal and generates attitudes that are not only based upon stereotypical profiles of the mothers but also ignore their vulnerabilities and needs. Ultimately this is counter-productive because it deters drug-using women from attempting to seek help.

Although awareness of women's needs has risen considerably in the UK over recent years, the organisational response from drug and maternity services has been slow. Since pregnant drug users form an increasingly large high-risk population, the need for measures to improve the quality of care for them has become urgent. However, there is evidence already that services can rise to the occasion in meeting the needs of pregnant drug users. At present this is found most in inner-city areas with significant drugs problems where they cannot be ignored. Lack of experience is closely associated with judgemental attitudes and hostility and not only undermines the quality of the care available, but is transparent to women who are already primed and sensitised to it in advance. An understanding of the histories and lifestyles of drug-using women and the pressures on them can endow their carers with insights that underlie truly professional discharge of a service that is judgement free. What has been lacking so far is information that can lead to views that are not distorted by prejudice or limited by conventional stereotypes. The aim of this book is to provide such information.

Acknowledgements

We would like to thank the women who participated in the research that underpins this book for their patience in staying with the project over such a long period of time and for their readiness to talk about their lives. We found their accounts illuminating and believe they will help to improve services for other mothers in the future.

No less illuminating were the observations of the service providers involved in the research. They offered alternative perspectives that increased our confidence in the veracity of our data. Despite the pressures that most were experiencing, they spared the time to talk at length about their observations and were willing to reflect on them with reference to the service they were supplying to drug-using women.

We are also very grateful for the contributions to this book from practising professionals. They provide descriptions of their services that will be valuable to those who seek to establish specialist services or wish to improve them.

Finally, thanks are due to the Department of Health, UK, for providing the funding for this work. The views expressed in this book are those of the authors, however, and not necessarily shared by the Department of Health.

The research base

SUMMARY

The research on which this book is based had two principal goals. The first was to document the experiences of women drug users during pregnancy, through childbirth, and into the early months of the child's life. The second was to describe the parenting strategies of drug users and the hazards faced by their children as a result of their parents' use of illicit drugs. The latter used data on drug-using parents selected from a number of our drug misuse projects that sampled different user groups. Both studies were commissioned by the United Kingdom Department of Health Task Force to Review the Effectiveness of Services for Drug Users, the grant-holders were Hilary Klee, Marcia Jackson and Suzan Lewis for the first, and Hilary Klee for the second. The views presented in the chapters that are the product of these studies are those of the authors and not necessarily of the Department of Health.

More specifically, the aims of the pregnancy study were to:

- Identify the clinical and social problems experienced by pregnant drug users and mothers.
- Identify their needs during pregnancy and early motherhood.
- Record changes in drug use over time.
- Document:
  1 their perceptions and experiences of maternity services and
  2 their expectations and experiences of social service interventions.
- Reveal current thinking on clinical treatment protocols for pregnant drug users among health care professionals.
- Document a range of service providers' views and experiences of drug-using pregnant women.
- Provide an analysis of the structural relationships between service providers – the nature and extent of liaison and communication – and their views of these relationships.

The aims of the parenting study were to:

*   Reveal the approaches to parenting by drug users.
*   Highlight the hazards for children and examine the parents' responsiveness to them.
*   Document parents' own efforts to protect their children.

The needs of women drug users have been neglected in the past by service providers. The majority of them are of child-bearing age and yet relatively few present to services. As a result, little is known about their lives at this particularly critical time. The longitudinal nature of the pregnancy study offered an opportunity to observe many aspects of the women's lives as they came to terms with the pregnancy and adapted to the arrival of a new baby. These data are supplemented here by observations on how the women's needs were being met by drug and maternity services. It is the 'customer' perspective that drives this research strategy, not least because the women's views have not so far been heard and disseminated. However, the views of service providers add additional insights into the difficulties of the task they face, and in this book the contributory chapters by practitioners on the changing nature of service provision help to identify ways they can be overcome.

From another perspective, child protection is the focus of increasing public concern in Europe and the United States. Many interventions by the authorities are associated with parental drug misuse. More babies are being born to drug-using women and higher proportions of their children are taken into care than in the general population – their home environment is regarded as potentially more hazardous to children born and reared there. In addition to possible damage caused through neglect, if not direct abuse, by parents who use drugs, there may also be the detritus from communal drug taking and injecting, and role modelling of drug users who do not conceal their activities. The stereotype of the 'junkie' parent, like most stereotypes, may be the product of ignorance and prejudice, but although it is challenged at times, it has not been subject to objective analysis. The data on parenting expanded the scope of the pregnancy study, which provided data up to approximately 18 months after the birth of the child, by examining data from parents with children of all ages. The data extracted from these studies were restricted to their parenting practices and examined qualitative data on parenting from diverse research samples to evaluate the evidence.

THE PREGNANCY AND EARLY MOTHERHOOD STUDY

The sample comprised pregnant drug users recruited through drug agencies, antenatal clinics, drugs outreach workers and through networking drug-using groups in the community. In anticipation of an attrition rate of approximately 20 per cent over the course of the research, some over-recruitment was built in. This rate was fairly low for longitudinal research among drug users but was based partly on our previous experience in this region of rates of 30 per cent, and the expectation that this group would be less mobile because of their children and therefore easier to track. A target of 50 respondents remaining in the cohort after six months was set. By the second interview, the sample had reduced from 64 to 51, most ($n = 9$) lost through relocation, and was 50 at the third interview. The rate of attrition was higher at the fourth interview largely because the extended period between interviews led to loss of contact, particularly with those at some distance or who had relocated. Thirty-two respondents were interviewed. In view of the decrease in sample size at this time, analyses of critical variables over time used data from the first, second and third interviews only, in order to avoid possible distortion of results through factors that could underlie this loss.

Semi-structured interviews were conducted with respondents by an experienced research worker (Marcia Jackson) and recorded on audiotape. These were subsequently transcribed for qualitative analyses. The women were visited in their homes at regular intervals by the researcher to record ongoing experiences in their lives, including those arising from their interactions with service providers. Home visits offered a more relaxed environment for the interviews and facilitated the development of a high level of rapport as well as opportunities for direct observation of the women's domestic context and lifestyle. The women were interviewed first during their pregnancy; then within a month of childbirth; then six months later. After an extension to funding provided by the Department of Health, attempts were made to contact respondents for a final interview. At this stage the children were between 18 months and two years old.

The research instrument

The range of questions was broad and included closed questions where previous research or pilot work had allowed a range of responses to be identified in advance. These yielded immediately quantifiable data for quantitative statistical analyses. Open questions yielded more detailed 'insider accounts' of experiences and attitudes. Such questions are more appropriate where prior information is low and they were used in three ways: to inform interpretation of statistically analysed data; to use in the formation of categories of responses that could be quantified; and to generate new ideas for further exploration. The first interview was comprehensive in its coverage: questions included, *inter alia*: current drug use; current treatment if any; physical and mental health; contraception; attitudes to pregnancy and childcare; experiences of antenatal care; expectations concerning the birth; interactions with health and social welfare professionals and attitudes towards them;

informal support from partner, family and friends; and expectations concerning the future use of drugs. The second interview focused on the period
in hospital and current health and care of the infant but also included questions on antenatal care, use of drugs in the final month of pregnancy, and
postnatally, contact with health professionals and social workers and support
from partners and family. The third and fourth interviews were concerned
with the mother's health and coping behaviour; informal support from partner and parents; contact with health professionals and social workers; the use
of drugs by mother and partner; and the anticipated future use of drugs. The
interviews lasted between an hour and a half and two hours.

Analyses

With a sample of 50 respondents about whom little was known we believed
that it was appropriate to focus as much on the qualitative analyses of
themes and critical issues as on standard quantitative parametric and non-
parametric significance tests of associations. Quantitative data and analyses
appear in full in *Illicit Drug Use, Pregnancy and Early Motherhood* (Klee,
H. and Jackson, M. (1998) available from the authors). Findings referred
to in these chapters are significant at or beyond the conventional level of
5 per cent. Thematic analyses using three independent judges were used on
verbatim material transcribed from taped interviews. In reporting verbatim
material all names contained within them have been changed to protect the
identity of respondents and their children.

The location for both this research and the parenting study was the same:
the north-west of England. The area comprises the Greater Manchester area,
Liverpool and its suburbs and other large towns in the region. This is an
area well known in the UK for the severity of its drug problems.

Sample characteristics

Mean age of the women was 25 years, range 18 to 35 years. For 28 per
cent it was their first baby and for 32 per cent it was their second child.
Forty per cent had more than one child. Nine mothers (18 per cent) had
children in care or looked after by relatives. Thirteen (26 per cent) reported
previous miscarriages and 10 (20 per cent) abortions. For the majority (72
per cent) this was an unplanned pregnancy, three-quarters (74 per cent)
used no contraception, 20 (40 per cent) believed they could not become
pregnant. Twenty (40 per cent) of the sample had seriously considered
aborting the current pregnancy.

The preferred drug of the majority (57 per cent) of the women was
heroin and 54 per cent of these consumed it during pregnancy, for 23 per
cent it was amphetamine and 38 per cent consumed it during pregnancy,
and 8 per cent named cannabis as their first choice, 67 per cent consuming

it during pregnancy. All of the respondents had both illicit and licit drugs in their repertoires. Amphetamine users and heroin users did not overlap in their preferences. No one consumed alcohol more than occasionally. All smoked cigarettes. Forty-one (82 per cent) were in treatment at the time of the first interview.

A high proportion (60 per cent) had been injecting prior to their pregnancy but this reduced to 18 (36 per cent) after becoming pregnant. Some injected in the early weeks or months when they were not aware that they were pregnant and two of these women subsequently stopped. Nonetheless, this means that over a quarter injected drugs during pregnancy.

Forty-four women had a regular sexual partner at the start of the study; the majority of them were drug users, 64 per cent using hard drugs and 20 per cent using only 'soft' drugs, mostly cannabis. Fifteen (34 per cent) partners were injecting.

Health care and social services

A small supplementary study was added to the main study comprising health care and social workers ($n = 49$) from the eight hospitals and five drug agencies in the areas from which the women were drawn. Thirty-four were maternity staff: hospital, community, and drug liaison midwives; special care nurses; obstetricians and paediatricians. Fifteen were drug workers and social workers. A more ambitious coverage was beyond the resources of this study.

Mixed methods of data collection were used: individual interviews and focus groups. These generated accounts of the professionals' experiences of drug-using pregnant women and mothers, and their views of the service provided to them, that were subjected to qualitative thematic analyses. Sampling across a heterogeneous range of experience yielded views that were influenced by direct experience on the one hand and those that were indirectly derived on the other. This was important since the stereotypes of drug-using women are strong and likely to occur generally across most occupational groups. In this case, the impact of such prejudgements was likely to affect the service available to the women. There are significant limitations to the degree of extrapolation from such a small sample and although some useful comparisons are made, they should be regarded as offering indications of the nature of deficiencies in services for pregnant drug users and should not be used as estimates of their prevalence.

THE PARENTING STUDY

Our research on health and drug misuse over the years included in the samples a high proportion of parents, and data on parenting were acquired serendipitously. Much of this was unguided by questions, but certain themes and issues reliably arose across all projects. We were commissioned by the Department of Health to perform a retrospective analysis of these data. These were undertaken as a first step towards an understanding of the nature of risk factors in the home environment and any protective factors that may exist. The studies used were undertaken between 1990 and 1998. They yielded samples of different categories of drug users comprising heroin or polydrug users and primary amphetamine users that yielded an aggregated sample of 240 parents.

In all studies of drug users the methods were the same: semi-structured interviews conducted by research workers, mostly located in respondents' homes and recorded on audiotape. Respondents were encouraged to elaborate their responses and it is these responses that form the basis for the qualitative data reported here. They were supplemented by field notes. The additional data are used in Chapter 10 on Drugs and Parenting and also inform the observations on child protection and prevention initiatives covered in Chapter 20 on Policy and Practice.

Further statistical details on the pregnancy study can be found in Klee, H. and Jackson, M. (1998) *Illicit Drug Use, Pregnancy and Early Motherhood* SRHSA, The Manchester Metropolitan University, and on the parenting study in Klee, H., Wright, S. and Rothwell, J. (1998) *Drug-Using Parents and their Children: risk and protective factors* SRHSA, The Manchester Metropolitan University, both available from the first author.

The changing context
Women, drugs and family life

This first part attempts to construct a context for the information that is to come later and comprises three chapters that focus on complementary topics: current attitudes to women who use illicit drugs, gender differences in drug use, and the concepts of motherhood that prevail in contemporary society. They are components of the broader picture, and the themes that emerge in subsequent sections of this book may be understood more fully by having a greater awareness of their implications.

The first chapter presents background material on drug-using women, locates them in the history of changing patterns of drug use and associated public health issues, examines public attitudes towards them, what keeps them in a drug lifestyle and what the consequences may be for their children.

In the second chapter, Samantha Wright provides a more detailed picture of women's use and experience of drugs by comparing them with men. These are particularly important benchmarks in evaluating their experiences when they present to drug treatment and antenatal services. The neglect of women's needs becomes more apparent when they become pregnant.

The third chapter by Suzan Lewis explores contemporary images of motherhood that drive so powerfully public attitudes towards mothers. These are perhaps epitomised by the 'squeezy mum' image that has appeared in TV advertising for half a century. The idealised and romantic nature of popular stereotypes leads to demands that many women cannot meet and that are particularly unrealistic for drug-using women.

Chapter 1

Women, family and drugs

Hilary Klee

This book is about women who use illicit drugs, get pregnant and become mothers. It reveals that a stressful and possibly hostile social environment awaits a drug-using woman when she becomes pregnant. It is a world in which her dependence on drugs on the one hand, and unattainable rosy concepts of motherhood on the other, will set constraints on her behaviour and require major changes in her life. Whether welcomed or not, the pregnancy is likely to cause strain on her personal and interpersonal resources that must be faced and overcome in order to ensure the delivery of a healthy baby and its normal social development.

MOTHERS WHO USE DRUGS

A range of factors is likely to contribute to the ease with which a drug-using woman negotiates the path through her pregnancy and hospital confinement. They include the wider context of trends in drug use and the social and political responses to them that mould public opinion. In the last two decades there have been developments in the ways that illicit drugs are used that have resulted in societal consequences of global proportions. Within this period the start of the AIDS pandemic occurred, which is not only decimating populations in Africa and Asia but continues relentlessly to invade new territories (UNDCP, 2000). Injecting illicit drugs was, and still is, a part of this new and apparently unstoppable 'plague' and has become a serious public health issue. The threat of viral transmission has raised the spectre of drug users as a source of terminal disease. Their actions in sharing their injecting equipment are seen as potentially lethal, not only for other drug users in their communities, but for anyone who has sexual contact with them. An already unacceptable form of behaviour which was not responding to threats by the state and stigmatisation by the public was demonised further when drug use became associated with AIDS.

For women to use street drugs seems to plumb an emotional reservoir of distaste and fear in the public, perhaps because of the role they are expected to play in society as caring wife and mother. The implications for family life are serious and justifiably cause much concern. However, it is interesting that a wide range of attitudes have been exposed towards women drug users that can be positioned on a dimension of tolerance, with liberals at one end and the savagely punitive at the other. Internationally the balance seems heavily in favour of the latter. Sadly, the issues associated with drug use evoke powerful emotions that encourage a degree of polarisation that seems intractable to resolution or compromise.

There are also the 'innocent victims' of drug-using mothers: their children. Revelations of foetal damage were seized upon in the US by news media that were keen participants in the 'War on Drugs' and obsessed with crack-cocaine users (see Reinarman and Levine, 1997). Already blamed for escalating crime figures, this was censure that could be attached most specifically to women. The sex industry, regarded as another aberrant aspect of womanhood, is a major source of funding a drug habit for female drug users that can involve risk of sexual transmission of HIV and hepatitis C through unprotected intercourse. However, it is the vertical transmission of disease from seropositive mother to child that seems to have been particularly influential in revealing public opinion on drug-using pregnant women, and this became one of the most emotive issues in HIV epidemiology.

Reactions to women using drugs are generally negative in all nations but risks of drug-induced damage to the child, combined with transmission to them of HIV, resulted in public actions in the US that resembled mediaeval witch hunts in Europe. The start of the 1990s saw a media-fuelled panic about 'epidemics' of cocaine use during pregnancy. Crack babies, it was predicted, 'present an overwhelming challenge to schools, future employers and society' (Murphy and Rosenbaum, 1999). Crack mothers were demonised; it was widely reported that they were indifferent to their children or directly abusive. Punitive legislation followed and criminal prosecution enacted in several states that resulted in their incarceration (Boyd and Faith, 1999; Centre for Reproductive Law and Policy, 1996), the publicity helping to perpetuate stereotypical representations of drug-using mothers in public consciousness. Irrespective of the risks of HIV, as female drug misuse continued to increase, women were criticised for bringing children into the world already damaged by their mother's drug habit. It is suggested that the hostility was made worse by selective reporting of clinical data on the postnatal effects of cocaine use (Zuckerman et al., 1998) which favoured negative outcomes with little regard to more positive fine detail concerning their severity or longevity.

Typically the discourse surrounding drugs was and still is densely populated with condemnatory and stigmatising judgements on women's behaviour. An otherwise useful study on social workers' views of child neglect and abuse (Reid and Macchetto, 1999) frequently lapses into emotional, if not incendiary language: 'A devastating tornado of substance abuse and addiction is tearing through the nation's child welfare and family court system leaving in its path a wreckage of abused and neglected children, turning social welfare agencies and courts on their heads and uprooting the traditional disposition to keep children with their natural parents.'

Reactions to the rising number of pregnant drug users have been more muted elsewhere and the approach to containment of the negative consequences of illicit drug use in several European countries is guided by the philosophy of harm reduction. This is a perspective that is 'more pragmatic and less idealistic, more reality based and less moralistic, and more focused on what *could* be done rather than what *should* be done' (Rosenbaum and Irwin, 1998). Public attitudes towards pregnant drug users and drug-using mothers in Europe may be similar to those in the US, but there seems to have been no research on this topic.

STIGMATISATION: COUNTERPRODUCTIVE CONSEQUENCES

Perhaps the most wide-reaching and long-lasting effect of the apparently merciless judgement of drug-using mothers by the press, the law and the public has been their increasing reluctance to approach medical services (Guerra, 1998; LGDF/SCODA, 1997; Mounteney, 1999; Sheridan, 1995) (see also Chapter 2). This can only add to the health risks for their children and for themselves. The view that there may be reasons for women turning to drugs has rarely been considered. Many women presenting for drug treatment report histories of childhood abuse and domestic violence (Ludwig and Anderson, 1989; Miller *et al.*, 1989; Nelson-Zlupko *et al.*, 1995; Roth, 1991; Russell and Wilsnack, 1991) and drug-using women tend to be victims of violence throughout their lives (Amaro *et al.*, 1990; Bollerud, 1990; Miller, 1998). Research that could produce insights into the consequences of such histories from the women's perspective has been comparatively rare. In the US, NIDA[1] has mounted diverse re-search programmes on women's use of drugs, but the value of in-depth social studies, while having a long history, has only slowly become recognised (Boyd, 1999; Colten, 1980, 1982; Murphy & Rosenbaum, 1999; Rosenbaum, 1981) and researchers who seek the views of drug users are still relatively rare in the American literature.

Despite the universally hostile attitudes to the use of drugs of dependence by women, and the correspondingly punitive consequences of transgressions, female drug use has been rising for some time (UNDCP, 1994), though perhaps undetected in many areas. The trend was described by a working group of the Council of Europe in 1996 in a way that hinted of surprise and concern '. . . in recent years drug use amongst women in

Europe has been undergoing dramatic changes . . . with women rapidly progressing towards similar levels of drug misuse as seen amongst men' (Council of Europe, 1995). The proposal for treatment services to address women's needs has received much support, but the ongoing debate has yet to be translated into policy and evidence-based practice. It is to be hoped meanwhile that a restrained and realistic view of drug use among women will prevail and that the needs of drug-using mothers will be met without prejudice

SELF-MEDICATION BY WOMEN

Increasing use of illicit drugs by women is partly accounted for by a tendency for women to self-medicate (Khantzian, 1985) their anxiety, depression and fatigue with drugs. The universal role of women as carers and protectors assigns to them heavy responsibilities (Glenn, 1994). Women are critically involved in the health and well-being of others. Even as children it is usually the female child that is expected to respond to family needs when these exceed the capacity of the mother (UNDCP, 1994). Perhaps such responsibilities, combined with greater familiarity with home-based treatment of domestic ailments, have contributed to the tendency for them to diagnose and self-treat. This has a long history that goes back to the 1950s and 1960s when prescriptions, first for sedatives and then amphetamine-based stimulants, were easily acquired, the latter over the counter (OTC). Advertisements at the time were aimed largely at women (Kandall, 1998) who were more likely to receive prescriptions than men. Kandall concludes his observations on female drug dependence with the assertion that 'a significant component of the problem of female addiction has come, and still comes from the inappropriate and excessive medicating of women by physicians and pharmacists, and through self-medication'. Should problems arise in maintaining legal supplies, strategies are widely used by both men and women that take the form of fraudulent statements. Most commonly reported are those made to doctors that allow them to obtain prescriptions from a number of clinics; and the nature of the symptoms being experienced which require heavy painkillers or sedatives. There is also a long history of collusion by physicians in private medicine who exploit this market. The drugs may change, but the practices continue. The limits imposed on benzodiazepine prescriptions once their dependence potential was revealed has now resulted in high profits for companies manufacturing fluoxetine (Prozac) which is prescribed significantly more often for women than men (Kramer, 1993). Self-medication through OTC drugs and the diversion of prescribed drugs to be shared by family members is a strategy that carries even less risk of detection for women than turning to illicit supplies or street drugs.

The attraction of pharmaceutical substances is understandable. They are safer than illicit drugs, have recognised therapeutic value, are pure, and the side effects are known. They do not carry the stigma of illicit drugs. Some have euphoric psychoactive effects, particularly if used in large quantities. Common examples are some anxiolytics, and OTC drugs that contain pseudo-ephedrine and codeine. Anorectics for weight control are amphetamine based and their use, mostly by women, is increasing worldwide (UNDCP, 1996) helped by liberal prescribing in 'health clinics' that results in diversion on to the illicit market. Most anorectics induce the usual positive effects of amphetamine on mood and energy, as well as suppressing appetite, which are an added bonus. Women diagnosed as overweight or obese and prescribed amphetamine have been known to respond to the termination of the supply by their doctors by going on to street supplies, resulting in some cases in significant dependence and absorption into the drug subculture (Klee, 1997). Amphetamine in another form (methylphenidate) is prescribed to improve the behaviour of 'difficult' children with ADHD (Attention Deficit Hyperactivity Disorder), and alleviate consequent family stress. Although particularly widespread in the US, this is increasing rapidly in Australia and there are signs of a similar trend in Europe (UNDCP, 1996). In all cases there is a risk of diversion on to the illicit market. The easy availability of drugs with psychoactive as well as therapeutic properties combined with the increasing use of the Internet for information and purchase, allows people to by-pass the normal controls imposed by GPs. This is a large 'grey area' of abuse about which very little is known.

PARENTING: CHANGING FAMILY PATTERNS

A trend that will affect parenting of future generations is the departure from the tradition of two-parent families. 'There has been substantial growth in lone parent families over the last 25 years. Lone parents headed 22% of all families with dependent children in Great Britain in 1995' (*Social Focus on Families*, 1997). The trend seems almost wholly due to a rise in the proportions of lone mothers, since the proportion of lone fathers has remained about the same.

There seem to be several features that are shared by lone mothers and drug-using women, most notably economic disadvantage and its consequences in family dysfunction and social isolation. There are many factors associated with lone parenting that are said to contribute to family dysfunction, for example: lone parents generally have much lower incomes; they depend more on state benefits and 'tend to be more likely to be living in overcrowded and poorer quality accommodation than other families' (*Social Focus on Families*, 1997).

The UK trends in family structure seem to be following those of the US which has a higher proportion of single-parent families than any other developed country (Weinraub and Gringlas, 1995). Research there showed that children of single-parent families are more likely to have difficulties with emotional and psychological adjustment, school performance and educational attainment and more likely to have behavioural problems than children of two-parent families. Similar patterns can be seen in drug-using families (Reder and Lucey, 1995) and in particular, that children are at high risk for later substance misuse themselves (Tarter and Mezzick, 1992).

Economic disadvantage seems fundamental to an understanding of these patterns and affects many other aspects of home life that may not be so obvious but are also typical of women living in deprived circumstances. For example, though a higher proportion of income is often spent on food, diet may be more restricted, with degrees of malnourishment associated with this. Diet and weight problems are very common features of heavy drug use, though this may be more to do with self-neglect. Social isolation can become a significant source of stress within the family for whom employment opportunities are limited. Peck and Plant (1986) argue that unemployed people may turn to drugs to restore purpose in their lives and suggest that 'drug use fulfils many of the social and psychological needs that are normally met by employment'. Family discipline and parental control may then be disrupted and lead to criminal activity. A higher proportion of teenage children from lone parent families report having offended (*Social Focus on Families*, 1997) and problems such as child custody and children taken into care are particularly pronounced. Fears of removal of children into care are, as we shall see throughout this book, a major influence on drug-using mothers that leads to a reluctance to approach helping agencies.

THE CHILDREN

The problems associated with social disadvantage and isolation among drug-using women perhaps become most marked during pregnancy and can influence their parenting behaviour. Health and attachment problems in mother and child cannot be related to drug consumption in a straightforward way: 'Poor pregnancy outcomes in women drug users may be due not so much to the drugs as to the underlying socio-economic deprivation or the effects of drug use on lifestyle' (Hepburn, 1993; also Chapter 17).

Associations between child neglect or abuse and substance dependence among parents have been claimed many times. They are implicated in an increasing number of children entering foster care in the US (Famularo *et al.*, 1992). While there is extensive evidence of risk most particularly to mental health (Velleman, 1992; Velleman and Orford, 1993) a clear and simple relationship has not been found (Mounteney, 1998). Substance abuse, poverty, psychiatric problems and domestic violence all feature in such analyses in a complex way and not in terms of cause and effect (Sheridan, 1995). Does substance abuse, like many other factors, contribute to family dysfunction that is associated with child neglect and abuse? The guidelines from the Institute on the Study of Drug Dependence on child-care by drug users assert 'Drug use does not itself indicate neglect or abuse' (Mounteney, 1999).

Addicted women's parenting has been characterised by neglect, physical and emotional abuse, excessive control and punishment, inconsistent discipline and lack of emotional involvement (Mayes, 1995). It is suggested that features of the home environment and maternal characteristics are more powerful in shaping child development than is exposure to drug use per se (Kumpfer, 1998) and include, *inter alia*, poor family relationships, maternal mental illness and diversion of family resources into maintaining drug supplies. However, a recent study (Suchman and Luther, 2000) that looked at the relationships between maternal addiction, child maladjustment and socio-demographic factors in determining parenting behaviours, concluded that socio-demographic factors such as poverty, education and unemployment contributed as much, if not more than, maternal addiction.

The evidence from parents themselves is generally unavailable since empirical studies of parenting by drug users have not often been reported in published literature. This is understandable since drug-using parents attempt to remain hidden to avoid the attention of the authorities. Traditionally the literature on drug use and parenting has focused on the effects of drug use on the unborn child, largely based on US data (Deren, 1986; Hawk, 1994; Zellman, 1993), and research on parenting by alcoholics. Research on drug-using parents is a much more recent phenomenon.

In the UK the problem of damage caused to infants by drug-using mothers has been mainly associated with accidental deaths of children through the consumption of methadone that is prescribed for a parent, or through cases of child neglect. There appear to be no statistics on such events. Media coverage is fairly low key but this does not mean that underlying emotions are not strong, only that they are revealed at a more private and personal level. The existence of such judgements is one reason for writing this book since they exert an effect on the health and welfare of drug-using women and their children that is damaging to them and self-defeating for those who provide services to them.

PERPETUATING A CYCLE OF SUBSTANCE MISUSE – THE NEED FOR SERVICE INTERVENTION

There has been much discussion concerning the perpetuation of family dysfunctionality across generations. In studies of adults' early attachment experiences, significant links have been found between how a mother views her own history, and the quality of her attachment to her baby (Burns and Burns, 1988) which sets up a multi-generational cycle of drug misuse and family dysfunction that needs to be broken (see Kumpfer, 1998). Hoffmann and Su (1998) investigated the relationship between adolescent and parental drug use and found the adolescents to be at increased risk of stressful life events, peer drug use and less emotional attachment with parents. They suggested that a cycle of drug use could develop that is characterised by poor family relations and greater influence of drug-using peers. These observations tended to support the view that parental drug use effectively pushed the child away from close family involvement (Stice and Barrera, 1995).

In the face of the number of interconnected problems revealed in the literature, of which drug dependence is only a part, the main goal of services in the US is increasingly seen as developing interventions that prevent family dysfunction and the exposure of children to damaging lifestyles and stress. Procedures that offer more than just treatment for substance abuse are needed according to Sheridan (1995), for example a procedure that incorporates parenting skills (National Children's Bureau, 1994) and does not deter parents from approaching health and social services (see Chapters 17 and 18). However, the achievement of effective interventions that are popular with drug-using parents will not be easy.

The LGDF (Local Government Drugs Forum) and SCODA (Standing Conference On Drug Abuse) in the UK produced new guidelines in 1997 for those working with drug-using parents and advised: 'Families with a drug-using parent need to be able to ask for advice and help, without fear of being drawn inappropriately into the child protection system' (LGDF/SCODA, 1997). While the sentiment is laudable, the delivery of a service that avoids such casualties is not yet with us, despite the efforts of many dedicated professionals. The most serious problems internationally appear to be the lack of training and clear unambiguous policy, which are issues taken up in Chapter 20.

Another major impediment to service improvement is the lack of empirically based data on parenting by drug users. The possible removal of children is a powerful sanction that is feared by many drug-using parents, induces deception and concealment and underlies their reluctance to seek help. An approach is required that assures them of support rather than punishment. To be effective, the intervention has to be seen by parents as credible; offered by those who understand their problems and who will not judge them. Not only the nature, but the delivery of such information will need to be acceptable, for example a high proportion of parents would want to avoid the perceived stigmatisation of attendance at a drug clinic. Researchers and policy makers need to listen to what is said by the targets of health interventions. This is a strategy that has been absent from medical research in the past. Research on illicit drug users can be difficult, sometimes dangerous and often frustrating, but that is no excuse for ignoring their views. More eclectic research methods will produce detailed and varied data sets that can improve our understanding of drug use and dependence and its social consequences. Qualitative data are particularly useful at this stage in providing insights. The ever-changing patterns of illicit drug use require a comprehensive approach that is sensitive to changes in the perceptions and behaviour of drug users and the context in which they live. There can be few needs for this sort of research investment that are greater than those of drug-using mothers.

REFERENCES

Amaro, H., Freed, L., Carbral, H. and Zuckerman, B. (1990) Violence during pregnancy and substance use. *American Journal of Public Health* 80(5), 575–579.

Bollerud, K. (1990) A model for the treatment of trauma-related syndromes among chemically dependent women. *Journal of Substance Abuse Treatment* 7, 83–87.

Boyd, S. (1999) *Mothers and Illicit Drugs: Transcending the Myths*. Toronto: University of Toronto Press.

Boyd, S. and Faith, K. (1999) Women, illegal drugs and prison: views from Canada. *International Journal of Drug Policy* 10, 195–207.

Burns, W.J. and Burns, K.A. (1988) Parenting Dysfunction in Chemically Dependent Women. Chapter 12, in: I.J. Chasnoff (ed.) *Drugs, Alcohol, Pregnancy and Parenting*. The Netherlands: Kluwer Academic Publishers.

Centre for Reproductive Law and Policy (1996) *Punishing Women for the Pregnancy During Pregnancy*. CRLP: New York, US.

Colten, M. (1980) A comparison of heroin-addicted and non-addicted mothers: their attitudes, beliefs and parenting experiences, in: *Heroin-addicted parents and their children: Two reports*. National Institute on Drug Abuse Services Research Report, 1–18. Department of Health and Human Services, Washington DC: Government Printing Office.

Colten, M. (1982) Attitudes, experiences and self-perceptions of heroin-addicted mothers. *Journal of Social Issues* 38(2), 77–92.

Council of Europe (1995) *Women and drugs: Proceedings of the seminar held in Prague, 1993*. Strasbourg: Council of Europe Publishing. ISBN 92–871–2838–3.

Deren, S. (1986) Children of Substance Abusers: A review of the literature. *Journal of Substance Abuse Treatment* 3, 77–94.

Famularo, R., Kinscherff, R. and Fenton, T. (1992) Parental substance abuse and the nature of child maltreatment. *Child Abuse and Neglect* 16, 475–483.

Glenn, E. (1994) Social constructions of mothering: a thematic overview, in: E. Glenn, G. Chang and L. Forcey (eds) *Mothering: Ideology, experience and agency*. New York: Routledge.

Guerra, P. (1998) Linking parental substance abuse and child maltreatment. *Counselling Today*, August.

Hawk, M.A. (1994) How social policies make matters worse: the case of maternal substance abuse. *Journal of Drug Issues* 24, 517–526.

Hepburn, M. (1993) Drug use in pregnancy. *British Journal of Hospital Medicine* 49(1), 51–55.

Hoffman, J.P. and Su, S.S. (1998) Parental substance use disorder, mediating variables and adolescent drug use: a non-recursive model. *Addiction* 93(9), 1351–1364.

Kandall, S.R. (1998) Women and addiction in the United States – 1920 to the present, in: C.L. Wetherington and A.B. Roman (eds) *Drug Addiction Research and the Health of Women*. National Institute on Drug Abuse, Washington DC: Government Printing Office.

Khantzian, E. (1985) The self-medication hypothesis of addictive disorder. *American Psychiatry* 142, 1259–1264.

Klee, H. (1997) *Amphetamine Misuse: International Perspectives on Current Trends*. Chapter 3. The Netherlands: Harwood Academic Publishers.

Kramer, P.D. (1993) *Listening to Prozac*. New York: Viking Penguin.

Kumpfer, K.L. (1998) Links between prevention and treatment for drug-abusing women and their children, in: C.L. Wetherington and A.B. Roman (eds) *Drug Addiction Research and the Health of Women*. National Institute on Drug Abuse, Washington DC: Government Printing Office.

LGDF/SCODA (1997) *Drug-using parents: policy guidelines for inter-agency working*. London: Local Government Drugs Forum and the Standing Conference on Drug Abuse.

Ludwig, G.B. and Anderson, M.D. (1989) Substance abuse in women: relationship between chemical dependency of women and past reports of physical and/or sexual abuse. *The International Journal of Addictions* 2(8).

Mayes, L. (1995) Substance abuse and parenting, in: M. Bornstein (ed.) *Handbook of Parenting, Vol. 4: Applied and practical parenting*. Mahwah, NJ: Lawrence Erlbaum.

Miller, B.A. (1998) Partner Violence Experiences and Women's Drug Use: Exploring the Connections, in: C.L. Wetherington and A.B. Roman (eds) *Drug Addiction Research and the Health of Women*. National Institute on Drug Abuse, Washington DC: Government Printing Office.

Miller, B.A., Downs, W.R. and Gondoli, D.M. (1989) Spouse violence among alcoholics as compared to a random household sample. *Journal of Studies on Alcohol* 50, 533–540.

Mounteney, J. (1998) *Children of Drug Using Parents*. Highlight Series No. 163. London: National Children's Bureau/Barnardo's.

Mounteney, J. (1999) *Drugs, Pregnancy and Childcare: A guide for professionals*. Drugs Work No. 6. London: The Institute for the Study of Drug Dependence (ISDD).

Murphy, S. and Rosenbaum, M. (1999) *Pregnant Women on Drugs: Combating Stereotypes and Stigma*. New Jersey, US: Rutgers University Press.

National Children's Bureau (1994) *Drug Misuse Highlight Series 7*. London: NCB.

Nelson-Zlupko, L., Kauffman, E. and Dore, M.M. (1995) Gender differences in drug abuse and treatment: implications for social work interventions with substance abusing women. *Social Work* 40, 45–64.

Peck, D. and Plant, M. (1986) Unemployment and illegal drug use. *British Medical Journal* 293, 929–932.

Ramsey, M. and Partridge, S. (1999) *Drug Misuse Declared in 1998: results from the British Crime Survey*. Research Study 197. London: The Home Office.

Reder, P. and Lucey, C. (eds) (1995) *Assessment of Parenting: Psychiatric and psychological contributions*. London: Routledge.

Reid, J. and Macchetto, P. (1999) *No Safe Haven*. National Center on Addiction and Substance Abuse (CASA): New York, Columbia University.

Reinarman, C. and Levine, H. (eds) (1997) *Crack in America: Demon Drugs and Social Justice*. Berkeley: University of California Press.

Rosenbaum, M. (1981) *Women on Heroin*. New Brunswick, NJ: Rutgers University Press.

Rosenbaum, M. and Irwin, K. (1998) Pregnancy, Drugs and Harm Reduction, in: C.L. Wetherington and A.B. Roman (eds) *Drug Addiction Research and the Health of Women*. National Institute on Drug Abuse, Washington DC: Government Printing Office.

Roth, P. (ed.) (1991) *Alcohol and Drugs are Women's Issues*, Vol. 1. New York: Women's Action Alliances and Scarecrow Press.

Russell, S.A. and Wilsnack, S.C. (1991) Adult survivor of childhood sexual abuse, in: *Alcohol and Drugs are Women's Issues*, Vol. 1. New York: Women's Action Alliances and Scarecrow Press.

Sheridan, M. (1995) A proposed intergenerational model of substance abuse, family functioning and abuse/neglect. *Child Abuse and Neglect* 19(5), 519–530.

Social Focus on Families (1997) Office for National Statistics. London: Government Statistical Service.

Stice, E. and Barrera, M. (1995) A longitudinal examination of the reciprocal relations between perceived parenting and adolescents' substance use and externalizing behaviour. *Developmental Psychology* 31, 322–334.

Suchmann, N.E. and Luther, S.S. (2000) Maternal addiction, child maladjustment and socio-demographic risks: implications for parenting behaviors. *Addiction* 95(9), 1417–1428.

Tarter, R. and Mezzick, A. (1992) Ontogeny of substance abuse: perspectives and findings, in: M. Glantz and R. Pickens (eds) *Vulnerability to Drug Abuse*. Washington DC: American Psychological Association.

UNDCP (1994) *Women and Drug Abuse*: A position paper by the United Nations. Vienna: UNDCP.

UNDCP (1996) *Amphetamine-Type Stimulants: A Global Review*. UNDCP Technical Series No. 3. Vienna: United Nations Drug Control Programme.

UNDCP (2000) *World situation with regard to drug abuse*. Commission on Narcotic Drugs, Economic and Social Council of the United Nations, New York, E/CN.7/2000/4.

Velleman, R. (1992) Intergenerational effects: a review of environmentally oriented studies concerning the relationship between parental alcohol problems and family disharmony. *International Journal of the Addictions* 27(3), 253–280.

Velleman, R. and Orford, J. (1993) The importance of family discord in explaining childhood problems in the children of problem drinkers. *Addiction Research* 1, 39–57.

Weinraub, M. and Gringlas, M.B. (1995) Single Parenthood, in: M.H. Bornstein (ed.) *Handbook of Parenting: Volume 3*. New Jersey, US: Lawrence Erlbaum Associates.

Zellman, G.L. (1993) Detecting pre-natal substance exposure: an exploratory analysis and policy discussion. *Journal of Drug Issues* 23, 357–387.

Zuckerman, B., Frank, D. and Brown, E. (1998) Overview of the effects of abuse and drugs on pregnancy and offspring, in: *Medical Developments for the Treatment of Pregnant Addicts and their Infants*. NIDA Research Monograph 149, Washington DC: Government Printing Office.

Chapter 2

Women's use of drugs

Gender specific factors

Samantha Wright

This chapter presents an overview of the literature on gender differences in illicit drug use. There are three main parts. The first comprises research findings on gender differences in drug use itself, the second outlines the social context of women's drug use and the impact that gender roles have upon women's experiences of drug use, and the third assesses gender differences within the various stages of the treatment process (access to treatment, patterns of help-seeking, experiences of service provision, treatment outcomes, and female clients' needs), describing how the male orientation of treatment services disadvantages female drug users. While much of the literature in this chapter emanates from the United States, and some of the research concerns problematic alcohol use, there are likely to be many similarities to women's experiences of drug use within the UK.

THE IMPORTANCE OF GENDER SPECIFICITY

Women have often been overlooked in the study of substance abuse. Lex (1991) has attributed this to three commonly held assumptions about women drug users: that they constitute an insignificant proportion of the substance dependent population; that they share the same characteristics as male drug users; or that they have psychological and social problems that make them too problematic to study.

These assumptions can be challenged. First, recent drug surveys suggest a convergence in the prevalence of drug use among young men and women (Parker and Measham, 1994; Ramsay and Spiller, 1997). Second, research has revealed many gender differences which deny the validity of the view that men and women's drug-using lifestyles can be regarded as equivalent. Such differences occur within many aspects of drug-using behaviour including: initiation into drug use and the escalation of drug use (Anglin *et al.*, 1987b; Hser *et al.*, 1987a and b), and patterns of help-seeking and treatment outcomes (Copeland and Hall, 1992; Fraser, 1997; Hughes *et al.*, 1997). Finally, although research has reported relatively high levels of psychological and social distress among female drug users, this may be attributed to the selection of research samples from within treatment populations. It has been suggested that female drug users in treatment differ significantly from those in the community (Kline, 1996) and it may be that most women only overcome the barriers to seeking treatment when they are experiencing severe difficulties.

Studies of female drug use have also revealed several under-researched issues which are important to service provision for both male and female drug users, for example: the use of benzodiazepines, the impact of violence in drug using behaviour, and the effect of interpersonal relationships on both drug use and its treatment (Broom, 1995). Nevertheless, the development of effective drug services for women remains restricted by a limited under-standing of female drug use, and many women continue to be deterred from presenting to drug services (Copeland and Hall, 1992; Copeland *et al.*, 1993). Thus, women's relatively small representation among drug service clientele should not be assumed to indicate that they are less likely to use drugs (Broom, 1995).

Much of the research to date has focused on alcohol or opiate users. It has commonly reported on treatment populations, and as a result, there is a paucity of literature regarding non-opiate users and drug users in the community (Klee, 1993; Powis *et al.*, 1996). Given the specific attractions that stimulant drugs hold for women (Klee, 1993, 1997a), combined with the barriers to seeking treatment, it is understandable that women are under-represented in drugs research.

GENDER DIFFERENCES: DRUG USE

Prevalence

It has been traditionally assumed that women are less likely to use illicit drugs than men; either because they are less likely to violate social codes, or because they have alternative patterns of breaching norms such as unmarried motherhood and prostitution (Freedman, 1980). The stereotypical illicit drug user is often perceived as being a disaffected young man in his early twenties (Taylor, 1993), with women thought to be more likely to (mis)use licit drugs. However, it seems that for young men and women the prevalence of illicit drug use is converging. The British Crime Survey revealed similar rates of reported drug use for male and female 16–19 year olds: 48 per cent of males and 42 per cent of females had used drugs; and 23 per cent of males and 15 per cent of females reported using them in the preceding month (Ramsay and Spiller, 1997). In a survey of 15–16-year-old school children in the north-west of England, girls and boys reported being offered and having tried illicit drugs in equivalent numbers: 72 per cent girls and 70 per cent boys were offered drugs, 47 per cent girls and 47 per cent boys had tried them, and 24 per cent girls and 28 per cent boys had tried them in the preceding month (Parker and Measham, 1994).

Initiation

It has been suggested that women are more likely than men to report being initiated into drug use by their partners, rather than by their peers (Almog et al., 1993; Hser et al., 1987b). However, this may not be so common (Rosenbaum, 1981). The stereotype of passive women pressured into using drugs by their partners is undermined by women who report taking an active role in their initiation into drug use and injecting, sometimes despite their partner's unwillingness or disapproval (Klee, 1996; Taylor, 1993).

As with men, women often start to use heroin out of curiosity, seeking excitement and euphoria (Rosenbaum, 1981; Taylor, 1993), trying to counteract tedium and depression (Rosenbaum and Murphy, 1990), or perhaps seeking diversion from problems within their personal relationships (Taylor, 1993). Drug use can offer a structure to their daily lives, whilst drug dealing can provide access to money, status and identity (Taylor, 1993). There can be many reasons for starting to use drugs that include: family problems (including their partner's substance abuse), low self-confidence, peer pressure, and the alleviation of symptoms such as depression and physical pain (Copeland and Hall, 1992).

Sustained use

In the US, Liu and Kaplan (1996) have examined gender differences in attributions for drug use. The young men in their survey reported using drugs to enhance feelings of self-importance and power, to improve social bonding, to influence others, to reduce boredom, or whilst anticipating or experiencing trouble. The young women reported that they used drugs when beset by personal problems, to deal with their anger and tension, or to self-medicate feelings of depression or worthlessness. These rationalisations for behaviour reflect gender-role characteristics, so it remains unclear whether women use drugs under different circumstances than men, or whether the gendered nature of social development influences individuals' perceptions of the reasons for their drug use.

However, although drug use may initially improve women's feelings of low self-worth, this is a counterproductive strategy. Continued use often results in the loss of self-esteem (Kline, 1996), and new problems that are associated with the drug-using lifestyle, for example: the financial cost; the removal of children into care; and perhaps a decline into a chaotic state which may involve needle sharing, violence, crime, prostitution and unprotected sex (Rosenbaum, 1981; Rosenbaum and Murphy, 1990; Taylor, 1993).

Drug preference

It is suggested that higher proportions of women use stimulants rather than opiates (Klee, 1993; Powis et al., 1996). Women are attracted to amphetamine in particular because it is relatively inexpensive, is perceived as non-addictive and therefore less stigmatising, and because of a variety of useful effects: suppressing appetite, enhancing confidence, boosting energy, facilitating social interaction, and disinhibiting sexual behaviour (Klee, 1996).

Whilst it is often assumed that heroin is the most 'dangerous' drug, there are additional problems associated with stimulant use. In comparison studies of female amphetamine and heroin users, the amphetamine users reported more social and sexual activity, a greater disposition towards casual sex, and less perception of HIV risk (Klee, 1993). Due to the opiate orientation of most treatment services, amphetamine users have few opportunities to seek help for problematic aspects of their drug use, and any difficulties that they face may remain untreated for many years (Klee and Wright, 1999).

Susceptibility to drug-related harm

Due to physiological differences, the safe level of substance use for women is less than that for men. Women's bodies contain different proportions of fat and water to those of men, which affects both absorption rates and the cumulative impact of alcohol, cannabis and some benzodiazepines. Female fatty tissue distribution and their tendency to have smaller, less prominent veins make it more difficult for women to find injectable veins (Hsu, 1995), whilst hormonal changes caused by the menstrual cycle, pregnancy and the menopause alter the effects of drug taking for women (Blume, 1990; Lex, 1991). Female substance use has been related to breast cancer and gynaecological dysfunction (Blume, 1990; Lex, 1991). However, the impact is under-researched and is likely to be related to other environmental factors such as nutrition and the experience of trauma (Lex, 1993).

It is often assumed that women consume drugs more moderately than men, although once dependent on illicit drugs, gender differences in patterns of use decline (Almog et al., 1993; Rosenbaum, 1981). However, compared to men, women's drug-using careers may be 'compressed', with women becoming drug dependent, and seeking treatment sooner than men (Anglin et al., 1987b; Hser et al., 1987a). Perhaps because of equivalent levels of drug use, women tend to develop health problems associated with substance use more rapidly than men, a feature known as 'telescoping' (Lex, 1991; Powis *et al.*, 1996).

GENDER DIFFERENCES: THE SOCIAL CONTEXT OF DRUG USE

Experience of trauma and psychological distress

The experience of victimisation, whether childhood or adulthood sexual/ physical abuse, is relatively high among drug users (Bennett and Lawson, 1994; Blume, 1990; Copeland and Hall, 1992; Hien and Scheier, 1996; Root, 1989; Swift *et al.*, 1996). Women drug users have more often been found to report poor backgrounds than their male counterparts, reporting higher rates of: school drop-out and poor parental relationships (Holsten, 1985); medical or psychological problems (Kosten *et al.*, 1985); family disputes (Robbins, 1989); and psychological or personal safety issues arising from childhood sexual abuse (Copeland and Hall, 1992).

The negative consequences of drug use for women may be exacerbated by the structure of gender relations. For example, the higher rates of family discord reported by women may be influenced by factors such as: expected gender appropriate behaviour; social disapproval and the stigma of women's drug use; and other family members' problematic substance use (Robbins, 1989). Davis and Dinitto (1996) have attempted to disentangle gender effects from drug-using effects in acounting for differences between male and female drug users. In their study, gender was found to be associated with reports of: family problems, sibling substance use, parental psychological problems, outpatient psychiatric treatment, and suicide attempts. Drug use, on the other hand, was related to reports of: parental divorce, current family problems, parental substance use, sibling substance use, and anxiety. Women's substance abuse itself was associated with having relatives who use drugs, and histories of attempted suicide.

Sexual partnerships

Illicit drug use by women is less socially acceptable, and more stigmatising than men's (Lex, 1991; Rosenbaum, 1981; Underhill, 1986), with women not only labelled as 'deviants' for their drug use, but additionally for breaching society's definitions of feminine behaviour (Ettorre, 1992). One consequence of the social stigma of female drug use is that women are more restricted in their choice of sexual partners. In contrast to men who are more likely to be single or to have a non-drug using partner (Gossop *et al.*, 1994; Klee, 1993; Klee *et al.*, 1990; McKeganey and Barnard, 1992; Powis *et al.*, 1996), women's partners tend to be drug users. Even within drug-using cultures, women drug users induce disapproval, with male drug users reporting preference for non-using partners (Klee *et al.*, 1990; Rosenbaum, 1981).

Addiction problems may become more complex for female substance users with drug-using partners. Women with drug-using partners tend to report spending more time with them than men in similar relationships (Anglin *et al.*, 1987b). Such women may become dependent on their partner for drugs and/or economic support (Rosenbaum, 1981). Although the financial burden of drug use may be lessened by economic dependence on a partner, women have reported that their drug use, particularly the use of drugs on a daily basis, is attributable to their partner's influence (Anglin *et al.*, 1987b; Hser *et al.*, 1987a). Women within drug-using partnerships often face traditional gender role expectations, and may act as 'caretakers' to their partners, attempting to limit their partner's drug use or inadvertently increasing their own use to match that of their partner (Klee, 1996).

Women who inject drugs may face additional problems to those of male injectors. They are more likely than male injectors to have a partner who is also an injector, and to have received their first injection from their partner (Klee *et al.*, 1993; Powis *et al.*, 1996). The sharing of injecting equipment may be taken for granted within sexual relationships, making it difficult for women to refuse or negotiate sharing without causing offence in a way that indicates lack of trust in their partner (Barnard, 1993; Klee, 1997b). Injecting couples are also more likely to have 'open houses' where other drug users come to inject (Klee *et al.*, 1990). In such an environment women may find their drug consumption increasing, feel out of control and more dependent – factors associated with sharing injecting equipment.

GENDER DIFFERENCES: ACCESS TO AND EXPERIENCE OF DRUG TREATMENT SERVICES

Given the nature of some women's earlier histories that are outlined above, perhaps it is not surprising that many women seeking drug treatment have multiple complex inter-related problems which require attention, for example: histories of self-harming/suicide attempts, polydrug use, personality disorders, eating disorders, physical health problems, experience of physical/sexual abuse, dysphoria, psycho-sexual disorders, low self-esteem and psychological distress such as depression, guilt, anxiety and affective disorders (Blume, 1990; Copeland and Hall, 1992; Reed, 1985; Robbins, 1989; Ross *et al.*, 1988; Swift *et al.*, 1996; Underhill, 1986). Female drug users report greater use of mental health services and more benzodiazepine consumption than men (Wilcox and Yates, 1993). Root (1989) has proposed that some women's drug use should be interpreted as a 'post-trauma coping response' rather than as a primary problem.

The discussion in this section does not focus directly on the provision of services for drug-using women or mothers. This is covered in detail in other chapters. Instead it explores women's attitudes towards, and outcomes of, interactions with health professionals more generally, and in this context issues that are relevant to the provision of ante- and postnatal care for drug-using women will be identified.

Access to drug treatment services

The social stigma of being a female drug user may deter women from acknowledging their problems to friends and family (Lex, 1991), and has a significant impact on their help-seeking behaviour and treatment outcomes. As a result female drug users have less contact with counselling or health services than men (Lex, 1991; Rosenbaum and Murphy, 1990). In the UK, women comprise approximately a quarter of all notified drug addicts (Corkery, 1997) which may be an underestimate.

Four main factors have been suggested for women's relative under-representation in services. First, women may have less need for treatment, due either to a lower prevalence of problematic use than men (Powis et al., 1996); or their ability to fund drug use through prostitution or financial dependence on a man (Perry, 1979). Second, the social stigma associated with being a female drug user may deter women from seeking help (Copeland and Hall, 1992; Perry, 1979), particularly for drug-using mothers who fear professional intervention in their children's welfare (DAWN, 1994; Klee and Jackson, 1998; Kline, 1996). Third, women receive significantly less family support for seeking alcohol/drug treatment than men (Beckman and Amaro, 1986). This is probably related to women's relatively higher likelihood of having a partner who is a drug user and who may be reluctant to seek help, so that seeking treatment may threaten the future of the relationship (Rosenbaum, 1981). Finally, services may be inaccessible to women or inappropriate to their specific needs (Copeland and Hall, 1992; DAWN, 1994; Klee and Jackson, 1998).

Many potential barriers for women seeking to access treatment services have been identified, both for women drug users in general (for example, money/transport difficulties, cultural factors, fear of discrimination or sexual harassment from clients/staff, concern that re-entry to services would be interpreted as personal failure, fears about the harshness of the treatment programme, and a lack of social support) and for drug-using mothers in particular (for example, the pressure of negotiating multiple responsibilities and a lack of childcare provision) (Copeland and Hall, 1992; Fraser, 1997; Kline, 1996; Reed, 1987).

Seeking treatment

Like men, women tend to report seeking treatment due to a 'loss of control' over their use of drugs (Copeland and Hall, 1992; Klee and Wright, 1999; Taylor, 1993; Wright and Klee, 2000). However, they may have a wider definition of 'taking control' than men that incorporates interpersonal issues such as: improving personal relationships, challenging criticisms about their drug use, defending against their partner's abusive behaviour, and encouraging their partner to seek help (Fraser, 1997). Gender differences have also been revealed in drug service clients' identification of the need for treatment. The women in one US study (Kline, 1996) sought treatment due to distressing psychological problems, paranoia, hallucinations, blackouts, concern for their children, the shame of harming relationships, and feeling ashamed of involvement in prostitution, whilst the men had been motivated by a fear of violence and/or being killed.

Women are thought more likely to seek treatment for psychological difficulties, in contrast to men who tend to seek help for problems with social functioning (Gomberg, 1993; Robbins, 1989). Yet comparisons between men and women in treatment have revealed similar high rates of unemployment, broken relationships, and unstable accommodation. Lower rates of stable relationships are reported among the women (Copeland and Hall, 1992). These authors suggest that this may be due to men being less tolerant of their partner's substance use, or because the break-up of a relationship prompts women to present to treatment.

The experience of treatment services

Women face many problems once they are in treatment. This is largely a consequence of the high proportion of men attending such services, since theories of substance use have been developed based upon male samples, and most treatment models are male oriented (Fraser, 1997; Marsh and Simpson, 1986). Acknowledgement of the physical and psychological differences between men and women remains rare (Copeland and Hall, 1992; Kauffman et al., 1997), with the result that women's needs have not been addressed adequately (Ettorre, 1994; Hartnoll, 1992). However, there are efforts to improve this, which have become more pronounced over the past two to three years.

Women often report feeling guilty about drug use (Lex, 1991), and are thought to be more receptive to therapeutic strategies than men (Andersson et al., 1983). Studies of clients with alcohol problems suggest that women are more likely to attribute their problematic behaviour to life problems, but it is unclear whether this is a valid measure which may enhance the outcome of treatment (Reed, 1987), or a strategy to deflect censure (Allan and Cooke, 1986). Reed (1987) argues that a willingness to admit distress may increase motivation and enhance the success of treatment.

Treatment outcomes

It is generally thought that women tend to fare badly in treatment services. Female methadone clients have been found to have higher drop-out rates from treatment than men (Anglin *et al.*, 1987a), although treatment and retention outcomes are better within those services which offer childcare provision (Beckman *et al.*, 1984; Reed, 1987). Even where women's contact with services is similar to that of men, the content of treatment and its outcomes may differ for the two groups (Powis *et al.*, 1996). Despite such difficulties, female drug users appear to be more successful in abstaining from drugs than men, both within treatment services and acting independently (Holsten, 1985; Hser *et al.*, 1987a; Wright and Klee, 2000).

Holsten (1985) has argued that whilst the men's abstinence from drugs is largely related to the development of employment opportunities, women have additional routes out of addiction such as marriage and motherhood. In his sample of young psychiatric inpatients, the women stopped using drugs sooner than the men, with steadily increasing numbers of them becoming abstinent. Several social factors were suggested for the different treatment outcomes: the men generally remained single, whereas the women either formed new relationships or got divorced. The women were also more likely than the men to have built networks of non-using friends, established their own place to live, and found employment.

Unfortunately, women's successful treatment outcomes may be relatively short-lived. A meta-analysis of research conducted on alcohol treatment services found that whilst women exhibited better results 12 months after initiating contact, it was the men who showed greater improvement later (Jarvis, 1992). Research on treatment outcomes requires a more long-term focus if the factors determining client success are to be explored fully.

Treatment needs

One of the aims of this book is to explore female drug users' attitudes towards and experiences of pregnancy, early motherhood and both ante- and postnatal health care. Although this chapter has a wider remit in focusing on the differences between male and female drug users, many women's experiences of service provision detailed in this chapter are relevant to the development of services for pregnant drug users and those with children. This section summarises briefly the basic requirements which have been identified for service provision to female drug users, and then focuses specifically on issues pertinent for drug-using women who have children.

Many differences between male and female substance users are related to gender itself, as opposed to drug use patterns, and a different approach is required in order for treatment services to be able to address this. While the provision of single sex services and childcare facilities is considered essential by some observers (Copeland and Hall, 1992; Fraser, 1997), services remain inadequate unless accompanied by actual procedural changes. Services which address the needs of non-parenteral and stimulant users would attract more female drug users, as there are relatively high proportions of women within these groups (Klee, 1993; Powis et al., 1996). Higher proportions of female clients are also thought to attend services which are linked with generic health services, or which provide telephone lines staffed by women (DAWN, 1994). Additional examples of possible service development include: women-only groups, one-to-one counselling, the use of non-confrontational techniques, access to female workers, outreach services, relapse prevention work which promotes social network building and the provision of a safe environment within which to address personal and psychological problems, particularly those arising from physical and sexual abuse (Copeland and Hall, 1992; Copeland et al., 1993; Rubin et al., 1996).

In Australia, it has been found that a specialist women's service (SWS) attracted groups of female drug users who rarely approached traditional mixed-sex services (TMS). They had chosen the single-sex service because it was women-only and because it provided childcare. These women tended to have serious and complex problems, and included: women with dependent children; polydrug users; women who had been sexually abused in childhood; women whose mothers had abused substances; women who had lost custody of their children, and lesbians who were presenting to services for the first time (Copeland and Hall, 1992). After six months, the women attending the SWS showed greater improvement in both depression and self-esteem than the women attending the mixed-sex service – findings which endorse the need for individual counselling, women-only groups, and the acknowledgement of sexual assault within a safe environment (Copeland et al., 1993).

The social stigma experienced by female drug users tends to lower their self-esteem (Swift et al., 1996). This may persist through recovery, and in order for women to counter their feelings of worthlessness, treatment and relapse prevention work which empowers women within a safe environment are advocated, using techniques such as encouraging self-empathy, and inclusion in treatment decisions to encourage the expression of personal needs. In this way women can increase their self-esteem, overcome social stigma, alleviate feelings of guilt and stop feeling responsible for problems outside their control (Markoff and Cawley, 1996; Schilit and Gomberg, 1987). In summary, women tend to benefit from supportive and empathetic counselling (Markoff and Cawley, 1996; Miller et al., 1980), and male treatment models which emphasise confrontation and the breakdown of denial are less appropriate for them (Reed, 1987; Underhill, 1986).

A more holistic approach towards working with drug users has been recommended, so that the social context of female drug users' lives can be recognised within treatment services. Many methods have been advocated for achieving this, for example: recognising women's multiple responsibilities which may impair their ability to keep appointments (Fraser, 1997); offering opportunities to examine relationship issues (Finkelstein, 1996); providing couple counselling for clients with drug-using partners (Nichols, 1985); addressing the interaction of drug and sexual risk taking (Powis *et al.*, 1996); and supporting women in building supportive social networks (Finkelstein, 1996; Schilit and Gomberg, 1987). Lex (1993) also suggests that services should address the social influence that women's partners have, the effects of being raised in substance abusing families, the experience of life stressors, socio-economic factors, psychological co-morbidity, and reproductive issues. In addition, for some clients, services may find it appropriate to evaluate their psychological states, assessing for conditions such as borderline personality disorder, affective disorders, bulimia, anxiety, sexual disorders, sexuality problems, dual diagnosis, and depression (Blume, 1990).

Issues related specifically to gender can be pertinent to those delivering services to female drug users. Finkelstein (1996) discussed how sexual behaviour may interrelate with women's drug use and their experience of treatment. For example, women may experience guilt due to their sexual behaviour whilst intoxicated, they may use drugs to block out memories of sexual abuse, and they may experience problems with sexual dysfunction when trying to abstain from drug use. Female clients may wish to address these issues within the treatment setting, or may wish to explore other experiences, such as: sex-role stereotyping, sexuality issues, body-image issues, fears regarding sexual harassment, the lack of social support for seeking treatment, histories of prostitution and experiences of sexual or physical violence (Copeland and Hall, 1992; Nichols, 1985; Reed, 1987; Swift *et al.*, 1996).

Clients' experiences of violence are traditionally thought to be peripheral to primary treatment for addiction (Fraser, 1997), yet women are more likely to relapse if violence and sexual abuse issues are not dealt with (Root, 1989). The provision of a safe physical and psychological treatment environment within which to explore these issues is important, particularly as women may be experiencing ongoing domestic violence (Fraser, 1997). Although co-operation between substance misuse and domestic violence agencies can be problematic (Bennett and Lawson, 1994), there is a need to ensure that workers are adequately trained to work with abuse and that appropriate interventions are offered which match treatment to the immediacy and severity of individual need (Swift *et al.*, 1996). Workers need to be confident in validating women's experiences, and in referring them to specialist services if required. Whilst basic identification and discussion of trauma is thought not to interfere with treatment, more intense exploration of such sensitive issues requires a safe therapeutic environment (Hien and Scheier, 1996), as inappropriate support may cause their clients damage, potentially leading to relapse (Swift et al., 1996).

Additional service requirements have been identified for women with children. Although parenting and child custody concerns are often not addressed in traditional mixed services (Colten, 1980; Swift et al., 1996), the acknowledgement of childcare needs, and the development of parenting skills could be an important element of service provision (Copeland et al., 1993; Klee et al., 1998; Swift et al., 1996). The provision of residential childcare would benefit drug-using parents who are seeking treatment, as many mothers currently have to relinquish care of their children prior to accessing services (Kline, 1996; Swift et al., 1996), and women have reported leaving treatment earlier than wished due to inadequate childcare provision (Copeland et al., 1993). However, services also need to be wary of focusing solely on women's relationships and their 'caretaking' roles, as female clients may wish to focus on developing self-reliance and independence (Fraser, 1997; Perry, 1979).

SUMMARY

There are relatively few differences between male and female drug users which relate to specific patterns of drug use, with the main difference being that women are less likely to inject drugs than men. However, it may be that as more young women use drugs, gender differences will decline even further, especially for dependent drug users where consumption patterns are very similar between men and women.

Many of the differences between male and female drug users relate to gender as opposed to substance use (Davis and Dinitto, 1996), so that differences in substance misuse mirror societal differences between men and women (such as parenting responsibilities, and the negotiation of intimate relationships). It is often the social context within which women use drugs which determines the gender differences in both drug-taking behaviours, and the differential consequences of drug use for women. In particular, the greater likelihood for women to have a drug-using partner, and the greater responsibility for childcare that most mothers face increase the risks of drug use for women.

The common male-oriented treatment provision focuses too heavily on individualistic factors, ignoring the more social aspects of female drug use, for example the influence of drug-using partners on women's drug use, childcare responsibilities which impede attendance at appointments and experiences of sexual or physical violence (Fraser, 1997). Since they are in a minority, women often fare badly in treatment, with their needs being seen as additional to 'standard' service provision. This means that economic considerations may preclude services from adapting to meet the requirements of their female clientele, despite evidence of the degree of unmet treatment need among women (Swift *et al.*, 1996). Women often accept that clinics 'cannot' adapt services to their needs, and either do not seek treatment for their drug use, or stop attending services when their needs are not met (Fraser, 1997).

At present there is no coherent strategy to attract women into services, with services for women being developed on an ad-hoc basis. Yet for services to be able to meet the needs of female drug users, they need to acknowledge gender explicitly in the design of treatment programmes (Rubin *et al.*, 1996). In particular, services need to address the growing prevalence of problematic stimulant and non-parenteral drug use – where women constitute a higher proportion of drug users, and where there is currently a dearth of service provision (Klee and Wright, 1999; Powis *et al.*, 1996).

Although research into women's drug use has expanded over recent years, further work is required to elucidate many important issues, for example: the social influence of male drug users over their partner, the interaction of drug and sexual risk-taking (Klee, 1997; Powis *et al.*, 1996); women's patterns of consumption and the social meaning of their drug use (Broom, 1995); the relationship between psychological health, drug use and treatment outcomes (Lex, 1993; Swift *et al.*, 1996); and women's patterns of help-seeking and ways of using services (Hunter and Judd, 1998). Indeed, a gender-sensitive approach towards understanding drug users could be used to inform the development of enhanced services for both men and women (Broom, 1995), and is particularly important for women whose lives are being directly influenced by gender issues such as pregnancy and motherhood.

REFERENCES

Allan, C.A. and Cooke, D. (1986) Women, life-events and drinking problems. *British Journal of Psychiatry* 148, 462.

Almog, Y.J., Anglin, M.D. and Fisher, D.G. (1993) Alcohol and heroin use patterns of narcotics addicts: gender and ethnic differences. *American Journal of Drug and Alcohol Abuse* 19(2), 219–238.

Andersson, B., Nilsson, K. and Tunving, K. (1983) Drug careers in perspective. *Acta Psychiatrica Scandinavia* 67, 249–257.

Anglin, M.D., Hser, Y. and Booth, M.W. (1987a) Sex differences in addict careers: 4 treatment. *American Journal of Drug and Alcohol Abuse* 13(3), 253–280.

Anglin, M.D., Hser, Y. and McGlothlin, W.H. (1987b) Sex differences in addict careers: 2 becoming addicted. *American Journal of Drug and Alcohol Abuse* 13(1 + 2), 59–71.

Barnard, M.A. (1993) Needle sharing in context: patterns of sharing among men and women injectors and HIV risks. *Addiction* 88, 805–812.

Beckman, L.J. and Amaro, H. (1986) Personal and social difficulties facing men and women entering treatment. *Journal of Studies on Alcohol* 47, 135–145.

Beckman, L.W., Babcock, P. and O'Bryan, T. (1984) Meeting the childcare needs of the female alcoholic. *Child Welfare League America* LK111, 6, 541–546.

Bennett, L. and Lawson, M. (1994) Barriers to cooperation between domestic-violence and substance abuse programs. *Families in Society: the Journal of Contemporary Human Services* 75, 5, 277–286.

Blume, S.B. (1990) Chemical dependency in women: important issues. *American Journal of Drug and Alcohol Abuse* 16, 297–307.

Broom, D.H. (1995) Rethinking gender and drugs. *Drug and Alcohol Review* 14, 411–415.

Colten, M.E. (1980) A comparison of heroin addicted and non-addicted mothers: their attitudes, beliefs and parenting experiences, in: *Heroin-addicted Parents and their Children*, 1–18, NIDA, Rockville: US Dept. Health and Human Services.

Copeland, J. and Hall, W. (1992) A comparison of women seeking drug and alcohol treatment in a specialist women's and two traditional mixed-sex treatment services. *British Journal of Addiction* 87, 1293–1302.

Copeland, J., Hall, W., Didcott, P. and Biggs, V. (1993) A comparison of a specialist women's alcohol and other drug treatment services with two traditional mixed-sex services: client characteristics and treatment outcome. *Drug and Alcohol Dependence* 32, 81–92.

Corkery, J.M. (1997) *Statistics of drug addicts notified to the Home Office, United Kingdom, 1996.* Home Office Statistical Bulletin, Issue 22/97. London: Home Office Research and Statistics Directorate.

Davis, D.R. and Dinitto, D.M. (1996) Gender differences in social and psychological problems of substance abusers: a comparison to non-substance abusers. *Journal of Psychoactive Drugs* 28(2), 135–145.

Drug and Alcohol Women's Network (DAWN) (1994) *When a crèche is not enough. A survey of drug and alcohol services for women.* London: Drug and Alcohol Women's Network, GLASS.

Ettorre, E. (1992) *Women and Substance Abuse.* New Brunswick, NJ: Rutgers University Press.

Ettorre, E. (1994) Women and drug abuse with special reference to Finland: needing the 'courage to see'. *Women's Studies International Forum* 17(1), 83–94.

Finkelstein, N. (1996) Using the relational model as a context for treating pregnant and parenting chemically dependent women, in: B.L. Underhill and D. Finnegan (eds) *Chemical Dependency: women at risk.* New York: The Haworth Press.

Fraser, J. (1997) Methadone clinic culture: the everyday realities of female methadone clients. *Qualitative Health Research* 7(1), 121–139.

Freedman, A.M. (1980) Drug Dependence, in: H. Kaplan *et al.* (eds) *Comprehensive Textbook of Psychiatry.* London: Williams and Wilkins.

Gomberg, E.S.L. (1993) Women and alcohol: use and abuse. *Journal of Nervous and Mental Disease* 181, 211–219.

Gossop, M., Griffiths, P. and Strang, J. (1994) Sex differences in patterns of drug taking behaviour: a study at a London Community Drug Team. *British Journal of Psychiatry* 164, 101–104.

Hartnoll, R. (1992) Research and the help seeking process. *British Journal of Addiction* 87(3), 429–438.

Hien, D. and Scheier, J. (1996) Trauma and short-term outcome for women in detoxification. *Journal of Substance Abuse Treatment* 13(3), 227–231.

Holsten, F. (1985) The female drug abuser: has she a shorter way out? *The Journal of Drug Issues* 15(3), 383–392.

Hser, Y., Anglin, M.D. and Booth, M.W. (1987a) Sex differences in addict careers: 3 Addiction. *American Journal of Drug and Alcohol Abuse* 13(3), 231–251.

Hser, Y., Anglin, M.D. and McGlothlin, W.H. (1987b) Sex differences in addict careers: 1 Initiation of use. *American Journal of Drug and Alcohol Abuse* 13, (1&2), 33–57.

Hsu, L.N. (1995) *Drugs and Gender Issues. Gender in Development.* 9 January 1995, UNDCP: Focal Point on Women.

Hughes, T.L., Day, L.E., Marcantonio, R.J. and Torpy, E. (1997) Gender differences in alcohol and other drug use among young adults. *Substance Use and Misuse* 32(3), 317–342.

Hunter, G.M. and Judd, A. (1998) Women injecting drug users in London: the extent and nature of their contact with drug and health services. *Drug and Alcohol Review* 17, 267–276.

Jarvis, T.J. (1992) Implications of gender for alcohol treatment research: a quantitative and qualitative review. *British Journal of Addiction* 87(9), 1249–1261.

Kauffman, S.E., Silver, P. and Poulin, J. (1997) Gender differences in attitudes toward alcohol, tobacco and other drugs. *Social Work* 42(3), 231–241.

Klee, H. (1993) HIV risks for women injectors: heroin and amphetamine users compared. *Addiction* 88, 1055–1062.

Klee, H. (1996) Women drug users and their partners, in: L. Sherr, C. Hankins and L. Bennett (eds) *Aids as a Gender Issue.* London: Taylor and Francis.

Klee, H. (ed.) (1997a) *Amphetamine Misuse: international perspectives on current trends.* The Netherlands: Harwood Academic Publishers.

Klee, H. (1997b) Amphetamine injecting women and their primary partners: an analysis of risk behaviour, in: J. Catalan, L. Sherr and B. Hedge (eds) *The Impact of AIDS: psychological and social aspects of HIV infection.* The Netherlands: Harwood Academic Press.

Klee, H. and Jackson, M. (1998) *Illicit Drug Use, Pregnancy and Early Motherhood: an analysis of the impediments to effective service delivery.* Report to the UK Department of Health Task Force to Review Services for Drug Misusers.

Klee, H. and Morris, J. (1994) Crime and drug misuse: economic and psychological aspects of the criminal activities of heroin and amphetamine injectors. *Addiction Research* 1(4), 377–386.

Klee, H. and Wright, S. (1999) *Amphetamine Use and Treatment: a study of the impediments to effective service delivery. Part 1: Access to treatment services.* The Manchester Metropolitan University, Manchester: SRHSA.

Klee, H., Faugier, J., Hayes, C., Bolton, T. and Morris, J. (1990) Sexual partners of injecting drug users: the risk of HIV infection. *British Journal of Addiction* 85, 413–418.

Klee, H., Morris, J., Ruben, S. and Prinjha, N. (1993) *Polydrug Misuse: health risks and implications for HIV transmission.* Report to the UK Department of Health. The Manchester Metropolitan University, Manchester: SRHSA.

Klee, H., Wright, S. and Rothwell, J. (1998) *Drug Using Parents and Their Children: risk and protective factors.* The Manchester Metropolitan University Manchester: SRHSA.

Kline, A. (1996) Pathways into drug user treatment: the influence of gender and racial/ethnic identity. *Substance Use and Misuse* 31(3), 323–342.

Kosten, T.R., Rounsaville, B.J. and Kleber, H.D. (1985) Parental alcoholism in opioid addicts. *Journal of Nervous and Mental Disease* 173, 461–469.

Lex, B.W. (1991) Gender differences and substance abuse, in: N.K. Kello (ed.) *Advances in Substance Abuse Behavioural and Biological Research*, Vol. 4. London: Jessica Kingsley.

Lex, B.W. (1993) Women and illicit drugs: marijuana, heroin and cocaine, in: E.S.L. Gomberg and T.D. Nirenberg (eds) *Women and Substance Abuse.* Norwood, NJ: Ablex Publishing.

Liu, X. and Kaplan, H.B. (1996) Gender-related differences in circumstances surrounding initiation and escalation of alcohol and other substance use/abuse. *Deviant Behaviour: An Interdisciplinary Journal* 17, 71–106.

McKeganey, N. and Barnard, M. (1992) *Aids, Drugs and Sexual Risk: lives in the balance.* Buckingham: Oxford University Press.

Markoff, L.S. and Cawley, P.A. (1996) Retaining your clients and your sanity: using a relational model of multi-systems case management, in: B.L. Underhill and L. Finnegan (eds) *Chemical Dependency: women at risk.* New York: The Haworth Press.

Marsh, K. and Simpson, D. (1986) Sex differences in opioid addiction careers. *American Journal of Alcohol Abuse* 12, 309–329.

Miller, W.R., Taylor, C.A. and West, J. (1980) Focused versus broad-spectrum behavior therapy for problem drinkers. *Journal of Clinical Consulting Psychology* 48(5), 590–601.

Nichols, M. (1985) Theoretical concerns in the clinical treatment of substance abusing women: a feminist analysis. *Alcoholism Treatment Quarterly* 2, 78–79.

Parker, H. and Measham, F. (1994) Pick 'n' mix: changing patterns of illicit drug use amongst 1990s adolescents. *Drugs: Education, Policy and Prevention* 1(1), 5–13.

Perry, L. (1979) *Women and Drug Use: an unfeminine dependency.* London: ISDD.

Powis, B., Griffiths, P., Gossop, M. and Strang, J. (1996) The differences between male and female drug users: community samples of heroin and cocaine users compared. *Substance Use and Misuse* 31(5), 529–543.

Ramsay, R. and Spiller, J. (1997) *Drug Misuse Declared in 1996: latest results from the British Crime Survey.* Home Office Research Study 172. London: The Stationery Office.

Reed, B.G. (1985) Drug misuse and dependency in women. *International Journal of the Addictions* 20(1), 13–62.

Reed, B.G. (1987) Developing women-sensitive drug dependence services: why so difficult? *Journal of Psychoactive Drugs* 19(2), 151–164.

Robbins, C. (1989) Sex differences in psychosocial consequences of alcohol and drug abuse. *Journal of Health and Social Behaviour* 30, 117–130.

Root, M. (1989) Treatment failures: the role of sexual victimisation in women's addictive behavior. *American Journal of Orthopsychiatrists* 59(4), 542–549.

Rosenbaum, M. (1981) *Women on Heroin.* California: Rutgers University Press.

Rosenbaum, M. and Murphy, S. (1990) Women and addiction: process, treatment and outcome, in: E.Y. Lambert (ed.) *The Collection and Interpretation of Data from Hidden Populations. NIDA research monograph. No. 98.* Rockville: US Dept Health and Human Services.

Ross, H.E., Glaser, F.B. and Stiasny, S. (1988) Sex differences in the prevalence of psychiatric disorders in patients with alcohol and drug problems. *British Journal of Addiction* 83, 1179–1192.

Rubin, A., Stout, R.L. and Longabaugh, R. (1996) Gender differences in relapse situations. *Addiction* 91 (Supplement) s111–s120.

Schilit, R. and Gomberg, E.S. (1987) Social support structures of women in treatment for alcoholism. *Health and Social Work* Summer, 12, 187–191.

Swift, W., Copeland, J. and Hall, W. (1996) Characteristics of women with alcohol and other drug problems: findings of an Australian national survey. *Addiction* 91(8), 1141–1150.

Taylor, A. (1993) *Women Drug Users: an ethnography of a female injecting community.* Oxford: Clarendon Press.

Underhill, B.L. (1986) Issues relevant to aftercare programs for women. *Alcohol Health and Research World* 2, 46–47.

Wilcox, J.A. and Yates, W.R. (1993) Gender and psychiatric co-morbidity in substance-abusing individuals. *The American Journal on Addictions* 2(3), 202–206.

Wright, S. and Klee, H. (2000) Developing drug services for amphetamine users: taking account of gender-specific factors. *Journal of Substance Use* 5(2), 122–130.

Chapter 3

Concepts of motherhood

Suzan Lewis

Images of motherhood are all around us; in the media, psychological and medical texts, childcare manuals, feminist texts, biographies and auto-biographies. These portrayals of motherhood communicate ideals and stereotypes. They tell us how mothers are expected to feel, think and act. But these images and the concepts of motherhood that underpin them are full of contradictions. Mothers are simultaneously idealised and blamed for not living up to society's ideals. Discourses of motherhood as natural and instinctive coexist with a discourse of professional expertise, and 'experts' clamour to advise on how to be a good mother. Mothers' own accounts also contain contradictions, with motherhood viewed as both 'heaven and hell' (Coward, 1997).

In this chapter we consider some of the overlapping and contradictory representations of motherhood portrayed in social scientific and professional literature, which both reflect, and are reflected in, popular culture. It is these contradictory and often oppressive notions of motherhood that form the backdrop to the experiences of the drug-using mothers that are described in later chapters.

MOTHERHOOD AS NATURAL, INSTINCTIVE AND FULFILLING

Motherhood is often regarded as women's destiny and ultimate fulfilment, the culmination of female identity. All women are expected to want to become mothers or to justify themselves if they do not have children (Woollett, 1991). Having a baby is romanticised as part of the 'happy ever after' myth, a far cry from the experience of most mothers, and increasingly rejected in favour of more realistic models. In this view of motherhood women are expected to provide unconditional love, to be nurturing and self-sacrificing, instinctively providing the best care for their children as enshrined in the cliché 'mother knows best', even with minimal support (Parker, 1997; Phoenix *et al.*, 1991). Caring for others is assumed to be something all women do; it is the essence of being female. As Gillian Dalley (1996) puts it: 'A view that holds women to be caring to the point of self sacrifice is propagated at all levels of thought and action; it figures in art and literature, it is the prop of official social welfare policies and it is the currency in which the social exchanges within marriage and the domestic sphere are transacted. It means that women accept the validity of this view as readily as men do' (21).

From this model of motherhood emerges the widespread assumption that mothers are or should be the primary carers of children. Mothers' primary child-rearing role, and the more marginal role of fathers, except in terms of economic provision, are frequently taken for granted as natural and right, despite the lack of evidence that children need exclusive maternal care (Tizard, 1991). This assumption relegates mothers' other activities and needs to a place of secondary importance and perpetuates the gendered division of labour in the family. Recent research has challenged some of the assumptions implicit in this view, for example by highlighting the significance of caring by fathers (Daly, 1993; Lewis and O'Brien, 1987) and by demonstrating how the taken-for-granted nature of maternal responsibilities influences decision making in families. For example, in making decisions about the distribution of childcare and economic provision, parents rarely consider the option of fathers being the main carers and mothers the breadwinners (Zvonkovik et al., 1996), even when this is economically and practically more viable or when the traditional approach is associated with great hardship (Lewis et al., 1999a). There have been some attitudinal shifts in relation to gender and parenting roles (Lewis et al., 1999b) but the ideal of the mother as the main and natural carer, subjugating all other activities to motherhood, remains powerful (Lewis, 1991; Lewis et al., 1998).

These assumptions also underlie the popular stereotype of mothers as content and fulfilled, bonding naturally with their babies at birth, and devoted and protective of them from then on. This stereotype is challenged by a large body of evidence that, while motherhood can indeed be rewarding, new motherhood is a difficult experience for many women (Boulton, 1983; Oakley, 1981). Nevertheless, the stereotype of mothers as adapting naturally to the demands of their role whatever their circumstances is not restricted to popular culture. There is a strong tradition of research in clinical psychology, which examines variables influencing adjustment to motherhood. This research tends to pathologise women who do not conform through appropriate bonding or acceptance of the motherhood role. Factors, which have been examined in relation to maternal emotional adjustment, include: mothers' personality; maternal age (Young, 1986); women's relations with their own mothers (Shereshefsky and Yarrow, 1973; Young, 1986); maternal self-efficacy (Pridham and Chang, 1992), and maternal preparedness for the reality of mothering (Coleman *et al.*, 1999). The emphasis on these individual factors fails to take account of social and material pressures that many mothers face. Although a few studies have also included situational factors such as social stress (Crnic *et al.*, 1983), and social support (Crockenberg, 1981), this line of research continues to reflect conventional assumptions about maternal responsibility and experience. For example, a recent study examining the relationship between the extent of realism in pregnant women's expectations of motherhood and the experienced reality of motherhood states 'an understanding of the multidimensional process whereby the primiparous woman *learns how to mother and accept the responsibilities associated with the role* is vitally important to the welfare of mother and infant' (Coleman *et al.*, 1999: 27 (our italics)). There is an implication here that there is a defined reality of good motherhood, which mothers must learn to accept, and for which they are blamed or pathologised for not accepting.

CONCEPTS OF THE 'GOOD MOTHER'

Despite the notion that good mothering is natural and instinctive, much of the research and writing on pregnancy and motherhood assumes that the needs of the child and mother are in conflict rather than interrelated (Woollet and Phoenix, 1991). This implies that mothers must be monitored to ensure that they measure up to experts' pronouncements on good mothering. Historically motherhood has been examined primarily in terms of its impact on children. An exclusive focus on children's needs, especially if they are assumed to be in conflict with the needs of mothers, renders mothers' own needs invisible or inconsequential. Until the late 1970s, when a number of feminist texts on motherhood first began to appear (e.g. Chodorow, 1978; Dinnerstein, 1976) mothers' voices were largely absent from debates on motherhood or good mothering, while children's perspectives were represented by adult 'experts' rather than by talking to children themselves. Recent research that does seek children's views (e.g. Moore *et al.*, 1996; Solberg, 1990) illustrates the interdependence of the well-being of mothers and children, and challenges some of the assumptions implicit in earlier representations of motherhood.

The research on 'good mothering' investigated maternal qualities and skills, which could be associated with positive child development, for example: maternal style that is controlling or child centred (e.g. Schaffer, 1986); and maternal sensitivity (Stern, 1977). This research remains influential and is often reflected in childcare manuals. Harriette Marshall, in an analysis of the content of childcare manuals, concluded that they place the responsibility for 'normal development' of children firmly on the mother, implying that she should be constantly available to care for and stimulate her child, thus inducing feelings of guilt by setting impossible standards (Marshall, 1991). Phoenix and Woollett (1991) argue that within the discourse of good mothering, mothers are expected to raise children in the 'right circumstances', and argue that the socially legitimated circumstances are in fact very limited; two heterosexual parents, preferably married, with the mother not too young or too old, and with mother as the caregiver and father as the breadwinner. Although receiving scant attention in previous research it can be assumed that the ideal mother would also be expected to take only legal drugs.

Notions of good mothering, with the embedded assumptions of the primacy and exclusivity of mothering, have fuelled debates about whether mothers of young children should undertake other roles such as paid employment outside the home (Lewis, 1991; Tizard, 1991). Debates about 'working mothers' (with the implication that caring for children is not work) stems from the work of John Bowlby and other developmental psychologists on mother–child attachment and separation. Bowlby's early research based on children in long-term care (Bowlby, 1953) has often been misinterpreted to imply that children will be psychologically damaged if they are not cared for exclusively by mothers, even though maternal separation per se has not been found to have any adverse effect on child development (Rutter, 1981). The focus on mother–child interaction and associated notions that motherhood is the most vital and demanding role in a woman's life is reflected in psychological research on the impact of multiple roles. This research has examined the impact of mothers' employment not only on children (Hoffman, 1979), but also on marriages (Staines et al., 1978) and on mothers' own well-being (Welch and Booth, 1977). The implicit, and sometimes explicit, view has been that motherhood is so all pervading that if mothers attempt to combine it with employment or other demanding activities, children and the family members will suffer. Multiple roles will then expose mothers to intolerable stressors and contribute to both physical and psychological distress. The evidence from these studies indicates that children are unlikely to suffer psychological damage if mothers work outside the home and indeed are likely to benefit from a variety of social contacts (Tizard, 1991). Furthermore, there is now much evidence that multiple roles, including motherhood and employment, tend to protect mothers' well-being, providing multiple sources of satisfaction (Crosby, 1987; Lewis et al., 1999a). Children benefit from mothers who are satisfied with their roles whether as full-time mothers or employed mothers (Hoffman, 1979). Nevertheless, these debates have often resulted in mothers being labelled as selfish or inadequate simply because they choose, or need, to undertake paid work; they have an identity and occupation other than motherhood. This has generated feelings of guilt and inadequacy in generations of employed mothers (Brannen and Moss, 1990; Lewis, 1991; Sharpe, 1984).

MOTHERHOOD AS WORK

Balancing the view of motherhood as instinctive, natural, joyful and women's ultimate fulfilment, a less idealistic view has emerged from studies which focus on mothers' experiences, treating women as individuals in their own right, and not only in relation to children. Motherhood is portrayed as hard work, often isolating and stressful, changing women's lives and involving great responsibilities. There are two research traditions that adopt variations on this view: one emphasises overload and stress, the other highlights the nature and extent of the work that mothers perform. The first approach examines maternal distress, particularly isolation, economic dependence of mothers without employment, fatigue, exhaustion and often depression (Graham and McKee, 1980; Oakley, 1981). While acknowledging that mothering can be very rewarding, this research also highlights the physically hard work of mothering and the emotional strains, particularly the anxieties and guilt, arising from feelings of inadequacy in relation to the impossible standard of the ideal good mother (which includes being content and unstressed). This view is not limited to social science research but is also evident in novels such as those of Fay Weldon who counteracts idealised and rosy notions of motherhood with more realistic images. Motherhood is shown to be stressful even in two-parent families, a factor that is often overlooked in discussions of lone parents, which often imply that mothers would be so much better off if they had a husband or partner. Although much of this literature has been criticised for being based on the experiences of white middle-class women (Featherstone, 1997), it has nevertheless served to challenge simplistic and romanticised views of motherhood.

The second approach to conceptualising mothering as work focuses on making visible the work that mothers do, which, it is argued, is often devalued. It challenges the assumed common sense, shared understanding of what motherhood involves. Rather than asking what mothers should do, that is, trying to identify good mothering, this approach looks at the everyday practices of mothering and argues not just that these constitute work, but that it is valuable and important work which should not be trivialised or underestimated (DeVault, 1991; Ribbens, 1994; Ruddick, 1989). This approach does not mystify such work as something that only mothers are capable of doing. Fathers too can undertake this work.

It has been necessary to examine the practices of mothering in this way because the work involved in caring is often viewed as a contradiction in terms, since care is assumed to be something done for love and therefore the antithesis of work (Dalley, 1996; DeVault, 1991; Trausdottir, 1991). This derives from a failure to make the conceptual distinction between 'caring for' and 'caring about' children (Dalley, 1996). 'Caring for' children involves the physical work of looking after them while 'caring about' a child refers to the feelings of love and affection for him or her. These two forms of caring tend to be blurred in discussions of motherhood (Dalley, 1996; Hooymans and Gonyea, 1995). The possibility of separating the two is rarely articulated except in discussions of 'deviant' mothers who defy norms by, for example, not caring for a child whom they nevertheless care about (Dalley, 1996). Thus if a mother allows someone else to care for her child, or gives up a child she cares about, because of emotional, economic or social difficulties, she is deemed unnatural. Because the caring for aspect of motherhood is deemed natural and inseparable from caring about the child, mothers are rarely acknowledged when outcomes are successful, but are frequently blamed if they fail to care for the child 'properly' (Hooymans and Gonyea, 1996).

This approach therefore makes visible the work involved in caring for children, usually performed by mothers, but which could equally be performed by fathers or others. Because of the focus on the nature and significance of this work but also the potential for overload and stress, it highlights mothers' needs for support, both practical and also often emotional, to enable them to achieve the best outcomes for their children and for their own well-being.

MOTHERHOOD AS A SOCIAL CONSTRUCTION

Recent research, which examines motherhood from mothers' own perspectives and recognises the interdependence of the needs of mothers and children, has begun to conceptualise mothers in relation to social structures and processes. Two major concepts of motherhood emerge from this trend: that motherhood is a social construction of impossible perfection that is internalised by all mothers, and a psycho-dynamic approach focusing on motherhood as an ambivalent state that results from society's failure to legitimise a range of maternal feelings.

Notions of motherhood and especially 'good mothering' can be regarded as social constructions that vary over time and place, and have important consequences for mothers and families (Kitzinger, 1978; Woollett and Phoenix, 1991). This can be illustrated in relation to national policies regarding maternal employment. Views on the employment of mothers of young children have changed over time and this is increasingly accepted and even encouraged nowadays although there has been little practical support for employed mothers of young children in Britain. Public childcare provision remains among the lowest in Europe (Moss, 1996), reflecting policy makers' ambivalence about mothers' employment, at least until recently and in contrast to countries such as France and the Scandinavian countries where it is taken for granted that mothers also undertake paid work and affordable publicly provided childcare is widely available

(Fagnani, 1998; Sandqvist, 1992). Even in Britain maternal employment is encouraged when it is deemed necessary for society. For example, during the world wars nurseries were opened to enable mothers to undertake the jobs vacated by the men at the battlefront. More recently, concerns about the growth of lone motherhood and the costs of financial support from public funds have resulted in efforts to encourage these mothers to seek employment and economic independence. Constructs of good mothering are not stable but changing and dynamic.

The model of socially constructed ideals states that women internalise societal expectations of motherhood and hence feel guilty if they cannot reach the standards imposed. Mothers have to deal with both external and internal forces. These coexist with contemporaneous directives for mothers to be active achievers in the public sphere. Raphael-Leff (1991) encapsulates this view when she states 'guilt-ridden modern day mothers find themselves engaged in a struggle – caught between the conflictual vectors of self-realisation and selfless maternal devotion, undermined by both external expectations and internalised demands in a society which idealises motherhood while under-valuing mothers' (393). A major task for mothers in this view is to negotiate ways of managing the disjunction between socially constructed ideals of motherhood and the realities of their lives.

AMBIVALENT MOTHERS AND SOCIAL PRESSURES

The impact of internalised ideals of motherhood is further explored by feminist psychoanalysts who focus on experiences of ambivalence among mothers. This approach is based on the observation that mothers are expected to experience only unconditional maternal love, to be child centred, ever responsive and sensitive to children's needs while denying their own needs and aspirations. It is argued that feelings of inadequacy and negativity are produced by this culture, but are also stigmatised. Society legitimates only a narrow range of maternal feelings and this excludes any feelings of maternal ambivalence (Hollway and Featherstone, 1997).

Feelings of maternal ambivalence have largely been pathologised in other approaches to motherhood. They are regarded as a failure to adapt to motherhood (Coleman et al., 1999). Feminist psychoanalytic writers, focusing on maternal subjectivity (Featherstone, 1997; Parker, 1997), not only regard maternal ambivalence as natural and pervasive, but also see this as the key to understanding mothers' experiences within contemporary society. What is unnatural, it is argued, is society's failure to recognise this ambivalence as natural. This creates the need for mothers to suppress these feelings rather than to be able to deal with them in a constructive way. According to Parker (1997): 'None of us find it easy to

truly accept that we both love and hate our children. For maternal ambivalence constitutes not an anodyne condition of mixed feelings, but a complex
and contradictory state of mind, shared variously by all mothers, in which
loving and hating feelings for children exist side by side. However, much
of the ubiquitous guilt mothers endure stems from difficulties in wea-
thering the painful feelings evoked by experiencing maternal ambivalence
in a culture that shies away from the very existence of something it has
helped to produce' (17).

Ambivalence can be a painful experience for mothers. To acknowledge
hating a child one loves, but who is totally dependent on the mother's care,
can be frightening. Parker (1997) makes a distinction between manageable
and unmanageable ambivalence. Manageable ambivalence, that is ambivalent feelings that the mother can accept and feel comfortable with, is a source
of creativity and insight. However, unmanageable ambivalence causes intolerable feelings of guilt and self-hate. Manageable ambivalence is difficult to
achieve in a society which denies mothers the right to feel anything but
unconditional love for their children.

This approach suggests the need for mothers to find ways of rejecting
impossible and contradictory social directives, to recognise mixed feelings about motherhood as natural, and to seek ways of mothering which
fit with their own capacities and circumstances.

THE IDEALISATION AND BLAMING OF MOTHERS

Stereotypes of mothers as naturally caring, nurturing, self-sacrificing and
wise, and the denial that they may feel any ambivalence about their role,
stem from the idealisation of motherhood. The stereotype of the perfect
mother is of course one that is impossible to live up to, even in the most
privileged of circumstances. It is particularly pernicious for those struggling to mother in abject poverty or in other extreme conditions and often
with minimal support. It is difficult, too, for those struggling to maintain
a drug habit or to overcome addiction. Feminist writers have criticised the
stereotype and explained imperfect motherhood in the context of patriar-
chal systems, which make women powerless (Dinnerstein, 1976). However,
Chodorow and Contratto (1992) argue that even in this approach there is
an implicit assumption that maternal perfection could emerge if only patri-
archy could be overthrown and mothers allowed to be their natural selves.

The ideal of the perfect mother also portrays mothers as being all
powerful. This power derives from the ability to determine how children
will develop. The popular notion that the mother–child relationship in
the first few years of life is crucial for a child's future psychological,
emotional and social development was derived initially from Freudian and

post-Freudian theory. It has exerted a strong influence on developmental psychology and also entered into popular received wisdom. Indeed some commentators have argued that this deterministic approach has become generalised to imply that early mother–child relationships determine the whole of history, society and culture (Chodorow and Contratto, 1992). Mothers are thus viewed as having the power to determine how their children will turn out, regardless of the social and institutional context in which they bring up their children, but are blamed if children do turn out to be less than perfect.

The other side of the stereotypical ideal that is portrayed in the media and academic texts is that when mothers are seen to be less than perfect they are regarded as unnatural and deviant. Because of the self-sacrificing ideal, mothers who are perceived as putting themselves first and whose behaviour conflicts with what is considered appropriate for motherhood are labelled as selfish, or even evil (Coward, 1997). For example, few mothers abandon their children, however difficult their circumstances, but those who do so are socially stigmatised. In contrast, fathers who abandon their children may be viewed as irresponsible, but their behaviour remains within the boundaries of social acceptability, especially if they continue to provide economically for the child. If mothers harm their children this is treated as beyond belief and mothers are vilified (Coward, 1997). Harm inflicted by fathers appears to be easier to accept; it is not condoned but fathers are not expected to be perfect. This blaming culture is nowhere more apparent than in discourses about lone mothers. Single mothers have long been stigmatised, and although there is considerably more tolerance now than in the past, they are often still regarded as problematic (Kiernan et al., 1998). Politicians and the media frequently represent lone mothers as problems and as the source of many other problems such as rising crime rates and male underachievement (Coward, 1997). In these discussions lone mothers are constructed as selfish or feckless, or as overassertive feminists, albeit many are divorced, abandoned, widowed or escaping from abusive relationships. They are blamed for 'depriving' children of an authority figure and of denying boys a male role model. Most recently political campaigns and media reports about 'Welfare to Work' characterise single mothers who claim benefits rather than seeking employment as lazy and scrounging from the state (Kiernan et al., 1998).

Negative stereotypes of mothers who do not conform to the ideal, such as single mothers or young mothers have been reinforced by psychological research, which shows a number of negative outcomes for children reared in these families (e.g. Simms and Smith, 1986). However, this body of research has been much criticised for its overly simplistic approach, isolating certain variables while neglecting other highly significant factors such as poverty or lack of support (Woollett and Phoenix, 1992). The effects of these social and structural factors cannot be separated from those of the conditions under scrutiny. A consequence of this concept of motherhood is that many mothers with intolerable burdens of responsibility, in need of support, whether physical, emotional, social or practical, are too often merely blamed for failing to conform to a stereotype of social acceptability.

Explanations of why mothers are idealised, and then denigrated if they fail to conform to the stereotype, often draw on psychoanalytic literature. For example, feminist psychoanalytic writers attribute the idealisation of mothers to the persistence of infantile fantasies, which they argue are the outcome of being mothered exclusively by one woman (the mother) who comes to represent the source of all good (and all evil) (Chodorow, 1978; Chodorow and Contratto, 1992). It has been argued that the denigration and criticism of mothers can be viewed as a defence against recognising that mothers are in fact not perfect (Parker, 1997) and that like any other large diverse group in society, they exhibit the whole range of human frailties. The more mothers exhibit socially unacceptable or stigmatised behaviour, the more they challenge the myth of maternal superhuman perfection, which explains resistance to the idea that substance-abusing women can also be good mothers. Substance-abusing mothers, who may also be lone parents or belong to other stigmatised groups, are only too aware that they do not live up to the ideal of the perfect mother (Taylor, 1993). Like countless other mothers they must struggle to cope with the feelings of guilt and inadequacy that myths of perfect motherhood generate. It is difficult to be a confident mother in these circumstances.

SUMMARY

A number of themes run through all the concepts of motherhood discussed above. The first is that society has enormous expectations of mothers. This chapter has examined some of the powerful stereotypes of the 'good mother' and the processes by which these become social directives to attain impossible standards. There are huge variations among mothers, not least in their social circumstances, and evidence that adequate mothering can take place in a range of social contexts (New and David, 1985). Labelling a mother as deviant because she does not fit the stereotype, due to substance abuse or other factors, can undermine her efforts to be a good mother, and obscure the support she needs.

A second theme is the widespread feeling of guilt and inadequacy as well as ambivalence among most mothers as a consequence of social pressures. All mothers must find ways of coping with these feelings. Substance abuse may be one way of coping, but it also perpetuates the gap between mothers' self-perceptions and their internalised ideals of the perfect mother. This highlights the crucial importance of non-judgemental support in helping them to manage these conflicts and do their best for their children.

Finally, when we look beyond the stereotypes and romanticising of motherhood it is clear that it is a highly demanding role. It is in the children's as well as the mothers' interests to recognise that mothers need support – physical and material, and also emotional – to help them manage the work of mothering and come to terms with the complex mixture of emotions that motherhood involves. Substance abuse is not in itself a barrier to good mothering, but the myth of motherhood perfection and subsequent feeling of guilt and inadequacy, which this produces among mothers, can reduce self-confidence and make it difficult for drug-using mothers to seek and then benefit from the support that is available.

REFERENCES

Boulton, M.G. (1983) *On Being a Mother.* London: Tavistock.

Bowlby, J. (1953) *Childcare and the Growth of Love.* Harmondsworth: Penguin.

Brannen, J. and Moss, P. (1991) *Managing Mothers. Dual Earner Families After Maternity Leave.* London: Unwyn Hyman.

Chodorow, N. (1978) *The Reproduction of Mothering.* Berkeley: University of California Press.

Chodorow, N. and Contratto, S. (1992) The fantasy of the perfect mother, in: B. Thorne and M. Yalom (eds) *Rethinking the Family. Some Feminist Questions.* Boston: Northeastern University Press.

Coleman, P., Nelsen, E.S. and Sundre, D.I. (1999) The relationship between prenatal expectations and post natal attitudes among first-time mothers. *Journal of Reproductive and Infant Psychology* 17(1), 27–39.

Coward, R. (1997) The heaven and hell of mothering: mothering and ambivalence in the mass media, in: W. Hollway and B. Featherstone (eds) *Mothering and Ambivalence.* London: Routledge, 111–118.

Crnic, K.A., Greenberg, M.T., Ragozin, A.S., Robinson, N. and Bashman, R.B. (1983) Effects of stress and social support on mothers of premature and full term infants. *Child Development* 54, 209–217.

Crockenberg, S. (1981) Infant irritability, mother responsiveness and support influences on the security of infant attachment. *Child Development* 52, 857–865.

Crosby, F.J. (1987) (ed.) *Spouse, Parent, Worker: gender and multiple roles.* New Haven, CT: Yale University Press.

Dalley, G. (1996) *Ideologies of Caring. Rethinking Community and Collectivism.* London: Macmillan.

Daly, K.J. (1993) Reshaping fatherhood: finding the models. *Journal of Family Issues* 14, 510–530.

DeVault, M.L. (1991) *Feeding the Family. The Social Organization of Caring as Gendered Work.* Chicago: University of Chicago Press.

Dinnerstein, D. (1976) *The Mermaid and the Minotaur.* New York: Harper and Row.

Fagnani, J. (1998) Helping mothers to combine paid and unpaid work – or fighting unemployment. The ambiguities of French family policy. *Community, Work and Family* 1(3), 297–312.

Featherstone, B. (1997) Crisis in the western family, in: W. Hollway and B. Featherstone (eds) *Mothering and Ambivalence.* London: Routledge, 1–16.

Graham, H. and McKee, L. (1980) *The First Months of Motherhood.* London: Health Education Council.

Hoffman, L.W. (1979) Maternal employment. *American Psychologist* 34(1), 859–865.

Hollway, W. and Featherstone, B. (eds) (1997) *Mothering and Ambivalence.* London: Routledge.

Hooymans, N.R. and Gonyea, G. (1995) *Feminist Perspectives on Family Care.* Thousand Islands, California: Sage.

Kiernan, K., Land, H. and Lewis, J. (1998) *Lone Motherhood in Twentieth Century Britain: from footnote to front page.* Oxford: Clarendon Press.

Kitzinger, S. (1978) *Women as Mothers.* Glasgow: Fontana.

Lewis, C. and O'Brien, M. (eds) (1987) *Reassessing Fatherhood: new observations on fatherhood and the modern family.* London: Sage.

Lewis, S. (1991) Motherhood and/or employment: the impact of social and organizational values, in: A. Phoenix, A. Woollett and E. Lloyd (eds) *Motherhood: meanings, practices and ideologies.* London: Sage.

Lewis, S., Kagan, C. and Heaton, P. (1999a) Economic and psychological benefits from employment. The experiences of mothers of disabled children. *Disability and Society* 14(4), 561–575.

Lewis, S., Smithson, J. and Brannen, J. (1999b) Families in transition in Europe. Young adults' orientations to work and family, *Annals of the American Academy of Political and Social Science* 562, 83–97.

Lewis, S., Smithson, J., Brannen, J., Das Dores Guerreiro, M., Kugelberg, C., Nilsen, A. and O'Connor, P. (1998) *Futures on Hold: young Europeans talk about combining work and family.* London: Work Life Research Centre.

Marshall, H. (1991) The social construction of motherhood: an analysis of child-care and parenting manuals, in: A. Phoenix, A. Woollett and E. Lloyd (eds) *Motherhood: meanings, practices and ideologies.* London: Sage.

Moore, M., Sixsmith, J. and Knowles, K. (1996) *Children's Revelations on Family Life.* London: Falmer.

Moss, P. (1996) Reconciling employment and family responsibilities: a European perspective, in: S. Lewis and J. Lewis (eds) *The Work–Family Challenge: rethinking employment.* London: Sage.

New, C. and David, M. (1985) *For the Children's Sake: making childcare more than women's business.* Harmondsworth, Middlesex: Penguin.

Oakley, A. (1981) *From Here to Maternity: becoming a mother.* Harmondsworth: Penguin.

Parker, R. (1997) The production and purposes of maternal ambivalence, in: W. Hollway and B. Featherstone (eds) *Mothering and Ambivalence.* London: Routledge, 17–36.

Phoenix, A. and Woollett, A. (1991) Motherhood: social construction, politics and psychology, in: A. Phoenix, A. Woollett and E. Lloyd (eds) *Motherhood: meanings, practices and ideologies.* London: Sage.

Phoenix, A., Woollett, A. and Lloyd, E. (1991) *Motherhood: meanings, practices and ideologies.* London: Sage.

Pridham, K.F. and Chang, A.S. (1992) Transition to being a mother of a new infant in the first three months: maternal problem solving and self appraisal. *Journal of Advanced Nursing* 17, 204–216.

Raphael-Leff, J. (1991) The mother as container: placental process and inner space. *Feminism and Psychology* 1(3), 393–408.

Ribbens, J. (1994) *Mothers and Their Children. A Feminist Sociology of Child-rearing.* London: Sage.

Ruddick, S. (1989) *Maternal Thinking: towards a politics of peace.* Boston: Beacon.

Rutter, M. (1981) *Maternal Deprivation Reassessed.* 2nd Edition. Harmondsworth: Penguin.

Sandqvist, K. (1992) Sweden's sex role schemes and commitment to gender equality, in: S. Lewis, D.N. Izraeli and H. Hootsmans (eds) *Dual Earner Families: international perspectives.* London: Sage.

Schaffer, H.R. (1986) Child psychology – the future. *Journal of Child Psychology and Psychiatry* 27, 761–769.

Sharpe, T. (1984) *Double Identity. The Lives of Working Mothers.* Harmondsworth, Middlesex: Penguin.

Shereshefsky, P. and Yarrow, L. (1973) *Psychological Aspects of a First Pregnancy and Early Post Natal Adaptation.* New York: Raven.

Simms, M. and Smith, C. (1986) *Teenaged Mothers and their Partners.* London: HMSO.

Solberg, A. (1990) Negotiating childhood: Changing constructions of age for Norwegian children, in: A. James and A. Prout (eds) *Constructing and Reconstructing Childhood: contemporary issues in the sociological study of childhood.* Basingstoke: Falmer Press.

Staines, G.L., Pleck, J.H., Shephard, C.J. and O'Connor, J. (1978) Wife's employment status and marital adjustment – yet another look. *Psychology of Women Quarterly* 3(1), 90–120.

Stern, D. (1977) *The First Relationship. Infant and Mother.* London: Fontana.

Taylor, A. (1993) *Women Drug Users. An Ethnography of a Female Drug Using Community.* Oxford: Clarendon Press.

Tizard, B. (1991) Employed mother and the care of young children, in: A. Phoenix, A. Woollett and E. Lloyd (eds) *Motherhood: meanings, practices and ideologies.* London: Sage.

Trausdottir, R. (1991) Mothers who care. Gender, disability and family life. *Journal of Family Issues* 12, 211–228.

Walkerdine, V. and Lacey, H. (1989) *Democracy in the Kitchen. Regulating Mothers and Socialising Daughters.* London: Virago.

Welch, S. and Booth, A. (1977) Employment and health among married women with children. *Sex Roles* 3, 385–397.

Woollett, A. (1991) Having children: accounts of childless women and women with reproductive problems, in: A. Phoenix, A. Woollett and E. Lloyd (eds) *Motherhood: meanings, practices and ideologies.* London: Sage.

Woollett, A. and Phoenix, A. (1991) Psychological views of mothering, in: A. Phoenix, A. Woollett and E. Lloyd (eds) *Motherhood: meanings, practices and ideologies.* London: Sage.

Young, R. (1986) Primiparas' attitudes towards mothering. *Issues in Comprehensive Paediatric Nursing* 9, 259–272.

Zvonkovik, A.M., Greaves, K.M., Schmiege, J. and Hall, L.D. (1996) The marital construction of gender through work and family decisions: A qualitative analysis. *Journal of Marriage and the Family* 58(1), 91–100.

Part II

Approaching motherhood

The pregnancy

Identifying the appropriate support for the care of pregnant drug users has occupied health professionals with increasing frequency over the last few years. This has coincided with the development of a better understanding of the medical problems that beset this group of women. Underlying these efforts is a belief that drug-using pregnant women do not get the help they need.

Part II examines in detail the experience of pregnancy in the sample of drug-using women participating in the study that is the basis for this book. The problems faced by the women, how they coped with them and who helped them are explored. There are issues raised by these observations that would apply to all pregnant women. However, for the drug-using woman there are additional concerns that will not be resolved easily and for which she will need extra help. Part II ends with a chapter that offers the perspectives of the professionals involved in the care of pregnant drug users who were interviewed as part of the research.

Chapter 4

Preparing for motherhood

Hilary Klee and Suzan Lewis

Becoming a mother is usually represented as a happy event, particularly if this takes place in what are socially constructed as the 'right circumstances', that is, as a married, non-drug-using woman. The research on the transition to parenthood has demonstrated that this can be a problematic period for parents, and especially mothers, whatever their circumstances. The birth of a child is a major life event, requiring substantial adjustment to changing roles and demands. As with other significant life events there may be an elevated risk of stress, physical and psychological illness and reduced satisfaction, but also the potential to learn new coping skills and for positive self-development.

ADAPTING

At one time researchers regarded the transition to parenthood as a crisis because of the extent to which new parents have to adapt to the profound changes in their lives (LeMasters, 1957). While this transition is no longer regarded as an inevitable crisis (Cowan and Cowan, 1995) it is clear that it can be a stressful time. Family stress is often indicated by a decline in marital satisfaction over this period (Moss *et al.*, 1986). At the individual level there is evidence of deterioration in mental health and particularly an increased risk of depression among new mothers (Elliott *et al.*, 1983). Although this applies to a minority of mothers, and other mothers can experience an improvement in physical and psychological health, depression in early motherhood can be severe and distressing. Some studies have attempted to predict which mothers are likely to be most at risk. The mothers' symptoms, life stressors, social support and marital adjustment before the birth have been identified as the most significant predictors of later adaptation (Cowan and Cowan, 1992, 1995). Thus mothers who are already vulnerable may risk an amplification of their difficulties during pregnancy and after having children.

Much of the research on adaptation after the transition to motherhood has been dominated by a medically oriented or individual deficit approach in which all postnatal difficulties are viewed as the result of hormonal or psychological deficiencies. The impact of the social and ideological context of mothering has been comparatively neglected. The evidence of increased stress or depression among mothers well into the early postnatal years, and similar observations for some fathers (Cowan and Cowan, 1995), casts doubt on whether this can be explained entirely in physiological or individual deficit terms. Brown and Harris (1978) first drew attention to the social origins of depression among mothers of young children. They found high rates of depression among mothers of pre-school aged children in inner London, and identified risk factors which included having three or more children, lack of a supportive relationship with a partner and lack of employment outside the home. Mothering in these circumstances could be isolating and stressful. Recent qualitative research has extended our understanding of women's experiences and of why many feel depressed or unhappy after the birth of a child (Mauthner, 1995; Nicholson, 1999). In such studies the women's accounts offer insights into the problems that many experience in adapting to new roles, demands and identities, and the impact on them of the myth of motherhood perfection, which makes it difficult for them to admit to mixed feelings. This can contribute to feelings of low self-esteem and depression and reduce women's confidence in themselves as mothers.

DRUG-USING WOMEN – A DISADVANTAGED GROUP

The transition to motherhood can thus be a difficult time for all women. Drug-using women may be a particularly disadvantaged group facing many additional anxiety provoking problems that test their ability to adapt and cope. Most will start out at a disadvantage in terms of their childhood models of parenting, their dependence on drugs, their current lifestyle, their social isolation, and possibly a sick and fractious infant with whom bonding will prove difficult. Each of these is a barrier to a trouble-free pregnancy and delivery, and when combined they can be overwhelming.

If becoming a mother is viewed as a dimension of crisis, then drug-using women are more likely to be located towards the upper extreme. This can be a perception that they develop early. News of the pregnancy rapidly generates a number of serious dilemmas that need resolving. In this study only half (48 per cent) reported that they were pleased when they were first informed. The reasons for any lack of enthusiasm were understood by several professionals working closely with them:

I think women who are drug users get a raw deal. No matter how people try . . . there's always some judgements made. When you see some of them they're so bloody guilty it's awful. Some have not known till late on in pregnancy . . . they're not sure if they want this baby or not and the whole situation is a mess. I think they're the unluckiest and the saddest people really. The options are so few as well . . . if a woman gets pregnant and she's not ready to stop . . . then it just makes them even more guilty and they set themselves to fail, and it's more guilt. One minute you're ticking over nicely then the next minute you've got everybody involved in your life. Some of the younger women have no experience with young children, they haven't a clue . . . it's not their lifestyle . . . it's frightening sometimes . . . they've never been near a baby.

Continuing the pregnancy

There is evidence that women are able to adapt more easily to pregnancy and motherhood if this is planned (Cutrona and Suhr, 1990). If the pregnancy is unplanned and unwanted, the drug-using woman is likely to experience great anxiety, even panic, and contemplate abortion. Approximately three quarters (72 per cent) of the sample in this study had not planned the pregnancy. There were many pressures towards termination that were admitted by the women, the most typical being: the expectation of damage to the foetus; the prospect of a problematic lifestyle change; the increased strain of an additional child; the break-up of a partnership; and doubts about the support available and exposure of their drug use to outsiders. Over a third (40 per cent) seriously considered abortion. The most common reasons for not aborting were that it would be 'emotionally stressful' or that it was 'too late'. Some women ruled it out as an option or were persuaded to continue because of their partner's response:

He wouldn't have let me terminate it anyway.

Is he really against that then?

No, he really wanted it as well.

* * *

How did you react when they said you were pregnant again?

Oh God, I didn't want it at first. I do now but not at first . . . but the guy I'm with at the moment, it's his first so he's all made up about it.

Multivariate analyses revealed that having a supportive partner was significantly associated with a positive attitude to the pregnancy (82 per cent compared with 56 per cent of those with more negative views) and rejecting an abortion (85 per cent compared with 52 per cent of women considering it). Many fathers supported the child's mother and several of them took their responsibilities very seriously:

How do you feel about becoming a dad again?

I'm happy about it. I just hope everything works out. I'm scared. A child is a big responsibility . . . it takes a lot of effort when they're growing up. If you're trying to cope with drug addiction at the same time, it's hard.

However, much of the women's faith in their partner's support rested, if the partner was a drug user, not only on the emotional and practical aspects of that support, but on him giving up drugs:

He knows I'm cutting down and he'll help me . . . but I've told him he's got to do it as well.

There were other strong influences in making decisions about the pregnancy. Another factor was the response of the woman's mother. A significantly higher proportion of those with a supportive mother had a positive attitude towards the pregnancy (67 per cent compared with 27 per cent of those with serious doubts). A mother could be a potent motivator, assuring her that she would be supported:

I wasn't going to have the baby but she [the mother] was all for it because she'd lost Derek who was adopted . . . and my brother's been in a lot of trouble and she lost his children [taken into care] . . . I really had the baby for my mum as well as myself.

In two-parent families, the success of any change in lifestyle that a baby would bring was heavily dependent on the support of the partner, particularly if relations with grandparents were poor. The women were asked what would make an ideal father; this woman summed up the main points:

Someone you could live with, someone who would get up in the middle of the night, someone who would give you a break when you're tired, someone who would take them out. Someone who would get involved in changing them and things like that.

There were other factors that contributed to the decision about termination. Several women had been powerfully affected by the scan, a standard hospital procedure:

I'd made the first appointment to sort out a termination, but because I was 12 weeks they sent me for a scan. When I saw the scan I changed my mind.

However, she now felt that she had no regrets:

Not now that I have her, none at all. But throughout carrying her I wondered if I had done the right thing. The main worry was I was frightened of her withdrawing . . . I didn't want to terminate the pregnancy because I didn't want her, I just didn't want her to go through that. When I decided to have her after all, I thought I would reduce and come off it, but it wasn't as easy as that.

Data from interviews that took place about six months after the birth revealed that mothers who had seriously considered abortion tended to be less happy with the baby in the early months (55 per cent were happy compared with 87 per cent of those who rejected abortion). These mothers were also more likely to have used heroin (60 per cent compared with 27 per cent) and to have injected drugs since the child's birth (45 per cent compared with 20 per cent). Predictably, perhaps, they were also more likely to have a non-supportive partner. It seems that their problems were still persisting during those first months, which confirms the validity of findings from work among non-drug users that any difficulties occurring before the birth tend to persist once the baby is born.

Some of the women had contemplated adoption if termination was not an option. While the scan was generally welcomed in providing reassurance that the foetus was making normal progress, under these circumstances it could make the dilemma much worse. This 21-year-old woman had contemplated adoption for a previous baby and her experience then acted as a strong deterrent for attending antenatal services this time. She was by this time eight months pregnant and being interviewed on the eve of her first appointment.

I was meant to be having Stuart adopted because I already had a little girl . . . I went to ———— [hospital] and they were giving me the scan and I asked him to turn the screen away because I didn't want to look because I wasn't keeping the baby. He wouldn't, and all the time he was doing it I was looking at the screen and he kept saying, 'Do you realise what you're doing to your unborn child?' And as he was feeling me stomach and everything he was saying, 'Well, there's his little head, there's his little leg' which, even if I was on drugs he shouldn't have done that. And I felt he was doing it on purpose . . . it was awful . . . I hated it.

She subsequently decided to keep the baby.

The consequences of delay

Decisions were needed early to ensure continuous care and attention to health during pregnancy. A major problem was the common delay in recognising the pregnancy. Since foetal damage is most likely at this early stage an extended delay meant increased probability of damage, particularly if street drugs were being used. A high proportion (42 per cent) was unaware of the pregnancy until the second trimester. This precipitated feelings of guilt and concern and also fears that they would be publicly blamed. There were likely to be other, less obvious consequences in that the time course for adaptation to the idea of a pregnancy was reduced. Several women seemed to be late in arriving at a full realisation of the implications, this woman was the most extreme in having her pregnancy confirmed just over three months before delivery and had been ambivalent about her emotions:

> I didn't know how I'd feel when I had him because I don't like babies, well I like kids when they're cheeky, you know, I'll bother with them then. I mean I was buying things but it was like it didn't register and then when I had him it was just a shock, and I didn't bother with him the first day, but I'm all right now.

> *It does take some getting used to.*

> Yeah, but I think it's just because I'd not had long to prepare for it.

Knowing there was an increased likelihood of abnormalities enhanced the importance of the scan and anxiety increased if the woman was asked to take an HIV test too. This woman felt pressured by the request:

> Yeah. It was a bit embarrassing to talk to somebody about it, and then you're frightened in case what the result's gonna come back like. It would be easier to just say, 'No I don't think I'm at risk' and turn my back on it, but then, I think I'd rather do it, I wouldn't want a baby with AIDS.

The perceived compatibility of drugs and mothering

The decision to proceed with the pregnancy did not help reduce the doubts about coping at this time. Drug management during pregnancy now became a highly critical issue and there was a deep fear of failure. Attempting to reconcile their drug use with the role of mother was a major source of anxiety. The change to a drug-free lifestyle had wide-ranging implications; if there was to be such a change then there were other decisions to be made that involved relocating in a different social structure and identifying a plan of action. Some resolution was needed, for example, about whether to continue to use street drugs or restrict consumption to prescribed drugs: how to use drugs and yet provide necessary care and attention for the child at the same time; how to avoid the critical appraisal of social workers who had the power to remove the child; and how to arrive at procedures or rules that safeguarded the child in the eyes of the professionals involved.

Almost all the women in this study were convinced that the child or children should come first and many thought that drugs and mothering did not go together. However, there were differences between amphetamine and opiate users here. For both, the temptation to use was likely to arise when they were under stress from the baby and unable to cope. However, the drugs produced quite different effects – energy was important to the amphetamine user:

> The energy is unbelievable, especially with me having the kids. I know people say that even without kids you need energy, but you . . .

> . . . *need more with kids?*

> Yeah, I think you do because you do a lot of running about – and you're up early so that it's brilliant when you get some energy to think I can take them out all day without thinking 'I've got a bad back' . . . and I've got tons of energy.

> *You said you never get aggressive?*

> No, I smack the kids very occasionally, but that tends to be when I haven't got anything. I'm a much more capable mother on whizz with them.

The women dependent on opiates were more likely to feel very ill until the level of their drug had been restored and withdrawal symptoms abated. They were less likely than amphetamine users to believe that it actively improved mothering:

> . . . if you've got a habit, when you get up in a morning . . . before you can even think about the children . . . you've got to think about getting yourself better, so I don't see how drugs can help somebody be a good mum.

Since drugs were seen as an antidote to stress, their use could increase because the mother could not cope with caring for the child. This was particularly acute for this lone mother:

> When you've got kids like and you're on your own, you can't – like normal people can sort of say, 'You mind the kids for a bit and I'll

go to bed for a couple of hours.' That's how it was when I was married . . . we'd swap over.

Withdrawal for both groups of users was not only unpleasant, it would be difficult to avoid it affecting the child:

> . . . I was dead quick-tempered like. But as soon as I'd done my methadone, then I'd be fine within minutes and be dead lovable. I think that's wrong . . . but you just can't help it sometimes.

A changed lifestyle

The idea that childbirth is an opportunity for women to stop using illicit drugs is widespread among both users and their carers. Even with high motivation, abstinence is difficult and the behaviour of a drug-using partner is a key factor (Farkas, 1976). Those without partners were similarly vulnerable to relapse, for different reasons. It seems that relapse prevention interventions in early motherhood are vital to sustain the efforts made during pregnancy and bolster the woman's good intentions. These may differ depending on the presence of a partner. It may even be easier to maintain a drug-free lifestyle without a partner, provided the support is replaced effectively.

There is evidence that socially isolated parents are more prone to neglect and abuse their children (Seagull, 1987) and lone mothers seemed particularly vulnerable to feelings of isolation in this sample. The prospect of being a single parent was of concern to some women without a partner although frequently this was their choice. The child appeared to be invested with additional meaning, which might have implications for the parent–child relationship later. This single parent of 19 years was concerned about her abilities, believing that there might be a feeling of helplessness when she had the baby:

> Living on your own and seeing no-one . . ., but I don't know really. Maybe colic, how will I react, how will the baby react. I don't want to panic, I want to know what to do about things like that, illness and things like that.

> *Do you think there will be any good things about having a baby?*

> Yes, having someone there 24 hours a day.

Most of the women (36: 72 per cent) saw the transition to motherhood as an opportunity to change their consumption of illicit drugs and methadone dose levels, since their motivation would be high. However, of those, 34 believed it unlikely that they would be able to abstain completely until the baby was born:

I think it'll make me get myself together and that, having another one.

Many formal guidelines on drug use and pregnancy (for example: Council of Europe, 1998; LGDF/SCODA, 1997; Mitchell, 1993) identify this period as an opportunity to change, and recommend that appropriate support is made available. Unfortunately, although many of the complexities of relapse prevention have been known for some time (Gossop, 1989), a full understanding of the pressures on a new mother with a history of drug use is needed if the necessary components of a support system are to be assembled. If these data are lacking, the results of this study suggest that the transition to motherhood for drug-using women will not include a transition to a drug-free lifestyle. It follows that the woman may be left yet again with a sense of failure and hopelessness, and her child faces the prospect of intergenerational transmission of all the associated disadvantages of a drug-using family.

COPING

It seemed remarkable that, despite their difficulties, just over half (57 per cent) of the women were quite confident they would cope with the newborn child. For those with children already this was largely the result of the earlier experience, although there were some who doubted that they would cope with the new baby because of those children and the existing drain on their energies. Sometimes confidence came through belonging to a large family, which had given them experience of living in an environment full of small children and learning from siblings and other relatives about how to manage them.

So how easy did you think it was going to be to adapt then?

Well, like I said, I've been brought up with babies, there's always been a baby at our house. I've been used to getting up and doing the middle feed or whatever for me mam when the kids have been staying. So that's not really a problem.

There were a few women who felt they were naturally endowed with the 'right' attributes. This woman reported a long-standing interest in child-care and was proud of her abilities:

When I was at school we did child-care for three years and I passed it every year. I've always been dead good with the kids . . . when I went to the college and worked with children and the old people, and the handicapped, they said I should look after the children because I was really good with them. I think I know all that I need to know, and the rest just comes naturally sort of thing.

There was a sense in which being a 'good mum' was a redeeming feature and in some way helped to restore self-esteem and confidence:

> I mean I'm really looking forward to motherhood. I've always had a good thing with kids, I mean I've always been good with children even when I wasn't into drugs, do you know what I mean. I'll cope . . . I'm a survivor me, I mean I've said to him [partner] you'll see a change in me when the baby comes . . . and if there's one thing I'm good at, it's getting babies to sleep because I used to help me mate with her nephew and one night we couldn't get him to sleep no matter what and both of us were trying, and then I went in and I got him to sleep. I don't know what it is . . . I think I'll make a really good mother and the drugs don't have anything to do with it.

Although there was optimism in many women's forecasts of the arrival of the child, it seemed at times very fragile. This volatility could be expected given their doubts about the effectiveness of their drug management and the unpredictable quality of the informal and formal support they would receive.

THE SUPPORT NEEDS OF PREGNANT WOMEN

The need for support to help new mothers towards positive adaptation is now increasingly recognised. However, it is important to identify the source and nature of support needed. Brown and Harris (1978) indicated the importance of a close confiding relationship and this has been widely interpreted in terms of support from a partner. But partners are unlikely to be able to provide all the support needed by new mothers at this time. Mothers need a range of support options. There is a need for practical, emotional, and relational support, not all of which can be provided by a single person. Support needs also vary at different stages. For example, immediately after the birth mothers particularly value tangible support and guidance, while at a later stage the support that comes from being integrated into wider social networks becomes more important (Cutrona, 1984). Support from their own mothers, health professionals and other mothers can all have beneficial effects on new mothers and their children (Cowan and Cowan, 1995; Oakley et al., 1996). Contact with other mothers and integration into the community can be crucial for helping new mothers to adapt. Women often withdraw from earlier friendships and social ties after having a baby and become more involved with other local mothers. Networks of new mothers can provide emotional and instrumental support to each other, sharing problems and helping out in numerous practical ways. However, contact with other mothers does not always reduce feelings of isolation and inadequacy, particularly for mothers who do not feel that they can be totally honest and confide their experiences and feelings (Mauthner, 1995).

Drug-using pregnant women and mothers face particular difficulties in obtaining support. The women will be inhibited about seeking help from partners and/or parents if they have kept concealed their use of drugs. Even if this is known there can be problems in getting such support. Our research suggests that many drug-using women are not in stable relationships with a partner. Most of those in long-term relationships have partners with drug-related problems of their own which threaten family stability. The relationships with parents are often strained and volatile following a family history that can include abuse, neglect and abandonment by parents and rebellion and deviance by the child. The highly restricted social network associated with the drugs lifestyle may be an alternative source of support, but this is likely to offer selective and dubious advice. These limitations raise doubts that there will be appropriate support available to help the woman make decisions that will reduce her anxiety and lead to the delivery of a healthy infant and a positive attitude to motherhood. Their need for support will be great but, sadly, it is likely that their sources of support will be limited.

While the reliability of informal support from partner, family and friends may be uncertain, the alternative of replacing or supplementing this with professional expertise is regarded as fraught with significant dangers and hence tends to be avoided. Fears of the consequences of exposure to health and social services may make it difficult for the women to confide their concerns to those who could provide information, reassurance and encouragement. The problems are not only considerably greater for the drug-using mother-to-be, their prospective resolution from the woman's point of view is likely to involve drastic consequences that may be both damaging and long lasting.

APPROACHING THE PROFESSIONALS

As the pregnancy proceeded the reluctance to approach the authorities and a preference for seeking help from social networks affected the mothers' decisions about how to prepare for the birth and the care of the newborn child:

> Yes, I've had loads of advice [about the delivery], everyone telling me which one to have.
>
> *Is this medical advice or friends?*
>
> Friends and sister.

An informed intervention by a sympathetic care-giver during this period could have helped. However, there were many who wanted to retain their independence and privacy:

> I'm not one for asking for help, I'd rather go on my own, I don't like people interfering. There's a social worker/midwife person coming round this afternoon, and I know they're there to help but, I mean, they ask you things and I think 'why?' I'd rather do things for myself and if I can't do it for myself then why should other people do it for me. I'm not one for asking for help I never have been, I'd rather do it on my own.

The majority (88 per cent) of respondents felt they had no need of professional help. There was strong confirmation of the well-established finding that drug-using mothers strive to avoid becoming involved with social workers because their children might be taken into care or they would persist in interfering in their lives. Analyses showed that there were factors significantly associated with such sentiments – a family environment heavily into drugs, the use of heroin throughout pregnancy, and reports of difficulty in coping with the baby.

This woman became indignant at the idea of social work intervention. There was a stigma attached to such interest:

> I wouldn't want dealings with them at all. I wouldn't like them to get involved with me and this baby. If they have reason to be, fair enough, but I wouldn't like the idea of them coming to my home, snooping around. Don't get me wrong, I've nothing to hide, I'd say come in, look at my home, look at my baby, look in my food cupboards and go away and don't come back. I wouldn't like dealing with them, even though some people do get things from them, I'd rather have nothing to do with them. I've seen too many girls be involved with them, take them into their confidence and then the same people come and take the kids away, because of things you've told them in confidence, not that they'd ever have any reason to take my kids away from me, that isn't the reason. I wouldn't like them around, I just don't see the point in them being around.

Eleven women had been in care as a child and therefore had first-hand experience of it. Mothers who had themselves been in care were more likely to report that they needed more help. They had irregular contact and/or poor relationships with their own mothers but were more likely to have contact with other mothers, which is regarded as an important source of support (Mauthner, 1995). Despite the expressed need for more help, even if their childhood social workers had been helpful, most of them did not wish to repeat their own history. This woman feared they would remove the child:

You saw them when you were in care?

Yes, but that stopped when I was sixteen.

How did you get on with them when you were in care?

All right. But that was different.

It was difficult for them to believe that services were not a threat even though they had been offered reassurance:

The only thing I'm worried about is social services, I've got it in me head an' I still have now that they'll take them off me because of what I'm doing even though I've been told by doctors and everybody 'your children are looked after all right . . . your house is okay, they look okay'. But because I'm a drug user an' all that . . .

The need for reassurance was high and some were keen to acquire information that would protect them:

I found out they can't take me kids off me because I've got food in me cupboard and me kids are well looked after and I've got electricity on. But they can be put on the 'at risk register' because they know that I'm injecting, so I don't let them know that.

There were some women, however, who seemed unperturbed:

I don't find them a problem.

If you needed some help with your kids would you consider turning to them?

Yeah, people have the wrong impression of what the social services do.

This woman was more aware of the real goal of social services and hence impervious to gossip:

I've heard all different things like they take your kids off you. I think if you need their help at some stage they're not gonna take your kids off you, they're there to keep families together, I believe that any way. I think it's just people who've been in homes that think things like that.

MODELS OF MOTHERHOOD

Maternal behaviour is usually thought to be learned by daughters from their own mothers (Chodorow, 1978); however, this assumes a reasonably positive mothering experience. Although the reluctance to seek professional help effectively removed one potentially valuable source of support, all of the women had very clear views of what parenting should be like which seemed to be based largely on their personal experience. The models they reported were informed by identifying the faults in their own experiences as a child.

The legacy of childhood experiences

Given the childhood history of many of the women it is unlikely that they would be keen to emulate the model of parenting that governed their own development or seek support and guidance from their own mothers. There was much evidence of deprivation: several had been in care; the home environment tended to be poor, sometimes violent and occasionally deviant. Some women were bitter about their experiences and laid the blame at their own mother's feet:

> I was dragged up . . . mum couldn't care if I got run over by a bus, that sort of thing. But I used to run wild, so my kids aren't going to be brought up like I was.

Others appeared to be more tolerant:

> I was brought up very strict by me nan [grandmother]. Like when I was born me mum couldn't cope, not that she couldn't cope, she was young. And she wanted me nan to look after me.

While parents were not always blamed for what was seen as their mistakes, clearly there was a perceived need to do better:

> Like my kids I tell them I love them and they have kisses and cuddles at night and everything. I never had that, and I've always said I'll bring my kids up differently.

There were, however, some women who took positive aspects of their mother's parenting as good examples. The women were asked what they thought made a woman a good mother:

> I think that just understanding them really. I think that you should stand by them . . . I don't know how I'd cope with prison and things like that . . . I couldn't handle that but I'd still be there. I couldn't ever turn me back on me kid, me mum's never done that with me.

There were women who felt wholly responsible for their drug dependence and regretted the impact on their parents. This woman now realised the implications for the future with her own baby daughter:

> *Do you think you'll bring your kids up in a similar way to what you were brought up then?*

> Most probably, I mean we were brought up right, I just hope she doesn't go off the rails like me.

Several women were intent on continuing their efforts at drug control during pregnancy after the child was born. Abstinence was a key feature of being a good mother for this woman:

> Someone who doesn't use drugs. If you use them, you don't have much time for the kids, and they're not getting what they should be getting, because it's wasted on drugs.

CONCLUSIONS

The transition to motherhood can be a difficult time for all women and especially so for a woman with a history of drug dependence. To achieve social acceptability in the eyes of the rest of society, it requires of her an extensive change in behaviour that starts as soon as the pregnancy is known. Her preparations for the child are not geared primarily towards the more rewarding aspects of accumulating the baby-oriented artefacts – clothes, cot, toys and so on. These are likely to be pushed into the background while she attends to the more urgent tasks of drug management and access to health care and support.

The impending event for her will affect personal and social relationships and precipitate an unwelcome curtailment of a key component in her usual coping strategy – her drugs. It is also likely to expose her to the negative judgements of people who are capable of removing her child. She may start out full of guilt about the drugs taken during pregnancy, whether this was inadvertent or not, and this is reinforced unless she can be reassured that she is doing all she can to avoid damage to the foetus. The support she receives at this time is critical, even more critical than for mothers who are not drug dependent. Service providers may need to play a much more proactive and positive role during her pregnancy and the early months of parenthood if the health of mother and baby is to be safeguarded. Blame at this stage is not only pointless, it can undermine her to the point at which she will abandon her efforts.

The aim of a trouble-free experience of motherhood, not dissimilar to the conventional picture promoted in the media, appears to be unrealistic, but is, nevertheless, often internalised and maintained by drug-using women despite the odds. Retaining motivation, hope and stability in facing the realities of what lies ahead should be the aim of all who are charged with the responsibility for her care.

REFERENCES

Brown, G. and Harris, T. (1978) *The Social Origins of Depression.* London: Tavistock.

Chodorow, N. (1978) *The Reproduction of Mothering.* Berkeley: University of California Press.

Council of Europe (1998) *Pregnancy and Drug Misuse: proceedings of symposium organised by the Pompidou Group.* Strasbourg, 1997. Strasbourg: Council of Europe Publishing.

Cowan, P.C. and Cowan, P.A. (1992) *When Partners Become Parents. The Big Life Change For Couples.* New York: Basic Books.

Cowan, P.C. and Cowan, P.A. (1995) Interventions to ease the transition to parenthood. Why are they needed and what can they do? *Family Relations* 44, 412–423.

Cutrona, C. (1984) Social support and stress in the transition to parenthood. *Journal of Abnormal Psychology* 93, 378–390.

Cutrona, C. and Suhr, J. (1990) The transition to parenthood and the importance of social support, in: S. Fisher and C. Cooper (eds) *On the Move: the psychology of change and transition.* Chichester: Wiley.

Elliott, S.A., Rugg, A.J., Watson, J.P. and Brough, D.J. (1983) Mood changes during pregnancy and after the birth of a child. *British Journal of Clinical Psychology,* 22, 295–308.

Farkas, M.I. (1976) The addicted couple. *Drug Forum* 5(1), 81–7.

Gossop, M. (ed.) (1989) *Relapse and Addictive Behaviour.* London: Routledge.

LeMasters, E.E. (1957) Parenthood as crisis. *Marriage and Family Living* 19, 352–355.

LGDF/SCODA (1997) *Drug Using Parents: policy guidelines for inter-agency working.* London: Local Government Drugs Forum, Standing Conference on Drug Abuse, LGA Publications.

Mauthner, N. (1995) Postnatal depression. The significance of social contacts between mothers. *Women's Studies International Forum* 18(3), 311–323.

Mitchell, J.L. (1993) *Pregnant, Substance-abusing Women.* Treatment Improvement (TIP), Series 2, Rockville: The US Department of Health and Human Services.

Moss, P., Bolland, G., Foxman, R. and Own, C. (1986) Marital relations during the transition to parenthood. *Journal of Reproductive and Infant Psychology* 4, 57–69.

Nicholson, P. (1999) Loss, happiness and postpartum depression: the ultimate paradox. *Canadian Psychology* 40(2), 162–178.

Oakley, A., Hickey, D., Rajan, L. and Rigby, A.S. (1996) Social support in pregnancy: does it have long term effects? *Journal of Reproductive and Infant Psychology* 14(1), 7–22.

Seagull, E.A.W. (1987) Social support and child maltreatment: a review of the evidence. *Child Abuse and Neglect* 11, 41–52.

Chapter 5

Antenatal care

Expectations and experiences

Hilary Klee

Although there is a wealth of research-based information on the medical aspects of pregnancy and infant morbidity among drug-using women, mostly from the US, there are no corresponding data on the social and psychological changes that occur at this time. Similarly, it is difficult to find any independent research on the use of antenatal services by drug-using women. Their reluctance to present to services, and their failure to keep appointments, has often been noted by health professionals. The reasons may have seemed so obvious that there was no need to explore them. As the only source of information these are not only insufficient, they are likely to reflect attitudes that are held by the practitioners involved.

This information vacuum has implications for the quality of care that is offered to pregnant drug users as they arrive at hospital labour wards in ever-increasing numbers (Chavkin *et al.*, 1991). Now women drug users are seen as deserving of special consideration. Fearing to reveal their use of drugs to the extent that they continue to avoid services when in advanced stages of pregnancy means that their own health and that of their offspring are at considerable risk (DoH, 1999: LGDF/SCODA, 1997).

FAILURE TO ATTEND

It is not only pregnant drug users who avoid antenatal clinics; there are demotivating constraints that can affect all women at this time (Murphy and Rosenbaum, 1999). Some of these are covered below. However, thematic analyses of responses to questions about their pregnancies yielded a variety of concerns among the respondents in this study that were wholly about how they and their babies would be treated by maternity staff – concerns that would not occur to most expectant mothers. It seems that there has been little improvement in this aspect of care: Rosenbaum reported similar fears among women in the US in 1979 (Rosenbaum, 1979; see also Irwin, 1995). Anticipated judgemental attitudes and criticism were deterrents to seeking antenatal care early and it seems that clinic appointments were rarely positive experiences. It is possible that their fears proved largely unfounded. Nonetheless there was much prospective anxiety and that some women did not seek information was perhaps the most revealing aspect of their state of mind at this time.

There were practical reasons for not attending for antenatal care. For example, clinics were avoided and appointments missed because of long waiting times, and some appointment times were difficult because of caring for other children. While this would apply to all women, the lifestyles of some of the respondents were difficult to reconcile with remembering to keep appointments, and there were additional disincentives, for example different doctors on each visit meant the woman might have to overcome the hurdle of talking about her drugs yet again. Nearly two-thirds (62 per cent) had missed an appointment, some had missed several. This was sometimes excused by diminishing their importance:

> they keep you waiting for hours, then just feel the baby, measure you . . . it's not a major crime to miss it.

For those with children, an existing family made life more difficult if there was no one to look after them, and it could be expensive:

> I only went once, once to the hospital and I didn't go to me doctors at all. I did have appointments to go to and that but I just didn't go.
>
> *Why was that?*
>
> It was too far.
>
> It worked out at four on the bus with all the kids. (partner intervenes)

The effects of past experience

Past experience had a direct effect on the willingness to attend services, a legacy that may take time to dissipate. Experiences were handed on to new mothers through the drug users' 'grapevine'. The information was generally negative:

> *Have you mentioned the methadone to the hospital?*
>
> No, I know I'll get treated different. My friends have been treated like scum.

Some of the women described practices that were insensitive and could be regarded as blunders in terms of patient care today. There were some that had occurred many years before that still affected their decisions. For this woman it ensured that she would conceal her use of drugs this time:

When I was having Neil [first child] you used to go to the reception
and there was a queue behind me and I had to pass them me file, and
you know when you see on the films it has 'Top Secret' written across
it? Well, right across it was 'Drug Abuser'. I was too honest in the
past, that's why I'm not saying nothing now. . . .

Discrimination and negative judgements

It seemed that by far the most important reasons for not attending were the
attitudes of the staff. The women were well aware of the judgemental and
often hostile attitudes towards drug-using mothers and, understandably,
wanted to avoid being exposed to them. Their general expectation of antenatal and ward staff was of negative discrimination and they were very
sensitive to it. The main complaint about maternity services concerned 'bad
attitudes'. Nearly a third (31 per cent) had experienced these and feared
meeting them again. It was a disincentive to be truthful for this woman:

Even if you smoke a cigarette they look as though they hate you
. . . God knows what they would do if I told them about the drugs.

Another woman felt doubly disadvantaged, and this may be typical of a
large number of drug users who are lone parents:

It would take a lot to get me there [antenatal clinic]. I'd only really
go if I thought there was something wrong and then I'd probably just
go to the doctor. They treat you like shit if you are a single parent
anyway.

There were others that were not so afraid, however, and decided to tell
staff about their methadone prescription:

How did you feel about that?

OK, it was just a computer thing. They just asked loads of questions
. . . I'd rather they know anyway because then they can look out for
things with the baby . . . rather than me not telling them and the baby
being sick and them not knowing why.

Women not subjected to hostility were, nonetheless, sensitive to the cues
that could give them away:

How did you feel about talking about it with them?

I was very embarrassed, but no-one seemed to look down on me. The
only time it bothered me was when they took blood from me, they

would put 'Danger, Infection' on the bottles, but that was the only thing really.

The dominant need of the women was to be treated just like any other patient, and when they encountered sympathetic treatment it was very much appreciated:

I was really worried about the consultant. I was told he was a bit off when he knew you were on methadone. He wanted you to have a hepatitis test or an AIDS test otherwise he wouldn't deliver your baby . . . that was the rumour that was going around. But as soon as I saw him he was great with me. Very loud and shouts a lot you know. Shouts, 'How are you on your methadone?' Shouts dead loud. But the thing is, we're all in individual cubicles so no one knows who he's talking to.

Great sensitivity was shown for the concerns of the mother at times:

Has anyone told you about what effect the methadone might have on the baby?

Yes, at the clinic . . . and I wanted to read up about it but they advised me not to because it might upset me too much.

It was a shock to find that you were labelled in some way. This woman believed that it affected the way she was treated:

the first thing they see when they open the file at the top is 'Mother on Methadone', and I could see a difference in the nurses in before they found out to after, the way they treated me . . . I was shocked at it but I expected it in a way. They sit and talk to you, and as soon as they find out you're a drug addict that's it, you're nothing. I think the nurses, they're there because they care about children, . . . and if they were being funny with me, well, I tried to understand it. I didn't expect them to be nice to me, but the way they were was just terrible, they didn't hide the fact, even when my boyfriend was there, they were the same with him, I couldn't wait to get out.

Most of the women with children could recount negative experiences associated with past attendance at an antenatal clinic. However, they were not always totally damning and were sometimes set in the context of more positive interactions. Criticisms were selective but with no particular group of professionals mentioned more than another:

Oh yeah, they were quite nice with me. It was paediatricians and the doctors themselves who were understanding. The people who can be nasty are the midwives. An oldish midwife came up to me and said, 'Oh yes, you're the one who's had heroin and methadone in the past aren't you?' And she pulled the screen down so people could hear, and I said, 'Can you keep your voice down, there might be someone here who knows me.' And she said, 'Well you shouldn't have done it.' She was a nasty one, it's hardly surprising really . . . but they've no right to treat you like that because they don't realise how hard it is.

The doctor were a bit sarcastic. He said, 'Well your veins are knackered' and he said 'you do know your baby will have to go to special care' . . . I know they have to tell you that but it was just the way he said it. The midwife, she were brilliant.

The women who injected their drugs were particularly concerned. There was an additional stigma attached to injecting, of which they were well aware, which was made worse by the possibility of the track marks on their arms being discovered:

he asked to do me blood pressure. I kept giving him this arm but he wouldn't take it, he said he wanted the other arm so I mean I felt a bit stupid, but I thought 'I can't be this close to the doctor if I can't tell him'. Anyway I told him, and he tried to tell me that was the reason I hadn't come on [menstruated] . . . because I was taking drugs. Apparently he's referred me to the hospital because I've had about ten letters, but I can't bring myself to go.

Why is that?

Because I know a girl and she was injecting and they made her take tests for hepatitis . . . they put a skull and cross bones on her cards and I'm not having that. I don't want that . . . I couldn't stand the dirty looks.

The first visit to antenatal was delayed for most of those with unplanned pregnancies, the extreme was eight months pregnant, despite reminders. One woman had not yet plucked up courage to attend:

Two midwives came three days ago. I wouldn't open the front door to them. They probably came to see why I hadn't been, because they'd been sending me appointments and I hadn't been, and I just wouldn't open the door. If my boyfriend had been in he would've opened the door. I just didn't want to. I was feeling down enough as it was and I thought they'd come to tell me off. They just put a note through saying would I try and make the next appointment. I'm gonna go, but I'm dreading it.

A few more experienced and less fearful women were proactive in working out a satisfactory arrangement for their antenatal care. Some were seen at home, others at an agreed location:

> They did give me appointments but I ignored them. I told the midwife who came out to see me that it was stupid going to different places [drug clinic and hospital] . . . so she said she would check the baby's heartbeat and everything else.

THE NEED FOR REASSURANCE

The desire by the women to control methadone consumption while pregnant was strong and based on the hope that the baby would not withdraw at birth. All the women subscribed to some extent to the conventional ideology of the caring mum responsible for the health and well-being of her children, seen also in other research (Boyd, 1999), and a great deal of guilt was associated with using drugs at this time. The women were acutely sensitive to the judgement of others, and for the child to be removed would be a sign to other mothers and nurses that their behaviour had damaged the health of their child. In some cases the guilt was then exacerbated by antenatal staff:

> They make you feel like if anything happens to the baby, it's your fault. I felt terrible when they said the baby might come out withdrawing.

The fear of the baby's removal was a strong and complex emotion and an inevitable component was the anticipated feeling of loss. Since drug management appeared to be a gamble, the probability of avoiding withdrawal was uncertain and the outcome for the infant was equally unpredictable. Hospital policy varied considerably and the women did not always feel they were getting accurate information in advance. Over a quarter (26 per cent) said they had no information about whether their baby would be taken into the Special Care Baby Unit (SCBU), 38 per cent were told that it may be removed and 28 per cent that it would receive standard care on the wards. It is difficult to judge the veracity of these accounts since many women were reticent about asking questions, but there were interactions reported that suggested that communication was very difficult:

> She said they would take the baby from me for two weeks to put into a Special Care Baby Unit to check, but I said I wasn't using any more. She said it takes about seven years to clear out of your system,

and it could come out the same as if I was still using. But it won't because I haven't taken any heroin.

For some women the anxiety was increased by memories of crises in a previous hospital confinement:

Is there anything that you're not looking forward to, any problems?

The way I get treated in the hospital. People keep reassuring me all the time, but until it happens I'm not gonna know . . . like when Sam [first child] was in special care me dad had a heart attack you see, with the stress and everything. I couldn't cope with it myself . . . I'd pick it up and walk out of the hospital – I wouldn't let them do it this time, I just wouldn't. Until that time comes I'm not gonna know.

For drug-using women the prospect of hospital confinement for an extended period is particularly stressful. Sustained effort would be needed to conceal their drug dependence in the unknown territory of a hospital ward. The respondents did not necessarily seek information to reduce the uncertainty by asking the professionals about the procedures. Some drug workers found their clients passive:

This will probably sound awful but they don't seem to sort of say, 'I'm using methadone what are the problems I'm going to find while I'm pregnant or when I go into labour?' I don't know if it's because they just accept that they're a drug user and the doctor is going to treat them in a safe way.

Rather than attributing the reticence to passive acceptance, others mentioned guilt and the need for concealment of their drug use from people who might censure them:

It's all to do with the guilt – they won't assert themselves . . . they don't ask certain things because it'll remind people about their drug use.

Some hospital staff shared this view and one nurse believed the defensiveness of some of the women was the product of a guilty conscience because they knew they were responsible for the baby's condition and did not want to be blamed:

They can be quite a bit on the defence . . . they know it's their fault that the baby cries . . . they're on the defence as if it's nothing to do with what they've been taking.

In some regions the communication of basic information by professionals was poor, perhaps not too much of a problem for patients able and willing to seek it out, but a potential hurdle for the more inhibited and less receptive. Twenty-six per cent of the women reported that no information on general procedures was offered to them, 43 per cent mentioned the administration of methadone, 28 per cent the care of the baby and 22 per cent the procedures followed by the Special Care Baby Unit. Sixteen women (32 per cent) said they needed further information. Reticence in asking questions deserves particular attention since there will be a significant number who will be suffering discomfort through their ignorance, but because of apparent compliance appear to be satisfied.

Compliance pays dividends for drug-using women in smoothing their interactions with staff that they believe may be critical. It should not be interpreted as an indication that they are well informed or that there is full compliance in all respects. The tendency to take control of their own lives, however unwise according to medical opinion, was strong. The compliance could be in principle, for example, in agreeing to reduce the methadone dose during pregnancy, but not as advised by their doctor in practice.

A part of the stereotype of drug users is that they are manipulative. It might be more helpful to regard some of their actions as the only empowering strategies they have at their disposal in a hostile environment, a skill practised over many years by some of the women. The respondents who reported no problems with judgemental attitudes on the part of their carers tended to be the more compliant: they were obeying the rules; they were showing remorse; they were trying to reform:

> No problems [with antenatal]. They even said at the antenatal how pleased they are with me . . . how well I've done. I might get treated a bit better.

> *We might as well talk about that then.*

> That's where it is . . . if they don't think you're trying, that's where they'll turn their nose up at you . . . because to be doing any job like that they think a lot about babies . . . it's their job. Then they go home to their families so it's their life isn't it? I tell them I'm ashamed and they seem to be nice with me and say 'you're doing well'.

A show of compliance was not always needed where attitudes among professionals were informed by greater experience. It seems there is less need to manipulate when they are on your side:

> *And how were they with you when you told them [about her drugs]?*

> All right . . . I said I felt a bit embarrassed about being pregnant and I was scripted on methadone and temazepam, and she said, 'don't worry

about it . . . the girls you get in here are in the same boat, on meth or whatever, it's just like an everyday occurrence now'. A couple of years ago it mightn't have been heard of, but now it's an everyday thing.

THE NEED FOR INFORMATION

Part of the service to pregnant women should be easy access to accurate and helpful information. A range of people could be approached for advice that might be alternative sources of information about what to do about drug use and what to expect the consequences to be for the baby. Consistency was a major problem. While issues of termination and abstinence from drugs gave rise to concern in the earlier months, there was much uncertainty later about breast feeding and the impact of methadone in the mother's milk on the newborn infant.

Breast feeding: an example of confusion

There were variations between hospitals on recommended practice on breast feeding, some regarding the continuation of small amounts as possibly beneficial in facilitating a less traumatic withdrawal by the infant, others strongly discouraging it. The discouragement was not necessarily direct, in this example it was fairly subtle:

> I did say to the nurse when I booked in I was thinking of breast feeding, and she said because I'd bottle fed the rest [of the children] I may as well bottle feed him.

The conflicting views by the professionals to whom they turned left the women at a loss:

> Everybody had different stories, the midwives were saying like they think that you could breast feed and it wouldn't affect it and then another one was saying, 'Oh no, it's just like alcohol, I wouldn't suggest it.' You know, in case the baby's getting methadone through your breast feeding.

On breast feeding, drug workers tended to believe that this was beneficial, which was in contrast to the majority of midwives who were not convinced on the advisability of effectively administering low doses of methadone:

> Now our clinic's point of view is that they should breast feed, it's the natural way to do it, the babies are getting all the antibodies from the

mum and yet methadone does pass through in the breast milk. So surely if the baby's going to withdraw that's going to reduce their withdrawal.

Perhaps because of the disagreement, there was caution among some health professionals when responding to the question. The issue was sometimes resolved by the women through network information or their own observations. This woman assumed that methadone passed through breast milk:

I don't know. I'll tell you something, I'm sure it does, you know why? . . . because I know a woman who was taking it [drugs] right? . . . and she has a little girl. She had it while she was taking and that baby used to scream until it got on the breast. And I mean proper screaming, not crying for food just really screaming and it would only settle down once it had been fed with the breast – not anything else.

The UK clinical guidelines (DoH, 1999) advocate breast feeding by drug users on methadone with the exception of women who are HIV or hepatitis C positive or using high doses of benzodiazepines (see also Chapter 17).

Asking the professionals

The unwillingness to seek information and advice from health professionals was due to many factors. It did not mean that the women were not interested – there were many who had preferred to read something rather than expose their need for information or ask someone who was not sufficiently knowledgeable or sympathetic to enable them to answer questions satisfactorily. Some women did not know what questions needed asking. In addition there was also a pronounced desire to escape the clinic environment quickly rather than prolong the experience with questions:

How happy are you with the care you've had in antenatal?

All right really. I suppose if I wanted more I should have asked, you know, but I just used to get in and want to get out.

In general the majority view was that communication was poor, that their needs should be known and clear information should be given:

Is there anything apart from the delivery you think you should have been told more about?

I think they should have told me more about like after the baby's born, and if I was still on meth what effect it would have on the baby, you know, like special baby care they should tell you more about that.

The need to ask was resented by this woman.

> I think they don't give you any advice, I think you have to ask for it, but I mean why should you ask for it? They should give you advice, you know what I mean? They should give it you, you don't ask for it.

There were additional problems in getting the attention of busy midwives that led to apathy in trying to get questions answered. The women's desire to escape appeared to be matched by a complementary need for the clinic conveyor belt to keep moving. These are not conditions that facilitate sensitive communication and considered advice. Hospital antenatal clinics came in for much criticism but even community midwives, more generally liked, seemed to have little time to help them sort out their problems:

> Barbara [the community midwife] is the only one that tells you things . . . but you have to go and see her. She'll explain if you ask her . . . she's had kids herself so she knows what she's talking about. A lot of it I've learned out of books . . . and other things I've been told by my mum.

While some of the complaints that they were not told enough about the birth and about their condition seemed grounded in the common problems of overworked staff in busy clinics, some women were not ready to receive information, particularly disturbing information, when they felt they could not cope with it:

> I didn't really listen . . . I thought I knew it all.
>
> *What were they saying to you?*
>
> I don't know, it went in one ear and out the other.

The women were given written information, some of it very detailed and they seemed to read it. Some also bought books and read those. However, it was evident that not all their needs were met and this seemed to be a consequence of deficiencies in service provision on the one hand and reluctance to approach them on the other.

EVALUATION OF ANTENATAL SERVICES

Forty-eight (96 per cent) of the respondents were attending antenatal clinics or were in contact with a community midwife during their pregnancy, although there was very wide variation in the timing of their first contact. They were asked for their evaluation of the service provided by the different groups of health professionals.

Confidentiality and communication

The majority (67 per cent) said they were satisfied with the care they received. Eighty-three per cent said that the maternity staff knew of their drug use. However, 21 (44 per cent) of those said they had felt annoyed or embarrassed that they had been informed. This was, however, expected by several respondents. There was regret voiced by this woman that a possible source of support had been effectively removed because of the sharing of information:

> *Did you trust the health workers' confidentiality?*
>
> No, not at all. Where children are concerned there is no confidentiality. I know that from what I've said to my social worker that's supposed to be confidential – they don't keep it that way. Now I just don't tell them anything that might get passed on.
>
> *Do you think there should be more trust?*
>
> I think there should be someone you can talk to without it being passed on.

There were many who seemed too unsure of the professionals with whom they came into contact to feel able to confide in them. Some had believed that all information was passed on as a matter of course:

> I thought they would just know. Because my personal doctor – she knew, I just assumed that it would be on the file. But I was reading a drugs leaflet in the smoking room and it said you have to tell them, the midwives and that, so you can get extra help.
>
> *So you assumed it would be on your records?*
>
> Yes. But I wasn't gonna go and tell the midwives . . . I don't think I would have done that because I know how funny they're gonna be.

Another woman believed that much was disclosed informally and without thought:

> I think they gossip about it amongst themselves. Last time this nurse was asking me about heroin and how I scored, I wouldn't tell her where, but told her the circumstances so she could understand that we need help and people are too frightened to ask for help in case they get busybodies interfering and their kids taken off them. She was flabbergasted, she said, 'We wish more people would tell us so we could help.' I said 'you want to get the nurses to keep their mouths shut, keep it amongst themselves and not have anyone else interfering'.

The perceived deficiencies of maternity services from the women's perspectives were not normally extended to their evaluation of drug workers:

What kind of relationship do you have with the drug clinic?

Pretty good . . . I get on with everyone . . . they all know what I've been through.

This was particularly the case with agencies with clinic sessions for pregnant drug users:

I think they're good . . . and they're very helpful. Like with Paul and Michelle, they're the pregnancy team . . . and we've built up a bond with them.

This woman had been accompanied to the hospital by a drug worker for her first pregnancy which she had found very helpful in getting the information she needed:

Last time it was easier though because I went with someone . . . you have key workers and that, and this girl was my key worker and she used to come with me every week and we got quite close and I used to tell her all kind of personal things. With her coming with me she used to ask them questions that I didn't think of asking. It was good that she came with me, I used to find it really helpful.

However, such attention was rare. The worker had taken on the role of advocate which made demands that would be too high for many drug workers burdened because of staff shortages and high case-loads.

PROFESSIONAL COLLABORATION

For many respondents, the questions on collaboration between agencies came as a surprise. The idea of collaboration had never occurred to them and though some reflected briefly on it, they had no information about whether this occurred or the form that it could take. Although confidentiality was an unresolved issue, there was a need for co-operation, particularly between drug workers and midwives:

I just think they [drug workers] would have a clearer idea of what your needs are. Especially I don't think most midwives know a lot about having an addiction and all that, it's a completely different thing to everything else, I think. Drug counsellors and them have a better idea.

Only in the areas that had been developing the service, through multi-agency pregnancy clinics or drugs liaison midwives, were the women aware of the relationship between different agencies and the effects this had on their treatment.

This woman had no problem with informing the hospital antenatal clinic of her drug use, aware that she would not be an unusual case. This was due to the links made between the drug agency and the clinic by a drug liaison midwife:

> *They weren't shocked or anything?*

> No, I think they're used to it in Liverpool, there is a lot of it about.

SUMMARY AND CONCLUSIONS

These accounts contained numerous complaints and, placed in the context of general provision of antenatal care, raise the question of how different these women are from non-drug users. A major difference was that positive feelings about the pregnancy were always tempered with doubts and fears of a very serious nature.

If it is unplanned the news of a pregnancy can be a very unwelcome surprise for many women, whether using drugs or not. Adaptation for a drug user would be particularly slow under these circumstances, despite the awareness of the need for rapid decisions, since there would be much conflict. Getting to the point at which pregnancy becomes a positive event depends largely, in this group of women, on the extent of the support available, both informal from partners, family and friends, and the formal professional care supplied by antenatal services.

Professional support was variable and sometimes threatening. This is sad since there was a powerful need among the women to be treated like everyone else, in a low key way and without special procedures. Their accounts tend to belie the notion that pregnancy is a time for rehabilitation, a view based on a poor understanding of the constraints on their actions. Such expectations can prove counterproductive when communicated to the women since they increase the pressure on them. In the absence of a supportive family, unless strong professional help is visible, acceptable and available, this may make matters worse. The next chapter deals with the issue that is of most immediate concern to drug users when they become pregnant, namely what to do about their drug use and what the implications could be for the baby, themselves, partner, family, lifestyle, not only in the short term but for the future. These are hard decisions at the best of times, when they are unexpected and need to be made quickly then the conflict is severe.

REFERENCES

Boyd, S. (1999) *Mothers and Illicit Drugs: transcending the myths*. University of Toronto Press: Canada.

Chavkin, W., Harris-Allen, M. and Oberman, M. (1991) Drug abuse and pregnancy: some questions on the public policy, clinical management and maternal and foetal rights. *Birth* 18(2), 107–111.

DoH (1999) *Drug Misuse and Dependence – Guidelines on Clinical Management* (Annex 5: Pregnancy and Neonatal Care). London: Department of Health, The Stationery Office.

Irwin, K. (1995) Ideology, pregnancy and drugs: differences between crack-cocaine, heroin and methamphetamine users. *Contemporary Drug Problems* 22, 613–638.

LGDF/SCODA (1997) *Drug Using Parents: policy guidelines for inter-agency working*. London: Local Government Drugs Forum, Standing Conference on Drug Abuse, LGA Publications.

Murphy, S. and Rosenbaum, M. (1999) *Pregnant Women on Drugs*. New Jersey, US: Rutgers University Press.

Rosenbaum, M. (1979) Difficulties in taking care of business: women addicts as mothers. *American Journal of Drug and Alcohol Abuse* 6, 431–446.

Chapter 6

Drugs and pregnancy

Hilary Klee

Hostility towards women's use of psychoactive drugs surfaces rapidly when they become pregnant. The only option, according to conventional wisdom, is for them to abstain from drugs immediately in order to avoid damage to the infant. Any alternative will put at risk the health and possibly the life of the innocent child. Since the predictability of damage is uncertain, it could be argued that this is the safest precaution. The lack of ambiguity is attractive and leads logically to certain actions and clear preventative messages to the woman. However, it is a specious argument that is uninformed by knowledge of drugs and their effects. Harm avoidance is not so straightforward and the foetus may be more damaged because of precipitate cessation of drugs than through the mother's continued drug use (Allen, 1991).

Inevitably there are serious health risks for the mother and her unborn child if she uses drugs. Mostly these derive from uncontrolled ingestion of street drugs of unpredictable composition and purity, and poor nutrition by the mother. The effect of using a mix of many drugs, with the potential for complex interactions, increases the risk. In addition there is uncertainty about the ways that pregnancy affects drug metabolism and how readily drugs cross the placenta to the foetus (Keith *et al.*, 1988), which appears to be particularly susceptible to teratogenic (malformation) effects in the first eight weeks of pregnancy (Finnegan, 1988).

Heavy opiate use induces menstrual abnormalities such as amenorrhoea which makes it difficult for the woman to know that she is pregnant. This is a hazardous feature for drug-using women given the importance of the early months of pregnancy in the development of the foetus, since chaotic and uncontrolled use at this time may have permanent effects. The subsequent adoption of health protective behaviour may come too late to avoid damage. Such dangers can be compounded by poor compliance with medical protocols considered necessary at this time and missed appointments at antenatal clinics. The solution is simple in theory: professionals should warn about mistaken interpretations of amenorrhoea, get women to use effective birth control methods and persuade them to attend antenatal services immediately pregnancy is suspected. In practice such methods have not always worked and an unknown proportion of drug-using women become known to services only when admitted to hospital in labour (LGDF/SCODA, 1997). There are, however, some negative consequences of labelling pregnant drug users as 'at risk'. Oakley (1992) suggests that they are likely to suffer mental health problems, particularly if they believe they cannot change their behaviour. In particular, the emotions that follow the news of a pregnancy that is unplanned seem to include guilt as a major component (Mondanaro, 1988), and the actions of the health professionals confirm her culpability. In this chapter the pregnant drug user's predicament concerning her use of drugs and her ways of dealing with it are explored.

DRUG USE: THE EARLY MONTHS

Over half the sample (55 per cent) had not been menstruating for some time and many of those who were reported irregular periods. Not surprisingly, they tended to believe that they were either infertile or that their drug habit prevented conception:

> I actually thought the methadone would stop me getting pregnant. I thought it would affect me like heroin. You can't get pregnant when you're on heroin.

Those in treatment were as likely to adhere to this belief as those not. However, many women in treatment had been warned by their drug workers but took the chance anyway:

> I should have known really. They say to you, even if you don't have a period you can still get pregnant. Everyone says that about all sorts of things don't they? I just didn't think I would.

Thirty-four per cent had reached 12 weeks or more gestation before they knew they were pregnant, some of these were unaware for much longer. Uncontrolled, periodic use of heroin is particularly hazardous during pregnancy since the foetus may be subject to fluctuating drug withdrawal and overdose. If the woman learns that she is pregnant late she will not automatically have associated missed periods with conception. The first two or three months, which are the most critical for foetal development, may be the most uncontrolled phase of her pregnancy.

Using street drugs

The news of the pregnancy meant that a decision was needed about drug consumption in the period up to the birth. The most urgent decision concerned the use of street drugs. The preferred drug of just over half of the women was heroin and 54 per cent of them had used it at some stage during pregnancy. A quarter were primary amphetamine users and 38 per cent consumed it during their pregnancy. However, all of the respondents were polydrug users with both illicit and licit drugs such as benzodiazepines in their repertoires. No one consumed alcohol more than occasionally. All were regular cigarette smokers.

There was a tendency for the use of street drugs to decline towards the end of pregnancy and persist for a short period after childbirth when it started to rise again. However, the number of women consuming amphetamine increased at this time. This is attributable to five women polydrug users replacing their drugs with amphetamine which they thought was safer.

Since you've found out about your pregnancy – your drug use, has it changed?

Yes. I've stopped everything but speed . . . really I need to have speed if I'm going out.

A high proportion of the women (60 per cent) had been injecting prior to their pregnancy but this reduced to 36 per cent after knowing they were pregnant. Two of these women subsequently stopped. Nonetheless, this means that over a third were injecting during pregnancy.

It is likely that delay in deciding about changes in drug use is emotionally disturbing in itself and that further stress may then occur when the time comes for action. Understandably, the prospect of radical change was intimidating to the women, even those who had planned the pregnancy. Some were reluctant to commit themselves to a particular goal during the early stages. Most women knew of the possible consequences of delay for foetal health but avoided decisions because of conflicting needs and demands. A few were not well informed, however, and this woman seemed unaware of the inherent dangers:

Do you think it does have any effect on your baby at all?

I don't know, I'll make sure it don't have none. I know it's all right saying that, but I'll try and cut down a lot when I'm about seven months. I mean I'm cutting down now, I want to stop, but if I can't stop I'll make sure that I totally cut down, make sure me arms are clean [currently injects] and I'll tell them how long it is since I've had it. It should be all right.

There were many such exceptions that did not bode well for success in abstaining from street drugs. The amphetamine users were particularly likely to believe they would not have a problem. This was part of a more general view. Several health professionals said that amphetamine per se did not produce abnormalities but that there was a significant risk of malnourishment. This woman was quite sure there would be no damage to the foetus, a view reinforced by her friends who had children:

So have you talked to any health professionals at all about the fact that you've taken the speed?

No. I'm ashamed of it really, especially with being pregnant. It won't do the baby any harm; I've looked into that. You've just got to make sure you're eating well.

Another young woman was exasperating her partner by her persistent delay in putting her objective of abstinence into action:

How are you coping with the pregnancy at the moment?

Fine. (respondent)

You just ignore it [partner to respondent]. We haven't made any steps in the right direction. We haven't done what we need to do. This week . . . it's Thursday and we've spent £180 since Sunday on heroin.

Good intentions

Irrespective of early delays, the majority of respondents were firm in their resolve to alter their use of drugs. Seventy-two per cent felt that pregnancy was a good time to stop using street drugs and a third aimed to become completely drug free. However, there was much concern about lapsing and returning to drugs postnatally. This woman was typically cautious in her attitude:

Do you think having a baby will help you to stay off the gear or away from street drugs and so on?

I always used to say if I was having a baby I would get off it . . . but it's easier said than done.

Women with experience of previous pregnancies were aware of their vulnerability to self-medication when under stress:

I can't say at the moment [if she will resume use], but you never know in the future. It's easy to get back into it – if everything is getting you down it's the first thing you're going to turn to.

The uncertainties were expressed by this woman who, like the majority, was tired of her lifestyle:

It's hard that, you know. I hope so, but it depends, you see, it depends how I feel. You can't say can you? I hope so, I mean I'll be here and me mum will be here. I've got to do it for myself haven't I, and the baby? I should imagine when I've had it I'll be so wrapped up in it, and it'll be summer and it'll be nice. I've had enough of it really.

Women with drug-using partners were familiar with the particular problems posed in having to take this into account:

Even if we stopped heroin we'd have to have some blow [cannabis] . . . we'd have to have something.

The likelihood of temptation arising from the social environment was viewed with some misgiving, and moving out of the area was often mentioned. Many respondents (43 per cent) felt their current accommodation was unsuitable – some were in temporary housing, or their home was too small or it was in a drug-using area and it would be difficult to control their own drug use. Moving away from the drug scene is regarded as the most effective solution for most drug dependent people and, if possible, service providers should try to facilitate a move:

I want to move away . . . I know there's drugs everywhere and ———— is dead small it's really easy to get involved with the wrong type of people.

Some women were concerned about increasing isolation if they stayed:

I don't want to stay in ———— the only concern they've got is about drugs . . . so I don't see anybody no more.

The potential negative influence of the social environment was very evident in this study. It was not used simply as an excuse for a prospective relapse:

What are you hoping to do once the baby is born, about your drugs, have you thought about what might happen?

I haven't thought too much about it, but I wouldn't be able to give them up altogether, to be honest, I really don't think I could. But I will try, I really will try. But I think it's harder in the environment you live in, if there's a lot of drugs about, or it's not far to go it is harder, but no matter where you go there are always drugs there.

METHADONE: ATTEMPTS TO REDUCE AND ABSTAIN

The majority (82 per cent) of the sample was attending a drug clinic by the later months of pregnancy, some of them newly referred. All primary opiate users were prescribed methadone, the standard heroin substitute. Nonetheless, there were risks to the foetus that most women sought to remove or reduce. The desire to control methadone consumption while pregnant was based on the hope that the baby would not suffer withdrawal symptoms at birth.

Multivariate analyses revealed that certain factors were significantly associated with success in reducing methadone during pregnancy: the successful women reported no mental health problems; were satisfied with the antenatal care they were receiving, were less likely to be heavy drug users; and were more actively engaged in preparing for the child.

No respondent stopped all use of methadone at this time, detoxification was considered ill advised by most of the physicians attending them (see Chapters 14–17 for a full discussion). Gradual reduction was an accepted strategy among drug workers and was certainly a preferred option for most women. However, there was often reluctance to discuss a reduction in dose with agency staff. Some women believed that if they asked to be reduced but could not manage to cope on lower doses, they would not be able to persuade the physician to restore the dose to the original level. This seems to be a common feature of other forms of substitute prescribing (Klee and Wright, 1998). In such cases it sets up a barrier to open communication between clients and workers that can have damaging effects if changes in methadone administration are concealed and clients independently vary dose levels.

There were some women for whom the ultimate target was complete abstinence. This respondent had made this her goal after receiving information about the hospital confinement:

What are you going to do for the next few months, carry on using 40 ml or try and reduce?

I'll carry on reducing. I want to get off it before the baby comes.

Did they say what would happen if you were still on methadone?

Yes, the baby would be in for about five weeks, that was why I want to get off it before that.

Another woman could see more clearly the pressures she would be under and was open in her dealings with the agency:

No. I'm not planning to [give up]. As soon as the baby's born I'm just going back on it [methadone].

Will they [agency staff] say anything to you?

I expect so, they're expecting me to get off it. It's really hard though being at home and coping with the kids, keeping the place tidy, it's a hassle without anything else. It'd be a lot easier if I could go in somewhere [an in-patient rehabilitation unit], but there's Darren [first child] to think about, and I don't want to leave him, it's a traumatic time for him.

Statements that revealed doubts about the translation of intent into action were very common. There were failures in the pasts of most women that introduced a degree of realism, however great the incentive to stop now:

I always thought that having a baby would make me do that [stop using drugs], but it's different when you're put in the situation . . . it's hard. I always used to say, if I was having a baby, I would do this and would do that, but it's easier said than done . . . now I am in the situation, it's different . . . I really don't know what I'm going to be like when the baby's born, I don't know until it's there.

Despite evidence of high motivation, it is unrealistic to expect all women to see the pregnancy as a time to seek a new, drug-free life if they remain firmly locked into their current social environment. Later analyses of data showed that their forecasts of the future were accurate in predicting problems in sustaining the reduced levels of methadone achieved during pregnancy. These developments are described in Chapter 11.

Professional advice

The advice given to most (45 per cent) respondents by drug workers, and the more knowledgeable antenatal midwives, concerning methadone was to reduce the dose gradually, although the advice varied, some suggesting that ultimate detoxification was best, some saying that there was no need to abstain. The conflicting opinions and statements about the unpredictability of outcomes were a source of worry and confusion to many respondents since they were seeking clear guidelines about how to avoid distressing symptoms in the baby.

I've asked, you know, what's the least I can be on for the baby not to turkey, some people are on 40 ml a day and it doesn't affect the baby and some people are on 10 ml and it does, so it's hard for them to tell.

It was particularly difficult for the women when health professionals disagreed between themselves:

Judy [drug worker] at the clinic said she'd seen babies turkey off 5 ml. And, there again, there's some mums on 40 ml and their babies haven't turkeyed.

So nobody told you that you should be getting down to a certain level?

The midwife – she sort of put pressure on me. She said, 'Are you still using methadone?' and I said, 'yes' and she said, 'Fifty ml is quite a lot. I told her what Judy had said and she sort of looked at me and said, 'Well . . . each to their own opinion'.

The advice about the process of reduction was more consistent, a sudden change was not recommended:

They've said to do it really gradually because if you do it too fast you might have a miscarriage. So I've just done it two ml a week. If I carry on the way I've been carrying on, I'm on twelve this week, I'm on ten next week, then on eight, then on six, and that's it. I should be off it three months before I have the baby, maybe before.

A variety of circumstances were reported that made it difficult to maintain the agreed reduction plan, or even to continue at the reduced dose level. Domestic and interpersonal problems tended to increase anxiety and habitual recourse to drugs had to be resisted if possible:

Yes, definitely. I wanted to get off it as soon as I found out but they said it would be worse for me and the baby . . . I had to get off it slowly. I haven't got long now . . . I was doing all right till he [partner] was made redundant and he was at home, and I couldn't do with the pressure of thinking about losing the house and everything. I told them to leave it [dose level] for the moment.

However, some women had assumed that they would have to give up their methadone and it was a great relief to be told that this was unnecessary:

They're great up there [antenatal clinic]. It was them who told me not to stop using the methadone because it was bad for the baby.

So who told you that?

It was the doctor himself, the specialist. He said, 'I'm not pressuring you . . . but advising you to stay on the script.' But at the end of the day, I wouldn't like to have it on my conscience if anything happened to the baby through me.

So have you stayed on the same level or reduced?

I've reduced it by 10 mls . . . it doesn't sound a lot, but it is.

For further discussion of this issue see Chapters 14 and 17.

Accessible sources of information

According to some of the health professionals interviewed, pregnant drug users tended not to ask questions. The respondents were asked why:

> *You said you don't really know what questions to ask?*

> Yes, because you don't know what they would give, or whether they know anything, because they've never said they know anything . . . so you don't know what to ask, like I say.

The drug-using network was a source of information often mentioned but not always influential in a woman's decision making:

> *Have you got friends with babies themselves and have they given you any advice?*

> Yeah, but you see they're on maintenance scripts. They said to me 'get a maintenance for when it's born'. I said 'yeah', but I don't want to be like that forever. That's what they said like, and how they cut it down until it were born sort of thing. I want to be able to not have anything.

One woman, having made a significant reduction in dose levels, was intent on finishing with methadone by the birth. She had seen the consequences of continuing on high doses of methadone for other women's babies and felt she had learned from them:

> I know a girl who said she was only using 20 ml, but she wasn't, she was buying it, she was on 50 ml, and when the baby was born it nearly died, and they treated her like dirt. I'm not being awful like, but she deserved it because she was only thinking of herself, not about the baby. It started having convulsions and everything. I think I've learnt by her. She always said, 'Don't do what I did, I made a big mistake.' The baby was on oxygen . . . she couldn't bring it home until it was about two months old. She had to go up every day, three times a day, to feed it. So I've looked at her and thought, 'I'm not going to be like her'.

INDEPENDENT ACTION

All of the women in treatment wanted authoritative advice on the use of methadone and if health professionals failed them, they asked their friends and drug-using associates. Some reduced their dose level even if advised against it by their drug clinic. This woman was typical of those who were not prepared to accept the advice of agency staff; she wanted to be drug free by the birth:

> They're not happy with me because I've come down, they say I've come down too quick. Nowadays you can be down to 40 when the baby's born, only down to 40 ml . . . you don't have to come down completely off it. But I'm not having that.

An attempt to control one's own destiny was understandable and at times implacable:

> *Have you got something planned out in your mind how you're going to cut yourself down?*
>
> Five ml a week. I know they're not happy with that but that's the way it's going.

The more experienced women were particularly confident that they were taking the right action:

> I done it myself last time [cut down] and I was all right. I took advice this time and I've got myself in a bit of a mess so I'm just going to stick to my own advice, listen to my own body like.
>
> *Did anybody talk to you about reducing?*
>
> No, they didn't want me to reduce because like with her being so small and that, they didn't wanna start messing about. That's all they were worried about, so they've just kept me the same all the way through and they said once you've had it we'll talk about reducing and that. You see I don't actually take all me meth anyway, I never have but I didn't tell them. It was just like if I did need it, it was there.

Conversely, this woman was reluctant to reduce her prescribed dose and feared pressure to do so:

> I'm staying on the same level. I haven't started reducing yet. I don't feel myself that I'm ready. I don't want to start saying I am to the people here at the drugs agency and make them think 'she's doing well', because it's like a lie then, isn't it?, and I'm not doing myself any good. Because if I start reducing myself and I'm not getting what I need, I'm going to start going getting money and scoring. I don't see the point in that. When I feel ready I will reduce, but I don't feel like I'm ready yet.

QUALITY OF INFORMATION: THE HEALTH PROFESSIONALS' PERSPECTIVES

The value of information offered to pregnant women was undermined if it was not consistent across expert sources. This was recognised by some health professionals. However, there were many issues on which views differed depending on who was being asked. Drug workers tended to recommend different action from maternity staff in many aspects of pregnancy and childcare, in particular the management of methadone administration during pregnancy and the baby's treatment for withdrawal symptoms, the drug workers tended to work at an individual level that took into account the circumstances of the woman's lifestyle:

> *Thinking about women on a methadone prescription, what kind of advice is given to them?*

> I think it depends on their situation, you know, what sort of support networks they've got, whether they've got a partner who's using and what they're likely to be doing about their drug use. For some women I think it's better that they stay on methadone and get down as low as they can rather than try and get off and then relapse. We do get a lot of women who do want to get off. I think they push themselves too hard, they want to be seen as drug free and sometimes that backfires.

Many women wanted to detoxify during pregnancy, but the experience of drug workers was that good intentions could be difficult to put into action without considerable help. However, it was no help to the women if they were faced with the need to judge between professional opinions about methadone regimes. The conflicting advice given to women about drug management during pregnancy sometimes led to independent and unsupervised changes on their part as we have seen.

We found differences between drug workers and maternity services on the prescribing of methadone to pregnant drug users, although most midwives preferred to leave this issue in the hands of the prescribing physician at the drug team. All agency staff believed that the use of street drugs should cease, and that sudden decrease or the abrupt termination of methadone was potentially damaging. Gradual detoxification was advocated by midwives with the aim of reaching a very low dose or abstinence by the end of pregnancy. Some of them were still convinced of a direct link with infant withdrawal, now generally denied by physicians:

> The more she takes, the more withdrawals this baby's going to have . . . and the more seriously ill it's going to be.

There were many midwives who were not prepared to have an opinion, however:

> I don't know [about withdrawals]. Special care is the best place to ask about that.

They were often asked for advice by their clients and were at a loss what to advise. Nonetheless, they gave their opinion and could be wrong, as one community midwife pointed out:

> In some cases . . . downright mistakes have been made . . . women have actually been given the wrong advice simply because the midwife felt she had to say something and didn't know what to say.

There was general recognition of the need for women to be given consistent advice to avoid causing confusion, but midwives in most hospitals tended to be ignorant of what other colleagues were advising. They were reluctant to accept the patient's word on this. One midwife believed that the patient might play one person against the other if conflicting information was given.

Drug workers were more confident about their advice, and tended to aim at stabilisation rather than dose reduction. They were more aware of the limits of control that could be exercised by their clients, in this case to the extent of being pessimistic about their capabilities:

> You're not going to get people to come off the drug . . . but we can stabilise them and prevent them stopping two days before the baby's due, thinking that will help.

A drug liaison midwife spoke of women trying to reduce too fast, not being able to maintain it and so increasing the dose levels again. The fluctuations were the problem, not the dose level:

> I believe they should stick to something specific whether it's at seven or seventy ml whatever . . . just stick at that. I would rather they didn't reduce if it means that they do reduce and use illicit stuff when they can't cope . . . the point of having treatment is to maintain the pregnancy and the equilibrium of the baby.

A paediatrician sympathised with women who made the effort to reduce despite the uncertainty:

> It's a puzzle, certainly the lower you get the less likely it is, but there's no doubt that some women on 80, 90, 100 ml of methadone who have babies that come out fine, and there are girls who try really hard

to get down to 5 or 10 and their babies have the full screaming match. It's very depressing and they need a lot of help afterwards because they feel terrifically guilty.

One social worker in a drug team was more radical and thought that if the women wished, they could detoxify without harm fairly rapidly, while agreeing that fluctuations were inadvisable. However, the local hospital apparently disagreed with this:

> They were getting really hysterical about her . . . saying she couldn't detox because it wouldn't be safe during pregnancy . . . and she was actually in the in-patient unit to do a detox . . . they'd really wound her up pretty bad.

Lack of resolution of the controversy was regretted by one consultant obstetrician who was a member of an agency team:

> Yes. I'm sure you realise that there's two camps – detox and the 'let's just stop it together immediately camp'. I don't know of anyone who's compared the two techniques.

The advice from health professionals was rarely consistent and the women had to judge for themselves whose advice they would take, if any. In the face of such inconsistencies there were doubts about the credibility of the information and the informer. The problem for services is that there has been conflicting research evidence on this issue for many years (Finnegan, 1988; Oloffson *et al.*, 1983; Shaw and McIvor, 1994). Nonetheless, it is still necessary to offer support, 'A pregnant woman needs, above all, to be convinced that the medical decisions she makes have been carefully thought through and that her decisions are the best under the circumstances' (Geller, 1991). Unfortunately this may not be acceptable; it is difficult to live with the uncertainty. As Hepburn (1993) observes, 'While women need clear, concise information, the limitations of existing knowledge should be recognised.'

The women's negative reaction to advice or information they received was very common. Their disappointment and disillusion were particularly unfortunate since so many of the women started out with expectations that their carers would have the answers. While the conflicts persist, some drug-using pregnant women continue to lack clear guidance from a credible source of information. The typical response is to turn to relatives, friends and their network of drug users for first-hand experience.

CONCLUSIONS

The solution to drug management during pregnancy in the absence of validated procedures and guidelines is currently under debate, research continues and various models of care are now being developed nationally in the UK. A similar process is under way elsewhere in Europe (Council of Europe, 1998). Meanwhile, it would be an improvement if there were some agreement on an individual's drug management that is known both to the prescribing physician and drug team on the one hand and to maternity services on the other. Better still if they are fully co-ordinated to present a common face to the anxious patient. Then, if the woman follows an instruction hoping to reduce the chance of the baby withdrawing and the baby nevertheless withdraws, she could be reassured that she does not bear the whole burden of responsibility. The guilt expressed by mothers of withdrawing babies is short lived according to some health professionals, but certain behaviours that are interpreted as signs of lack of caring may be equally well attributed to an inability to cope. A need to distance oneself is a self-preserving strategy for people who feel they are failing.

A critical issue in coping at a time of stress is the level of sustained support available to the woman through pregnancy and in the critical early months of motherhood. Chapter 7 deals with the two major sources of informal support at this time, her partner and her mother.

REFERENCES

Allen, M.H. (1991) De-toxification considerations in the medical management of substance abuse in pregnancy. *Bulletin of the NY Academy of Medicine* 67(3), 270–276.

Council of Europe (1998) *Pregnancy and Drug Misuse*, Proceedings of symposium organised by the Pompidou Group, Strasbourg, 1997. Strasbourg: Council of Europe Publishing.

Finnegan, L.P. (1988) Drug addiction and pregnancy: the newborn. Chapter 4 in: I.J. Chasnoff (ed.) *Drugs, Alcohol, Pregnancy and Parenting*. UK: Kluwer Academic Publishers.

Geller, A. (1991) Chapter 13 in: P. Roth (ed.) *Alcohol and Drugs are Feminist Issues: a review of issues*. NY: Women's Action Alliances and Scarecrow Press.

Hepburn, M. (1993) Drug misuse in pregnancy. *Current Obstetrics and Gynaecology* 3, 54–58.

Keith, K.G., MacGregor, S.N. and Sciarra, J.J. (1988) Drug abuse in pregnancy. Chapter 24 in: I.J. Chasnoff (ed.) *Drugs, Alcohol, Pregnancy and Parenting*. UK: Kluwer Academic Publishers.

Klee, H. and Wright, S. (1998) *Amphetamine Use and Treatment: a study of the impediments to effective service delivery. Part 2: Treatment and its outcomes*. UK: The Manchester Metropolitan University, SRHSA.

LGDF/SCODA (1997) *Drug Using Parents and their Children*. Local Government Drugs Forum and the Standing Conference on Drug Abuse.

Mondanaro, J. (1988) *Treating Drug Dependent Women*. Springfield, Ill: Lexington.

Oakley, A. (1992) *Social Support and Motherhood*. Oxford: Blackwell.

Oloffson, M., Buckley, W., Anderson, G.E. and Friis-Hansen, B. (1983) Investigation of 89 children born by drug-dependent mothers. *Acta Paediatrica Scandinavia* 72, 403–406.

Shaw, N.J. and McIvor, L. (1994) Neonatal Abstinence Syndrome after maternal methadone treatment. *Archives of Disease in Childhood* 71, 203–205.

Chapter 7

Informal support

Partners and mums

Hilary Klee

INTRODUCTION

Historically, practices in obstetrics and gynaecology have focused wholly on medical health care during pregnancy and childbirth and overlooked critically important social dynamics of this phase in a woman's life that will influence her physical and psychological well-being. As with any disadvantaged group, drug-using women have suffered disproportionately from the lack of understanding that is a consequence of such disinterest. Research is now showing that their health at this time is highly dependent on the informal support available from partners, family and friends. However, the particular needs of drug users have been under-researched, and information is limited about the nature of support they can expect. The paradox is that at a time when such stress would be self-medicated with drugs, a pregnant drug user is expected to abstain.

Social support comes in several forms (Cutrona and Suhr, 1990). It includes emotional support in terms of attachment to significant people in the social network, instrumental support such as practical and financial help and informational support that supplies the data on which her decisions can be based. Each type of support is necessary to ensure an adequate level of coping that will preserve the health of the mother and her child. If formal, professional help is not used, the informal support available to her at this time is critical.

An understanding of informal support networks could be helpful to health professionals in providing appropriate care for their patients. In particular the failure of those people closest to the drug-using woman to provide support at this time should signal the need for extra resources to be made available to her. In this chapter the most potent sources of support – partners and mothers – are explored.

PARTNERS

The conventional prescription for good parenting in most cultures is that there should be two parents in the home. Beyond this there is scope for variations that are not value free, two women are more acceptable than two men, for example. The desirable arrangement is one in which parents complement each other in their roles and responsibilities. Single mothers suffer from a bad image and drug-using single mothers are placed several levels below them in terms of acceptability to the public. A common view is that they would be better off with a partner, particularly if he is a non-drug user:

> the scenario necessary for *normal* mother–infant interaction presumes the presence of a supportive father and husband. In the case of a drug-abusing mother, the situation calls for an heroic father who can fill the roles of both mother and father when needed . . . Sad to say, in the case of drug-abusing mother the heroic father is a rare breed. More often than not the fathers of these children are absent or drug-abusers themselves.
>
> (Burns and Burns, 1988)

The view of the partner as hero is limited to men who, coping already with fatherly roles, will take on aspects of the woman's job. It is unlikely that a single female drug user with a family would be accorded the same accolade.

Forty-four respondents had regular partners. The relationships tended to be fairly stable; for over two thirds (69 per cent) it was three years or more and half were over six years. Most women (85 per cent) named their partner as the person closest to them in whom they could confide.

Partners who use drugs

Twenty-six partners were opiate dependent at the start of the project, and all were receiving a prescription for methadone. Fifteen (34 per cent) were injecting at the start of the study. Previous research has found that a drug-using partner can undermine a woman's efforts to give up or reduce her use of drugs (Farkas, 1976; Kaufman, 1985; Smithberg and Westermeyer, 1985) unless they agree to joint action and have the same degree of commitment (Pearson, 1987). Over half of the drug-using partners in this study were not intent on making any change to their own drug consumption, which for most was simply sticking to their prescription with some illicit drugs on the side. However, some couples made an agreement to take joint action on their use of street drugs and ten partners agreed to stop:

And did you use any street drugs in the last month?

About twice I think it was, I can't really remember now but I think it was about twice. Yes, because I remember me and Michael made this promise to each other that we wouldn't, you know like, we wouldn't entice each other into doing it, we'd sort of, like, pack it in. I know I still had three months to go but that was what we said. Because I didn't get me confirmation [of the pregnancy] till late did I? So from then we said that we'd just cut down, right down, which was good. So we did.

There were many who were uncertain whether the partner was capable of change:

I'll just have to see if he will cut down, he hasn't got the incentive that I've got being pregnant.

Many women had experienced good intentions that ended in relapse:

He said before I got pregnant, 'If you get pregnant I won't use it again.' But when it happened he did. But he doesn't like it, he's upset.

This woman felt that the child could be a motivating factor towards change in her partner:

He's got something to work for now and to stay out of prison for.

The history of some couples was one of a developing attachment that was associated with drugs and the lifestyle that went with it; the anticipated difficulties were clear:

I've known him all my life, but we've been living together four years. Sometimes I wish we hadn't bothered. He's always been into drugs and it's hard when there are two of you into it because if one has some the other wants some.

The past for some couples had been chaotic. This woman believed that the birth of the first child had been a major feature in their escape out of a cycle of self-damage:

I think if it hadn't been for him [first child] I'd have been dead by now. Between me and my boyfriend we were using a couple of grams each a day. Also looking a mess and loads of court cases. Getting my methadone scripts, and temazepam and valium on top of that and whatever gear I could get on top of that. He was in a bad way as well. He had to have enough gear so that he overdosed each time. He wasn't stoned unless he'd gone over. It was getting that way that the ambulance was here two or three times a week. They were getting really sick of it. He'd come round in the hospital and then ask for me and say he was going. The pair of us were in a right state. Having Mick has really sorted me out. Just before I had him I got this place. Having somewhere of my own has helped. I've got to keep straight for him and the new one. Not getting the tea ready, not wanting to get up in the morning – that's no good.

Twenty-eight (64 per cent) of the women were dependent solely on their partners for supplying them with drugs. This was often not a simple, instrumental relationship:

Yes I think it was the drugs that kept us together, then after a while I couldn't cope without him. I really relied on him, I got the money, he'd score and get the stuff together. It was a weird set-up. He says the best thing would be if we didn't see each other and I start seeing this straight guy and get myself together. He says that, but then he says he still wants to see me, and I still want to see him and I get all upset. I don't know whether I'm getting upset because he is so related to the drugs. I don't know whether it's him I'd miss or the drugs I don't want to say goodbye to. I'm all muddled up, I've tried and tried analysing it, and the more I do that the harder it is to try and disentangle the two.

This woman's drug use was more directly led by her partner's needs:

I do try and stick to me script strictly . . . my drug use really has always been centred around Pete, it's something that we do together. It doesn't really interest me when I'm on me own. I mean I have to have me methadone, I need it because I couldn't cope without it but I wouldn't go out of the door later on if there was only me here and buy something just because I wanted it, because I've never been like that.

A close relationship was sometimes too exclusive and could increase the woman's social isolation:

No, I don't trust nobody. I've confided in a few people and they've all shit on me so there's only me and him.

An agreement to modify drug use with a supportive partner is perhaps the most effective form of influence and a partner's continued use the most damaging. From statistical analyses we found evidence that the lack of a partner was significantly associated with the most damaging behaviour of all, that of continued injecting. The presence of a partner, even a drug-using partner, may be a restraining influence on the excesses of drug use among women at this time. Twenty per cent of partners strongly disliked the woman using drugs while pregnant. There was pressure from partners of women who were still heavily into street drugs, particularly if they injected:

It was James me new boyfriend, because he's dead against injecting.

Does he inject himself?

No, he can't stand it.

So what does he think about you injecting?

That's why I stopped, because of him. At first I'd do it behind his back but then I stopped.

Most partners were very pleased about the prospects of fatherhood and were said by the women to be sympathetic to their needs. However, the lack of enthusiasm of many partners to change their drug use has significant implications. Respondents realised that their own control of drugs was strongly influenced by their partners and that if the partner continued to use street heroin, it seriously undermined their own efforts:

So you're saying really, if it wasn't for the fact that it's brought in for you, you probably wouldn't really bother?

No. Because the way I see it is I've just got this house and there's loads what needs doing . . . and he's spending, what, £80 a day? I could've got that room done out in a week . . . carpets, curtains, wallpaper.

Although a high proportion of partners were reluctant to change their own behaviour, there were some who were more concerned about the respondent's health than the respondent herself. If known to health professionals involved in the care of such families, this could be a valuable resource:

When I was turkeying with Carol [first child] he wouldn't give me any gear. He was frightened. He doesn't force things on me, but he gets mad with me sometimes.

Many partners were keen to help to limit the woman's drug consumption, but some women were strongly independent, a characteristic that was prominent in Taylor's (1993) sample. Such women do not always co-operate in health protecting actions, as this partner's intervention shows:

[Partner] In one day she's taking valium, nitrazepam, methadone and heroin. That can't be doing the baby any good . . . and smoking as well! I just don't want you [addressing the respondent] to tell her [the interviewer] a load of rubbish about what you're taking. I'm worried . . . I don't want the baby to be addicted to heroin.

At the time of the interview this respondent was taking all her prescribed drugs over one or two days and was still using street drugs.

The supportive partner

Thirty-six (82 per cent) of the women with partners were living with them and the majority (64 per cent) reported that they provided emotional support and helped with the chores at this time. This varies from the stereotypic picture of the drug-using male that has, in fact, been supported in some feminist literature. He would be seen, even more than a woman, to be focused exclusively on drugs and the criminal activities associated with it.

Boyd (1999) found in her sample of 28 Canadian drug-using mothers that only five reported that their partners were supportive. In Taylor's ethnographic study of female injecting drug users in Glasgow (Taylor, 1993), partners were as likely to be exploitative as they were to be helpful. The relatively small samples used in these and our own study precludes any attempt to estimate the amount of help available to women from their partners. The disparity between them suggests that great variance is likely and the ratio is likely to differ with culture, class, degree of dependence and many other factors in the areas and populations sampled.

The drug-using partners in our research outnumbered those who used no drugs or only used 'soft drugs' ($n = 26$: 59 per cent compared with 18: 41 per cent), nonetheless this is a significant proportion of non-dependent partners in view of the reliable observations that drug-using women are unlikely to be found living with them (Gossop et al., 1994; McKeganey and Barnard, 1992; Powis et al., 1996). The impact of the partners' drug use on the women is taken up again in Chapter 11.

The absent father

Some partners were rejected completely – the pregnancy had not been planned and the women wanted no further contact with them, they preferred single parenthood:

I haven't seen him for months. When he came up to my house I couldn't get rid of him, no matter what I tried. He'd just sit on a chair and I'd go to bed and he'd still be there in the morning. Anyway, he said, 'I've come to see your mum' and I said, 'She's busy upstairs.' So she came down and said, 'What do you want?' . . . he said, 'Nothing' and she said, 'Good, because we don't want nothing from you either' . . . it's what I wanted to say but I didn't want to hurt his feelings. He's not a bad lad really, but he's not the right person for me.

Even when the woman had a partner, a high proportion of them were absent periodically when they went to prison. For the women the partner's absence was likely to raise problems.

He's in ———— [prison] for nine months. I go and see him every week. I get the train to Crewe, then the coach. I can claim one visit a month. It leaves me with nothing out of me benefit.

Will he be there at the birth?

Yes, if he's not back in prison.

Mostly, however, the separation had been wanted by the woman, simply because of incompatibility, in this case in terms of the drugs they favoured and their associated interests:

Is the baby's father around?

Yes, he lives round here. We split up before I found out I was pregnant. We just clash – he's a piss-head and I like raving.

It was not always the case that contact was severed with absent fathers. There were several women who were on reasonably good terms with them:

What does the baby's father think about your drugs?

He just said he'd help in any way he can. If I need to talk to him, he said just to phone him up, whatever time it is. He obviously wants me to get as low as I can for the sake of the baby. He tries to understand that it is very difficult. He's very good.

MOTHERS

Another potential source of support for a pregnant woman is her mother (Cowan and Cowan, 1995; Oakley *et al.*, 1996) who is often a strong influence on her maternal behaviour (Chodorow, 1978). All but one woman had a mother living, and 78 per cent were in contact with them, a third almost every day. Approximately two thirds (62 per cent) of the women had good relationships with their mother. The support they had from them was highest during pregnancy and tended to decline a few months after the child was born, which may have been due to disagreements about parenting behaviour. For those without a mother's support there were sometimes opportunities to replace this female support with their partner's mother or another relative, perhaps a grandmother or aunt. However, some of the respondents were relatively isolated and therefore highly dependent on their partner. Conversely, women without a partner were highly dependent on their mothers.

Mothers who don't know

A major barrier to accessing the support of a close relative is if the relative is unaware that the woman uses drugs. Forty per cent of the mothers knew nothing of their daughter's involvement with drugs. This created physical barriers as well as emotional ones – there was always a need for concealment and deception and open contact was restricted. Often the daughter did not tell her mother because of the damaging effect this would have. This woman's mother was a nurse and a considerable amount of deception had been needed to avoid discovery. The dilemma was intensely painful:

> *What do you think she would do if she found out?*
>
> I think it would destroy her, I don't think she'd disown me or anything like that . . . me dad doesn't know anything about the drugs, he'd disown me, definitely, but me mum wouldn't, she'd be upset. I wouldn't like her to find out.

The woman was particularly fortunate in that her partner and his family were also very supportive, but they too were not aware of her dependence:

> They've been the best . . . every time she's bought me a pram, she's been great. I don't know what I would have done without her to tell you the truth . . . and his auntie . . . but they don't know any thing about the drugs, they know John was into them but they don't know about me.
>
> *What do you think their reaction would be?*
>
> I . . . reckon if they find out the baby's turkeying [withdrawing], they'll know . . . but I can keep it from them so I'm not too worried about them . . . but my mum would know.

Some of those mothers who knew about their daughter's use of drugs gave their help wholeheartedly even though extremely concerned:

She doesn't like it at all . . . but she's not the sort of person to judge. She knows how easy it is to get addicted to something, but she doesn't realise what it's like. She comes with me to the hospital every time I go.

So how confident are you that you're going to manage?

I'll manage now I'm with my mum.

Vulnerable or rejected mothers

Despite the high level of support offered by some mothers, there could still be doubts about taking advantage of it. The mother's distress made the woman feel guilty which created an environment in which confiding about drug-related problems was inhibited. Forty per cent said they could not confide in their mothers.

I denied it to start with . . . then it came to light and she was annoyed and upset, but she gradually accepted it. She doesn't like it . . . she hates it but she'd rather look after us [brother also an addict]. She stands by us both. It's a shame . . . I feel guilty about my mum.

Half of the mothers were happy about the baby but for a large proportion (42 per cent) of the women, their mothers had little or no involvement in their pregnancy. Sometimes this was because of geographical distance, but 70 per cent lived within 30 minutes of their mothers and any lack of contact was mostly due to a breakdown in the relationship, often because of the daughter's use of drugs or criminal activities. The respondents tended to have complex histories that included family trauma: divorce was common, and physical and sexual abuse was also reported. Many women came from dysfunctional families and 52 per cent had siblings who used drugs. Divorce and separation were common and some had felt rejected when their parents separated. This woman was angry and also unforgiving about being abandoned by her mother:

My mum remarried when my dad walked out on us, about eight years ago, and I went into care because I was a daddy's girl. Her boyfriend used to abuse us and she chose him instead of me and my two brothers. They're heroin addicts now. She chose him instead of us and every time he used to see me he used to smack me so I just don't have anything to do with her.

However, it was sometimes the daughter who had broken all contact with the mother, blaming her for the childhood experiences that had such damaging effects:

I just blame her for everything that's happened. She had thirteen kids, no . . . fourteen, one died like . . . and every single one went into care.

Judgement by mothers

A mother's disapproval of her daughter's lifestyle could increase when hearing about her pregnancy since it was now fuelled by concern for the child. Some relationships deteriorated further:

> They don't come here a lot. We had a big argument when I was having Becky [first child] and she went to the doctor's telling them I was on heroin and to see if they'd take the baby off me . . . but they said 'she's getting help, there's nothing we can do'.

In contrast there were mothers who made every effort not to judge:

> *What's her reaction to you using drugs, is she supportive, does she understand?*

> At first she went mad and that but now she's accepted it sort of. She doesn't like it, she hates it . . . but me brother's thirteen and she's worried about him getting into it.

After perhaps years of deception there was some relief in being open and truthful. This inevitably carried a risk of alienation, and the extent of their honesty had to be governed by an estimate of the potential for damage:

> *What does she think of you being pregnant again?*

> She knows I'm on methadone. Instead of ranting and raving, she asked me in the car a few months ago whether I was still on methadone . . . expecting me to say no. I thought f*** this, why should I lie, so I said yes I am and she said, 'you want to get off it', but I said it was too hard. They don't know . . . she just says you shouldn't be on it. My dad is as bad and he said, 'I hear you're using needles', and I denied it. I know I'm lying, but I know they are worrying like f*** so I said to my sister, 'don't tell them because they worry'.

CONCLUSIONS

Partners play a pivotal role in the lives of pregnant drug users. Their support and their own use of drugs have a significant effect on the woman's drug management and health. However, partners may be absent, rejected or ignored. They may be incapable of changing their behaviour or unwilling to do so. Fathers in this sample were mostly supportive during the pregnancy and looking forward to the birth of the child. Their receptivity to change should be high at this time.

Mothers can contribute protective and sustaining emotional support and the benefits of experience, as well as practical help. However, estrangement arising from childhood events or the daughter's use of drugs is common, and the mother's ignorance of the woman's drug use or her distress can be barriers that severely limit mothers as a resource.

For pregnant drug users the informal support that is so critical for the well-being of both mother and child may be lacking or have negative features that risk further destabilisation in their lives. This suggests that compensatory professional support systems should be available. As a first step, new ways of assessing and meeting such needs should be developed that are fully informed by an understanding of the social dynamics of the mother's lifestyle. Social workers, health visitors, community midwives and outreach drug workers could all play a part in the analysis, diagnosis and remedial action necessary to help the dysfunctional family.

Although alternative sources of support may be found by the pregnant drug user, including a sympathetic drug worker or midwife, there is no real substitute for a person who is close and reliably on hand when needed. If there are known deficiencies they should be addressed. Ideally all sources of support should be mobilised and this requires that the potential contributions of partners and families should be explored and used to maximum effect. Where there are interpersonal problems, then family counselling could be an option aimed at increasing the integrity and strength of the bonds between them. Where they are affected by practical problems of housing, finances, legal matters and so on they are more likely to improve with help in their resolution. The severely dysfunctional family perpetuates dysfunction in the next generation of parents and effective interventions may need to be sustained over very long periods.

REFERENCES

Boyd, S. (1999) *Mothers and Illicit Drugs: transcending the myths*. Canada: University of Toronto Press.

Burns, W.J. and Burns, K.A. (1988) Parenting dysfunction in chemically dependent women. Chapter 12 in: I.J. Chasnoff (ed.) *Drugs, Alcohol, Pregnancy and Parenting*. The Netherlands: Kluwer Academic Publishers.

Chodorow, N. (1978) *The Reproduction of Mothering*. Berkeley: University of California Press.

Cowan, P.C. and Cowan, P.A. (1995) Interventions to ease the transition to parenthood. Why are they needed and what can they do? *Family Relations* 44, 412–423.

Cutrona, C. and Suhr, J. (1990) The transition to parenthood and the importance of social support, in: S. Fisher and C. Cooper (eds) *On the Move: the psychology of change and transition*. Chichester: Wiley.

Farkas, M.I. (1976) The addicted couple. *Drug Forum* 5(1), 81–87.

Gossop, M., Griffiths, P. and Strang, J. (1994) Sex differences in patterns of drug taking behaviour: a study at a London Community Drug Team. *British Journal of Psychiatry* 164, 101–104.

Kaufmann, E. (1985) *Substance Abuse and Family Therapy*. New York: Grune and Stratton.

McKeganey, N. and Barnard, M. (1992) *AIDS, Drugs and Sexual Risk: lives in the balance*. Buckingham: Oxford University Press.

Oakley, A., Hickey, D., Rajan, L. and Rigby, A.S. (1996) Social support in pregnancy: does it have long term effects? *Journal of Reproductive and Infant Psychology* 14(1), 7–22.

Pearson, G. (1987) *The New Heroin Users*. Oxford: Basil Blackwell.

Powis, B., Griffiths, P., Gossop, M. and Strang, J. (1996) The differences between male and female drug users: community samples of heroin and cocaine users compared. *Substance Use and Misuse* 31(5), 529–543.

Smithberg, N. and Westermeyer, J. (1985) White dragon pearl syndrome: a female pattern of drug dependence. *American Journal of Drug and Alcohol Abuse* 11(3), 199–207.

Taylor, A. (1993) *Women Drug Users: an ethnography of a female injecting community*. Oxford: Clarendon Press.

Chapter 8

Practitioner views of pregnant drug users

Marcia Jackson and Hilary Klee

This chapter will explore the views about pregnant drug users that have emerged from interviews with health care providers involved in maternity or neonatal care across north-west England. Research suggests (Davis, 1990; Lewis *et al.*, 1995) that drug users' willingness to approach health care services can be influenced by expectations and experience of the attitudes to drug use that they encounter among the practitioners they meet. The experiences of our pregnant drug users that are documented in earlier chapters have revealed a number of stressors arising from their interactions with staff. Those responsible for their care now provide their own perspectives on drug-using mothers. We try to present a balanced view of the attitudes of our professional informants, reporting accounts of members of a range of professions – obstetrics, paediatrics, midwifery, drug and social work – and noting the contrasts that occur among them.

THE UPTAKE OF SERVICES

It became evident from interviews with antenatal staff that drug users were often regarded as unlikely to be sufficiently concerned about their health during pregnancy to seek antenatal care:

> Some [drug using] women seem to come in with a real 'I can't be bothered' attitude . . . bored . . . don't want to know what you're talking about. And others come along and say, 'I know I shouldn't really be taking the stuff, and I've cut down, honest.' They come across all very earnest and like they really care. Sometimes it's difficult to know how much they do care because you know you've seen that kind of patient before and she hasn't even cut down and all the rest of it.
>
> (Registrar in obstetrics and gynaecology)

It was acknowledged, however, that drug users' reactions to advice and support varied. Practitioners felt that for some women, pregnancy could motivate a change in drug use:

> I have to say they are either motivated to reduce or not. You get the ones who are quite comfortable to take whatever they've been on for years. You've got others during pregnancy, it's a trigger to get off or get down to as little as they can.
>
> (Consultant obstetrician)

> A lot of them I've seen are already reducing and are trying their best. I think a lot of the women do think quite carefully about it because it's another person, it's their baby.
>
> (Registrar in obstetrics and gynaecology)

Rather than indicating a lack of concern for the pregnancy, late presentation was attributed by some to amenorrhoea (absence of menstruation), which can be associated with heavy drug taking and a consequent failure to recognise pregnancy in the early stages. For others it was a lack of structure in their lives that accounted for their apparent lack of compliance. It was acknowledged that this was not necessarily attributable solely to drug use. Several people said that they did not feel that drug users were any worse at keeping appointments than any other group of patients:

> I think they tend not to keep diaries, I think they don't keep track of time . . . I think one day is much like the next, isn't it? I don't think that's peculiar to this group, to drug users, I think that's true of a large number of people who are unemployed.
>
> (Consultant obstetrician)

Failure to attend was regarded more positively by others as a way of managing their own care:

> Why come out in the rain, on the bus, to sit in a clinic to be told everything's all right, because they know that after your second default that the midwife would pop around. I thought, they're not daft, they're wise.
>
> (Antenatal clinic midwife)

Regardless of the reasons for failing to take up care during pregnancy, drug-using women need encouragement to attend antenatal appointments. Discussions with drug users revealed that fear of encountering judgemental attitudes is a major deciding factor in whether or not they do so. Most health workers were well aware of this problem:

> I think sometimes they come late because they're frightened of being found out and thinking the babies will be taken off them.
>
> (Senior registrar in paediatrics)

The negative attitudes that were encountered during the interviews had often developed as a result of a poor experience with the client group in the past. Despite this, many respondents reported trying hard to take into account drug users' feelings of guilt and marginalisation, and aimed to be understanding and sympathetic to the needs of each woman as an individual. It was considered important for drug users to have the opportunity to talk openly and honestly with their team of carers without feeling they were being stigmatised or judged. Although this view was common across professional groups, some believed that their efforts would be fruitless. One nurse commented:

> You might as well talk to a brick wall.

With more insight, it was suggested that such patients are reluctant to ask for advice, being fearful of the consequences of disclosure. A social worker neatly summed up the feelings of many drug users:

> We come to you for help, and you take our children.

Furthermore it was suggested that maximum use of services is made by those who least need it:

> I think it's unfortunate that, sometimes the 'middle class', if we put it that way, healthy normal pregnant woman can often be quite demanding of doctors' time, because they've read this or that book and they want to discuss the pros and cons of things which in a health sense are pretty marginal . . . whereas the patient [group] we're talking about is one which is undernourished, abusing drugs, is living in terrible circumstances and has got major health and social problems. To me it seems to be more productive of my time to spend time with them rather than the other women who, whether I was here or not, are likely to have a normal pregnancy and delivery.
>
> (Consultant obstetrician)

Clearly there is a need to identify ways of encouraging disadvantaged women to make better use of antenatal care. It must be noted that one midwife believed that some staff are happy to maintain the status quo. She commented that well-motivated, healthy patients made for a more pleasant working environment and that by encouraging patients with a potential array of medical and social problems, the views and working practices of staff would necessarily have to be changed. It was felt that encouraging more 'needy' patients also increased the workload for an already overstretched workforce. Perhaps it is not surprising that efforts to develop services for pregnant drug users can encounter resistance.

PRACTITIONERS' VIEWS OF DRUG USERS' PARENTING CAPACITY

There was a range of attitudes towards drug users as parents. Drug users might be reassured if they were aware that not all health and social work professionals see drug use as a barrier to good parenting:

> I think people now recognise that you can be an excellent parent, or at least a good enough parent, and also continue to use drugs.
> (Drug team social worker)

> I think you have to make your mind up on each individual case.
> (Senior house officer, obstetrics and gynaecology)

Many workers were prepared to assess parenting skills on an individual basis and not purely on the basis of drug use. It was considered important to remember that all drug users are individuals with strengths and weaknesses just the same as non-drug dependent parents. This was a view held most markedly by drug workers:

> I suppose if I'm being totally objective . . . just looking from the outside, I don't think they make any worse or better parents than most people. They've still got the same potential for abusing their children physically, emotionally and whatever. So the potential's there but I don't think just because they're a drug user they need more supervision or anything like that . . . they are capable parents most of the time.
> (Drug worker)

Guidelines for social workers emphasise that drug use alone should not be used as a reason for intervention, though the issue remains controversial. The family circumstances must be taken into account. In most instances social workers found no need to intervene when drug-using parents were assessed:

> If she seems fine and she's attending antenatal, she wants to breast feed, she's bought things for the baby, she's got a warm home, then we'd hold this information on file [that she's a drug user] and until or unless you've got anything else, that's as far as it would go . . . we don't come from the basis that drug users can't be good parents, because they can be if it's controlled and they have support and they're getting the services.
> (Social worker)

However, staff were well aware that drug users were concerned that their parenting skills would be under scrutiny and deemed inadequate:

I think every drug user I've had has said, 'Am I going to have my baby taken away?'

(Community midwife)

Clearly such a fear can have major implications for a woman's willingness to discuss her drug use with people she sees as in a position to separate her from the child. The paradox of course is that unwillingness to share information with health workers is itself likely to attract attention:

they [drug users] say, 'I don't want to talk to them' [social workers]. And not wanting to talk to them is a sure-fire way of making them interested in you. Talk to them and then they'll go away.

(Drug worker)

Of great concern to many child-oriented practitioners was what might happen when the new-born babies of drug users went home:

They get the drug withdrawal symptoms and then after that they're more prone to sudden infant death, being bashed . . . and within the last year or two there have been several babies or toddlers who have actually been poisoned by methadone that the parents have been using, either given it deliberately or the child's come across the bottle and had a swig . . . When they get older they are more prone to learning difficulties, lack of concentration, bed-wetting and so on.

(Consultant paediatrician)

An assumption prevailed among service providers that most drug users have poor housing, little money, and no family support. For some drug users, as for many other women living in deprived circumstances, this is no doubt true, but it requires an individual assessment to determine whether or not a particular person's ability to provide adequate parenting is affected.

It was felt by some practitioners that drug users would probably not be concerned if their children played truant from school or fell foul of the law. Where these issues were raised in our interviews with drug-using women, there was often a determination that their child would be regular school attenders and respectful of the law. As with most parents, they wanted their children to achieve something from life.

ALTERNATIVE PROFESSIONAL PERSPECTIVES

Drug workers' views

Drug workers' attitudes towards pregnant drug users and their views on collaboration with other agencies tended to differ from the other health professions. Perhaps inevitably, they were more sympathetic and know-ledgeable about pregnant drug users, particularly those workers with special responsibility for women or for pregnancy. Some were ex-social workers with continuing responsibility for child protection and many were commu-nity psychiatric nurses (CPNs). They were aware of drug agencies' poor record of attracting women, and fear of social service intervention was seen as the major impediment to improvement. This was addressed by resolute maintenance of confidentiality that could, however, be at odds with the mission of district social workers. A belief among drug users that they would not automatically pass on information to social services was regarded as important by drug workers although the Children Act set limits. Efforts were being made in most agencies to provide a degree of reassurance to women, though it was difficult to get it across at times:

> Until we get a good service then the only information they'll have is what they hear from other women . . . and usually what they hear are the worst stories possible, and then they'll interpret that as the norm and in some instances what has happened [child taken into care] is right because the child was at risk, but if you can only get bits of information it's rather like reading the *Sun*.

> At the moment there's two women about to lose their children . . . I know the whole picture but the rest of the women don't . . . that's the tricky bit . . . you have to say it's not their drug use it's just everything else that goes with it . . . that's the problem especially if it's a small group . . . they all know each other so they'll quote who's lost a child and who hasn't.

Drug workers recognised the damage to the women's confidence in their carers if the information was not consistent across sources – there were many issues on which views differed depending on who was being asked. They were also more aware of the conflicts that ensued for women attending both the hospital and a drug agency:

> there was conflicting advice at the antenatal stage within the hospital, conflicting advice between the drugs team and the hospital . . . and then the antenatal service was not preparing the women, not giving the women reliable information on what they could expect postnatally both for them and for their babies. And that caused, I think, a lot of problems.

> There's a lot of fallacies going around that methadone makes babies deformed. I had a referral from a midwife from out of our area and I was asked if I would go and do an assessment for a termination. She was having twins – she'd had a miscarriage while she was away from home and she miscarried one of the twins and the midwife in

that hospital said, 'Oh you're on methadone, that's why you've had a miscarriage, because methadone deforms babies' [the woman went on to have a healthy baby].

Antenatal staff

Lack of experience among antenatal staff in some areas led to summary evaluations of their drug-using clients in terms of conventional stereotypes as we have seen. The stereotypes that emerged from the accounts of health professionals ranged from uncaring, neglectful mothers to poor unfortunates who are victims of circumstances beyond their control. However, there was evidence of empathy in some staff treating drug users that indicates a potential convergence with drug workers' views:

> There but for the grace of God . . . I can imagine if I'd had a bad day and somebody said 'Here, this will cheer you up' . . . I've never been offered it . . . I like a drink and if anyone told me I couldn't have a drink any more I'd think 'Who the hell are you talking to.'

The development of trust and support is essential for a successful relationship between patient and carer. However, the difficulty of achieving this with a drug-using client group was sometimes acknowledged:

> I do feel that sometimes they're frightened of disclosing it [drug use] because of the way we professionals will look at them.
>
> (Midwife)

From the perspective of the antenatal staff there were some difficult problems in delivering a good service. Establishing a positive interpersonal relationship was a major problem that occurred early. Several respondents mentioned the defensiveness of some women:

> I think they come in sometimes and they're a bit on the defensive because they think we're going to be off with them because of their problems. It all goes downhill from then on, I think.

This situation was exacerbated by poor communication between caregivers, which resulted in clients receiving conflicting advice (as discussed above). This could aggravate what was already a sensitive relationship:

> Very often mums will come in and they'll say, 'well, the drug team told me the baby will only be on special care for a week' . . . or, 'the drug team told me I can breast feed'. And the answer to all these is incorrect.
>
> (Midwife)

However, there were relatively few examples among antenatal staff of overt hostility and the common human tendency to turn negative inter-personal experiences into generalisations and stereotypes of the 'bad mother' was resisted by many of the maternity staff when they were inter-viewed. Often this involved giving some thought to the women's backgrounds or childhood:

> I feel very sorry for some of them. A lot of them are using drugs because they lost out on their childhood, they've been in care them-selves . . . they want to get out but it's so difficult.

Community midwives in particular showed tolerance and understanding, possibly because of more extended involvement with the woman in her home – saying the women had 'walked in the wrong path' and commenting on their isolation and the need for extra help:

> I'll do my best for her and if there's any problem then obviously she'll need a bit more help. You must have had a problem in the first place to start using drugs, mustn't you?

> I mean, they've tried to wean [themselves off drugs] . . . they've failed sometimes but they have tried. So that speaks for itself that they're thinking about the baby.

At times the sympathy blended into pity, which might help the relation-ship with the pregnant woman but could reinforce her feelings of helplessness.

> To some degree they try to make plans . . . I just feel that they can't help themselves.

There were comments from obstetricians about the rise in numbers of drug-using women presenting to services and the complexity of their needs. Despite some negative interactions, there were efforts to understand their problems:

> In my experience when they do come they are quite time consuming, not just from a medical point of view but there's all the other things happening to them, you know, they've got other illnesses, care of other children, court appearances, one thing and another.

While there was some sympathy for pregnant drug users who did not make use of antenatal services, less tolerant attitudes were also evident. It was felt by some that drug users tell lies at every opportunity, particularly regarding their drug use, and that they are unpredictable and unreliable:

You learn over the years that certain people can be very unreliable and they'll just tell lies, and you learn to take it all with a pinch of salt really . . . you have to be aware that anyone like that, who abuses drugs, is not one hundred per cent reliable.

(Ward midwife)

One consultant obstetrician was the most critical in believing them to be 'congenital liars'.

I'm sorry but I don't believe a word any of them say.

He recounted a variety of unrewarding experiences that had undoubtedly contributed towards his cynicism:

I went out of my way quite a lot to try and help as best I could and it all came to absolutely nothing. I realised afterwards – when you're into mainline drugs, you're a lost cause.

He was also concerned for the welfare of the child once it had left the protected environment of the hospital, a problem that might be avoided if there was open communication with mothers:

My greater worry [over that of Neonatal Abstinence Syndrome] is the care of the child afterwards . . . I've heard of cases where the mother's stoned out of her mind and the baby dies in the house . . . you see these cases in the press.

Paediatricians tended to be very concerned about early discharge from hospital:

I would say that my major worry is that a lot of mums are too fright-ened to admit to their drug use so that it may be that many mums nowadays are only in hospital a day or two, and that's not long enough to know they're withdrawing. We certainly hear now and then of a baby withdrawing at home and that frightens the life out of me because it can be quite severe.

(Consultant paediatrician)

Social workers

There were contrasts in allegiances between social workers in drug agencies, and hospital or district social workers. In drug agencies it was considered important that they protect the interests of their clients since no one else would. Among district social workers there was a corresponding focus on the child but also conviction that the image of the social services as automatically hostile to pregnant drug users needed to change if they were to become more effective:

> I think traditionally, social workers have not got a good image, and it only takes one woman at the pregnancy clinic to say 'those bastard social workers have taken my child, don't get involved with them'. But then, people don't know the whole story . . . how we've tried to work in a preventative way . . . we do give people opportunities and chances and people only hear the horror stories.

> We're trying to think of better ways of communicating . . . offering them support. We're going to try and have a lot of impact with the pregnancy clinic to try and alleviate some of the fears around social work . . . that we can be supportive and we can be of assistance. It's trying to work on people's image of social workers . . . we're going to try and make ourselves a bit more visible.

It was repeated many times that drug use was not a reason for children to be taken into care. It was also apparent that their reputation was felt to be undeserved, since there were many aspects of the service other than child protection. They denied the charge that they panicked and moved too precipitously:

> If they're chaotic and intoxicated they're not capable of caring but we wouldn't panic and just think 'they're drug users, they're pregnant, let's all panic around this one'.

There was a sense of unfairness about many of the criticisms levelled against mothers:

> Quite a few of them have already been in care and have very negative experiences of social services. Some women want help sorting out the practical things like finance . . . and others don't respond at all. Some are very cagey about what's happened and they want help but don't want to talk about anything that's happened previously . . . quite a lot still believe that just because they use drugs we're going to take the baby. There's a tremendous fear of social services it seems to me.

The implicit criticism that social workers' attitudes to drug users were based on stereotypes was challenged repeatedly and vigorously:

> Social services in this area don't get involved because of drug use . . . but if there's been some other incident or some other concern and drug use is known . . . that can be a factor.

A change in the social service image among drug-using women in treatment depended partly on co-operation with the drug agency personnel who were closer to the women. Services with inter-agency teams were in the best position to reduce or remove their fears and persuade mothers to see social work as beneficial. In regions where there were few links, or there was antagonism, the options were limited. District social workers found liaison to be generally easier with health visitors and midwives:

What sort of help is on offer to the women?

it would be whatever they come up with . . . housing . . . a few of the families I've worked with have had absolutely nothing for the babies . . . so it's getting them sorted out. Then there's the drugs side . . . liaising with the Community Drug Team (CDT) if necessary for prescription increases and stuff like that . . . and then there's child protection, if there's any risks.

What would that involve?

First of all you do a couple of computer checks to see if the family's named, and then if they've got any other children we need to liaise with the health visitor if the child's under five. Quite a lot of the families don't particularly want anything to do with us . . . which is fair enough . . . that's their right. And then we'd check with agencies to see if there's any reason for us to be involved. Sometimes we talk to the drug team but we don't seem to get an awful lot of information out of them because it's very hard for them to tell us anything because their confidentiality is for the client.

MOVES TOWARDS PROFESSIONAL COLLABORATION

There were maternity staff not versed in drug issues and drug workers unaware of hospital procedures and policies – they tended to be in regions where they had identified relatively few drug-using pregnant women, had less experience and hence felt little pressure to develop in this way. In areas where initiatives such as the appointment of drug liaison midwives had been pursued, the signs were that ignorance was unlikely to persist for long. A rapidly growing number of health professionals were enthusiastically involved in improving the service.

Removal of discrimination and prejudice was being actively addressed in one large drug agency in collaboration with local hospitals. A system of dealing with drug users had been developed that did not discriminate between them and other high-risk pregnancies. Two obstetricians saw the women, channelled to them by a liaison midwife:

it's steadily increased since the service was introduced . . . It was clear
that we were seeing a lot of drug users but we didn't know about it until
the babies withdrew on the postnatal ward. What we wanted was some
system that allowed people to 'come out' as it were and be happy to
talk about it with us. To do that we had to give them very personal care,
both at the midwifery and at medical level. We feel it's worked . . .
When we started the clinics we saw what people would regard as quite
stable drug addicts. That isn't the case any more . . . we see them but
we also see the more chaotic users, more social service involvement
. . . the proportion has gradually increased. You're more conscious that
there's always some really chaotic users, whereas three or four years
ago you used to wonder if there was really a problem here.

The agency personnel were proud of their record in attracting the women:

They've risen about ten-fold and I'd like to think it's because of the
package of services that's offered to the women. They know that
because of the non-judgemental way they're treated – not only by us
but by the social workers and maternity staff who are involved in the
team – that it's not automatic that you present as a drug user and
your children go into care.

It seemed to be a part of the philosophy of all new developments that
drug use should not be equated with inadequate parenting or lack of co-
operation, and that pregnant drug users needed extra support. They should
not necessarily be regarded as high-risk pregnancies but were likely to
present particular challenges to staff. Effectively this was a neutral stance
that attempted to sidestep the issue of personal evaluations of the patients
by applying generalisable principles that were free of moral judgement.

Collaboration between agencies brought into high relief the issue of
confidentiality. This was a major concern of the pregnant drug users and
was not only associated with avoiding social work intervention, but also
with the need to prevent their drug use being revealed to key people in
their lives. There were differing views and operationalised definitions of
confidentiality between care providers both within and between professional groups. Disclosure to non-professionals was regarded as a different
issue and was unambiguous. Examples of this were regarded as inadvertent breaches of confidentiality that arose from ignorance:

*So have there been occasions then where confidentiality hasn't been
maintained?*

I think it's lack of thought rather than people intentionally breaking
confidentiality. They discuss things without thinking who else is within
earshot – I think that's the main problem.

Without an agreed definition of confidentiality, communication between client and worker is likely to be strained. The law decrees that child protection must be paramount, but the perceptions by some of our women of overzealous reporting to social workers seemed to have a detrimental effect on the development of trust between clients and health care workers.

Policies were discussed by those staff in drug agencies with a high proportion of pregnant women and established links with the hospitals, but in a few districts the co-operation between drug agencies and the hospital was fairly minimal. The motivation to change was apparently poor according to this drug worker:

> I don't think they want to be talking to us really.
>
> *Why do you think that is?*
>
> I don't know. I think maybe there's a fear around how much drug use there is amongst women who are pregnant and if they start to identify it – it'll become a massive problem that they can't deal with. They don't know what to do with it anyway – they're not that well informed. So I think it's a case of 'we don't really want to open this can of worms', that's my view.

Liaison between drug workers and social workers was poor in some areas. From the social workers there was criticism of Community Drug Teams (CDTs) concerning their co-operation in providing information; however, this was tempered by an appreciation of their different roles:

> The CDT don't approach us – very rarely, health visitors are much more open but CDT wouldn't approach you.
>
> *You think they should a bit more?*
>
> They use their confidentiality and believe in it and keep to it and, in fairness, they don't work with the child. Our brief is with the child.

There seemed to be no satisfactory solution to this for the drug worker. While social workers were more single-minded about their information needs, drug workers seemed troubled by the strain of dual responsibility to their clients and their children. They were aware of the risks for children but needed to balance this against the dangers of alienating their clients to the point at which they would stop attending. There was evidence of poor relationships between district social workers and drug workers in the regions in which there was no formalised system of collaboration. This social worker was able to take the moral high ground having worked out the implications of lack of communication:

If it was a child protection issue and it was going to put the child at risk and other agencies were involved then they'd have to know. Which would be the same with the CDT, if they think a child's at risk they should be sharing information with us.

Which they're not doing?

Well, not really, no. I mean we've never had a referral from them and they probably do see a few things so that probably speaks for itself really, doesn't it?

While some district social workers seemed to have a very clear sense of priorities and moral obligations, for drug workers a breach in confidentiality could seriously undermine the trust that had been established, sometimes over a long period.

The relationships were not always antagonistic. In districts where it was good, with co-operation on both sides, there were opportunities to work on individual cases with greater freedom. This had often required an enlightened and proactive approach by the agencies:

I think the CDT have provided training across the Department as well as about drug substitution. They've been excellent and provided us with written stuff as well as chatting to us about different things.

(District social worker)

While there were examples of good practice in managing somewhat problematic alliances, the very different orientation towards drug misuse between the two professional groups frequently revealed itself:

I've had clients with young children who would say to you that they love them to bits, and they do . . . but they love the heroin as much. My argument is 'How much more do you love the children than you love the heroin?' Unless it's above it, it can't work. Very rarely can they say they want the children more than the heroin . . . which is very sad.

(District social worker)

There was a general consensus within maternity and social work settings that lack of confidence in dealing with the problems of pregnant drug users was exacerbated by limited liaison with specialist drug services. There was frustration from some of the health care workers at what appeared to be poor information sharing but, equally, there was concern about the lack of good basic knowledge about drugs.

DRUGS KNOWLEDGE, EDUCATION AND TRAINING

There were differences in the type of information that was important to maternity staff, drug and social workers. The maternity staff tended to want information on drugs, the social background of drug users and their require-ments of services. The drug workers wanted more information about the medical aspects of pregnancy, stimulant users and breast feeding. They did not report extensive knowledge of hospital procedures or even the need for this but simply telephoned if they required information for a client.

Low levels of knowledge about illicit drug use were very common among nursing staff. Questions about this revealed that the type and amount of training undertaken by staff varied considerably, but there was universal agreement that coverage of drug misuse during professional training was poor. Workers in all the professions, except drug specialists, reported lacking confidence when involved in the care of pregnant drug users. It was felt, particularly by some midwives and junior doctors, that having more knowledge about the use of street drugs would help to increase the credibility of health professionals amongst drug users:

> they think, 'well, if you don't know what we're talking about how can you help us?'
>
> (Midwife)

Few of the maternity staff interviewed had received any information on drug misuse in their initial training. This was associated with the length of time since qualifying. In those courses that included drug misuse, coverage had been fairly rudimentary and not very helpful, largely because the subject had not been taught by a specialist:

> We didn't have a specialist person. We just had one of the tutors give us a talk . . . and it wasn't very informative.

The English National Board *Guidelines for Good Practice* (1996) addressed the future training needs for nursing staff, with reference to post-qualification training. However, this makes heavy use of 'on-the-job' training and requires resources. Examples of post-qualification 'training' were given as: formal study days devoted to drugs and HIV; working alongside specialist drug and maternity services; and informal discussions with drug workers. We found that pressure on services meant that funding was limited for such training and of low priority.

There were also doubts expressed by antenatal staff about the value of courses and study days. For example, that research had not yet yielded enough useful information, and there were complaints about the nature of the information, which was sometimes difficult to understand and often American in origin. The standard day conference had been disappointing for this midwife, who was evidently concerned to appear knowledgeable to her patients:

> There have been days set up, training days for discussing women's issues, pregnancy and women, but I don't think any of the people running the training days actually know any more than what I knew before I went into the room. A lot of it is experiential learning. A lot of it is being as cute as what your clients are. When they tell you something, you treat it as if you know, you're very 'au fait' about it.

The lack of knowledge about drugs was seen as a real disadvantage by maternity staff and even potentially a hazard:

> I don't think we're given enough information really. I mean . . . new drugs come on the scene and we're left to try and work out what it is, what effects it's likely to have . . . we need more updating, perhaps every twelve months.

There were some aspects of drug use that were more urgent than others. For example, one area of ignorance that stretched across all services was the impact of drugs other than opiates on the pregnant woman and the foetus:

> Because we deal with opiate users every day we tend to sort of think of amphetamine users as being not so dangerous, but it scares you a bit more if someone's using amphetamine rather than heroin.

Some drug agencies were finding an increase of women with combined heroin and amphetamine problems:

> I'd be more concerned about amphetamine than I would be about heroin . . . They tend to be really underweight, undernourished, less well vitamin-wise and I think for me, ring far more alarm bells for a developing foetus than heroin does.

Amphetamine is a popular drug among women and relatively easy to conceal. Users are unlikely to be attending a methadone clinic. Stimulants should perhaps be given more emphasis when developing policy on education and training in drug use.

In other areas of knowledge the differences in views needed resolving. However, the validity of some of them was in question. One example was breast feeding. This drug worker had a practical approach:

my view is that if a woman was successfully breast feeding then it's ridiculous because she's on methadone to suggest she should take the baby off the breast and give it a bottle . . . so I stood my ground [with antenatal staff]. But I couldn't say to them 'Well, there's the evidence', it was just my opinion really.

(Drug worker)

There were other training needs identified. For example, knowing how to interact with pregnant drug users. One community midwife felt that coun-selling skills would be useful and a drug worker wanted skills for working with families. Although many health care staff said they dealt with drug users and non-drug users in the same way, some believed that special skills were required to ensure that the women retained contact:

A lot of midwives are very unsure about how to handle women that are drug users . . . they can alienate them and you may never see them again.

(Drug liaison midwife)

Training was being undertaken by drug liaison midwives partly to influ-ence policy as well as inform. One drug liaison midwife was going to update midwives on the wards and offer in-service training:

so that babies can eventually be looked after on the ward with the mum . . . for a normal baby who needs observing or who's with-drawing but not severely, then they can be left on the ward with mum.

Although such changes were not simple to put into effect and could be met with resistance, there were successes from this drug worker's point of view:

I was saying there was no reason for the babies to stay in special care for six weeks . . . they should be with their mother . . . there's bonding problems. And the maternity services looked again at their policies and decided that, even if the baby was withdrawing, they should be with their mother.

Apart from access to formal knowledge, the drug-using women themselves were mentioned as an important source of information by antenatal staff, particularly about the lifestyle, informal support and the ways that drugs were used. There was a willingness to learn from the clients:

I've learned a lot from the women themselves, who tell you about it. Probably you learn more from them than any other group.

(Community midwife, also other professionals)

Education and training were seen by many health care staff to have several advantages. For example, through being more knowledgeable they would be in a position to offer appropriate advice to their patients. This in turn would help build confidence and trust between them and hence lead to an easier relationship. From a wider perspective, raising awareness of issues around drug use within a service may go some way to help reduce stereotyping and hence break down prejudice.

CONCLUSIONS

An essential feature for the preservation and enhancement of maternal and child well-being is for health professionals to build trust with their patients and clients (Oakley *et al.*, 1996). Health care workers should be aware of how their own reactions can affect the relationship with the new parents, who may be coming to terms not only with parenthood but also the guilt of having taken drugs during the pregnancy and a baby that is experiencing withdrawal. The realisation that drug-using women can have a stable home life should encourage professionals when considering the viability of successful parenting and influence their attitudes to drug-using mothers.

While the needs of pregnant drug users have been officially recognised as requiring attention (English National Board, 1996; LGDF/SCODA, 1997; Mounteney, 1998), there was little visible support in terms of providing the necessary resources for the education and training of their carers. Well-informed staff are likely to be more confident and effective and it is of concern that so many professionals at all grades had some reservations about their ability to offer quality advice to drug-using women in their care.

Better collaborative procedures are also advocated yet poor communication and disagreements between departments and agencies continue to expose clients to conflicting advice. There was frustration at what appeared to be poor information sharing, and a desire for better communication between maternity, social work and drug agencies. Fortunately, many of the problems identified here are being addressed by a growing number of concerned professionals. The success of these services demonstrates just what can be achieved against the apparent odds with thought, planning, concern and an open mind.

REFERENCES

Davis, S.K. (1990) Chemical dependency in women: a description of its effects and outcome on adequate parenting. *Journal of Substance Abuse Treatment* 7(4), 225–232.

English National Board (1996) *Substance Use/Misuse. Guidelines for Good Practice in Education and Training of Nurses, Midwives and Health Visitors.* London: ENB.

Lewis, S., Klee, H. and Jackson, M. (1995) Illicit drug users' experiences of pregnancy. An exploratory study. *Journal of Reproductive and Infant Psychology* 13, 219–227.

LGDF/SCODA (1997) *Drug Using Parents and their Children.* Local Government Drugs Forum and the Standing Conference on Drug Abuse.

Mounteney, J. (1998) *Drugs, Pregnancy and Childcare: Drugs Work 6.* London: ISDD.

Oakley, A., Hickey, D., Rajan, L. and Rigby, A.S. (1996) Social support in pregnancy: does it have long term effects? *Journal of Reproductive and Infant Psychology* 14, 7–22.

Part III

Motherhood

The focus of Part III is the birth and subsequent care of the child in the home. A vivid picture of the mother's confinement in hospital is revealed in the first chapter. Arguably, the hospital ward is the place where she faces her most testing time. Her wish to avoid exposure of her drug use to staff and other mothers fuels her anxieties, which also include the prospect of the baby's withdrawal. Her efforts in reducing her drug use while pregnant may have been in vain and she could now attract more criticism from staff and return home with a baby that needs much attention and care. What is a 'happy event' to other mothers could be a stressful time for her.

Once home, the demands of the infant will be a priority and the degree of strain this causes may undermine her earlier resolution to avoid using illicit drugs. Relapse could perpetuate her dependence on drugs with potentially damaging consequences for her and her child. Is this really a 'window of opportunity'? Difficult issues surrounding drug use and childcare are raised. The nature of the potential hazards for the child at home and parental actions to avoid them are examined. Insights into individual cases are offered and provide an overview of the events in the lives of four women from their pregnancies and into motherhood. The section ends with a chapter by Julian Buchanan and Lee Young that provides many insights into how the issue of child protection has come to dominate social work practice.

Chapter 9

Hospital confinement

Hilary Klee

A dominant theme that emerged from the women's accounts of their ante-natal care was a desire to be treated like any other pregnant woman. Their rights and their special needs have been recognised by professional bodies and are appearing now in guidelines for professionals (e.g. LGDF/SCODA, 1997; Mounteney, 1999). However, the implementation of such a policy across health authorities has been variable and practices which are said to stigmatise drug-using women may still persist in some areas in the UK. It is likely that their reticence and/or avoidance of contact during the pregnancy means that they will not be well prepared for their time in hospital.

ADMISSION TO HOSPITAL

Hospital environments, despite efforts to make them comfortable and attractive, can be intimidating, and patients share with their carers the desire to make their stay as brief as possible. Maternity units differ from most others in their associations with a 'happy event' that heralds a change that is welcome to the majority of patients admitted there. Nonetheless, there are anxieties about the birthing experience and the health of mother and baby. The prospects for the pregnant drug user include outcomes that would add many other stressors to this list. In this study the women, particularly those who had poor antenatal experiences, reported appre-hension about the interactions with staff that confinement would entail. There appeared to be several sources of stress for a drug-dependent woman entering hospital: exposure to other mothers and staff; the need for conceal-ment of drug use from them; and their attitudes towards her and treatment of her. Heroin users in treatment tended to worry about the ways that methadone would be administered; the prospect of the baby withdrawing and of being taken away; dealing with visiting relatives; and finally, their 'performance' under the eyes of midwives and critical social workers. Such close attention is threatening for a woman who normally avoids it where possible. Unlike other mothers she could feel that she has to prove that she is competent if she is to keep her child. If the child were sick, it would be more difficult to cope. Such anxiety is a poor start to this period of major psychological adjustment.

Rejection and exposure

Pregnancy and childbirth is emotionally hazardous for drug-using women because they have to extend their contacts beyond those of their drug subculture and reveal themselves to people who are unlikely to be sympathetic. It was particularly while in hospital that women tended to be hypersensitive to the possibility of rejection. There was evidence that such expectations induced defensiveness and non-compliance. Mutual hostility between a patient and hospital staff could arise quickly.

Deteriorating relationships were more manifest in the interactions with less experienced staff. Hospital midwives on high dependency wards tended to acknowledge the stress to which the women were prone and also made realistic evaluations of the problems in dealing with them:

> Some are very concerned and worried about the signs of the baby withdrawing and they're very frightened. They don't like the hospital environment . . . they don't like being ordered around. If we say we're bathing the babies now, we're bathing the babies now and they don't like the regimented routine. They're glad to get away . . . they've rebelled against society and we're part of society. They're very suspicious if you're nice to them because they're used to being trodden down all the time . . . it's very hard.

Perhaps most encouraging were the comments by staff that the variations found among drug users in terms of their attitudes and behaviour were no different to the range they found among non-drug users. Such an acknowledgement must be an effort for nurses working in Special Care Baby Units who are closest to the baby's distress.

There were very different perspectives and insights into the patients and their needs in hospital. Drug workers, though having few illusions about some of their clients, were aware of their difficulties in coping with the discipline demanded by hospital staff at this time. Hospitals varied in their procedures and in their experience of caring for drug-using patients, however, and drug-user networks were familiar with them. As a result, many respondents had developed ways of avoiding the anticipated problems of exposure and hostility:

> One of the things that happened was that hospitals then began to develop certain reputations and the women would try and circumvent things, take things into their own hands as it were . . . discharge

themselves very, very quickly, denying they were using drugs . . . which was causing more problems both for them and for services.

(Drug worker)

The struggle to maintain control over their lives, apparent in their covert adjustments to methadone doses, was a recurring feature of women in this study. While not obeying the rules may be considered basic to the drugs lifestyle, this explanation is too simplistic and hence uninformative. Other reasons could be that the women feel they know better than their carers what is best for them, which is possible if the carers lack knowledge and experience. Another is to have freedom of choice – in this case choosing to avoid exposure because this is more important to them than the risk to their own and the baby's health, which they may discount as unlikely or even preferable to the alternative. Since concealment could be potentially hazardous the answer is to be aware of their priorities and take them into account rather than expect compliance.

Reception on arrival

The women's worst fears mostly dissipated when they were admitted. The majority of the women were happy about their reception on arrival at the labour ward: 24 (47 per cent) said it was 'excellent', 19 (37 per cent) 'good' and 8 (16 per cent) 'fair'. When asked if any staff were particularly helpful 41 per cent said that they had no problems with any of the staff. A third (35 per cent) picked out midwives as the most helpful. Only 5 (10 per cent) of the women said they did not find the staff helpful. Perhaps it should be borne in mind that the women tended to expect discrimination and although they were extremely sensitive to signs among the staff, they seemed easily satisfied if they were treated as normal patients.

The reality of the labour ward was mostly much more supportive than they had expected, and was appreciated. They were asked about the staff that dealt with them:

Really nice, really caring, they didn't treat me any differently from someone who wasn't taking drugs.

Were you concerned about what they would be like with you?

Yes, because of the antenatal visits. But it's not the same staff, I was really relaxed on the ward, I didn't feel left out or anything.

Some women were able to take occasional disagreeable encounters in their stride:

What was your reception like when you got there?

Great, I can't complain at all, they were marvellous. Like the methadone wasn't an issue especially like once they start talking to you a bit. I mean obviously you get one or two that have got this stereotypical image of what they expect you to be like and they treat you in that manner, but I wouldn't let people treat me like that, I'd stop them before it starts. There were only one or two nurses like that, but everyone else was great.

Maintaining medication

For the opiate-dependent women the regular supply of methadone was a potential source of anxiety along with concern about the way it would be administered. The fear of exposure, which had been a disincentive during pregnancy to attend antenatal services, increased for those entering hospitals that had not developed links with drug agencies. However, most (86 per cent) of the women were consulted about its use on the ward and for 73 per cent of those the arrangements were acceptable and discreet.

> *So presumably all the staff knew that you were on the methadone and there were no problems about that?*

Well, most of the staff knew. When I went in they came and said to me, 'You're on the methadone.' And they kept it all quiet and they got the pharmacist to come up and have a word with me about it.

However, the woman had been reducing her consumption independently during pregnancy. When face to face with professionals she relinquished control and resumed the higher dose without informing them.

> Because I was on 45 ml – when I was in hospital, I took the lot. I took the lot because you're supposed to, aren't you? So I did. For those couple of days I took it all. And I don't take it all usually, I only take 30. So I used to take 25 in the morning and 20 of a night. They used to say 'come and ask one of the staff' . . . you go in a little room on your own and they bring it to you in the room. It was all confidential, no one else knew . . . it was good.

Women in other hospitals tended to have different problems in establishing a satisfactory regime to their methadone administration. This woman experienced delays, which she found upsetting:

> At first I had my 5 ml in the evening, the next morning I'm lying in bed and I said to one of the midwives, 'Can I have my methadone.' And they said, 'Well we'll have to phone up.' And then about two hours later I said, 'Have you phoned them?' They said, 'Yeah, we're

waiting for a fax to come through with the amount of your prescription.' Another two hours, 'Has it come through yet?' 'Well, can you just hang on a bit, we're a bit busy at the moment.' I didn't get it until tea-time that day. They were really bad . . . each day I had to go up and ask for it, they didn't come and give it to me like when they come round with the drugs trolley.

Some antagonism occurred because of a lack of understanding of the respondent's methadone requirements:

> *What were the nurses and midwives like with you, did they know about the drugs?*
>
> Yes, they knew, they never spoke about the drug abuse to you, when I went up on the ward to have her I had to take my own tablets with me. They didn't speak to me about it, they were used to it. I think they looked down on what we did because of what we were doing to the baby. I know they thought I was a heroin addict. I had to ask for a tablet in the end because it was nine at night and I was supposed to have it in the morning. She told me I had to wait, and I said I wouldn't . . . so she didn't like it.

Confidentiality and exposure

The administration of methadone was a situation seen by the women to be one in which their drug dependence was likely to be exposed to other patients on the ward, and hostility was often precipitated in them by lack of sensitivity or understanding by some members of staff. Breaches of confidentiality occurred with inexperienced staff that tended to lead to loss of co-operation by the women:

> There was one night and one of the nurses hadn't been on the ward before . . . she came in and shouted in front of everyone – did I want my methadone? It upset me because everyone tends to look at you as though you're dirty and things like that.

The women were fearful of such disclosures, sometimes unnecessarily so. In this case the woman had automatically assumed that others in the ward would know what sort of medication methadone was.

Deficiencies in confidentiality were felt most acutely by those women whose relatives did not know of their drug use. This could be revealed to them through chance remarks by the staff and record sheets attached to their own bed:

> The file only has to be left one minute and someone could see it. They don't understand . . . they think that because you're hurting your

own body you shouldn't mind. My mum doesn't know nothing. She just knows I smoke ciggies. My brother knows but he wouldn't say anything because he knows it would hurt my mum.

Since about a third (36 per cent) of the women's mothers and over half of the fathers knew nothing of their daughter's drug use this is a serious source of anxiety for many drug users coming into hospital. It is likely to be an additional deterrent to booking into an antenatal clinic prior to delivery when the drug use may be revealed, the staff forewarned, and a formal record made.

There were health care professionals and systems of care, however, that were highly successful; non-discriminating, sympathetic and discreet; and there was a sense of relief and surprise as well as appreciation in the women's accounts. Such events had considerable impact on them, which is testament to the degree of prior conviction that women have about the way they would be treated:

> *Were you worried about confidentiality at all . . . the fact that they were talking about drugs?*
>
> No, not at all, they were really helpful. All the nurses knew, and when they told me he [baby] was going on the morphine they took me to one side and told me . . . they didn't want his dad to know . . . but I told them that he knew already. It was really good of them . . . but I told them that no one else knows. When my mum was here it was never mentioned.

The experiences of many women once they were in hospital were rather better than those anticipated during pregnancy:

> They knew I was on the methadone so they had to keep a close eye on him sort of thing. And the thing I liked is that they don't discuss it with you while anybody's there, they keep it very private. And your notes, they keep anything like that in a grey folder, which is closed. So nobody knows. It's all very confidential, which I liked because you don't want people knowing your business really. I think the nurses were lovely with me, I've got no complaints.

Hospital staff varied greatly in their attitudes and there were significant differences within and between the eight hospitals that we covered. Even in those hospitals that had developed a good working policy on confidentiality there were problems when new staff were not fully briefed. However, such hospitals received the most praise by respondents and had a reputation among drug users for having staff that were more experienced and sympathetic. Understandably, efforts were made by the more informed women to have their babies there.

INFANT HEALTH

Premature birth

The dominant pre-occupation of the opiate-dependent women during their pregnancy was the effect of their drug use on the foetus. Despite efforts on their part to reduce the risk of damage, they could not be sure until the baby arrived whether it would be affected. A common consequence of illicit drug use is premature birth. However, nearly two-thirds of the women (63 per cent) had a normal delivery and 57 per cent of the births were full term. Of the 12 women who gave birth prematurely four were three to five weeks early and eight were over five weeks. Few of the babies were underweight; the average was 6.49 lb (2.95 kg) with over a third above 7 lb (3.2 kg).

Rather surprisingly statistical analyses revealed a significant negative association between cannabis use during pregnancy and premature birth, that is, cannabis users were unlikely to give birth prematurely. Cannabis had been a popular drug prior to the pregnancy; 37 (74 per cent) had been using it. This reduced slightly to 33 (67 per cent) during early pregnancy and 26 (52 per cent) in the last month of pregnancy. The use of this drug was significantly associated with critical variables in several analyses. For example: it was associated with past suicide attempts and overdose; early lack of interest in pregnancy; and various health indicators of heavy use of drugs. The picture that emerges is one of a problem user. Nonetheless, this group were more likely to give birth full term. Its alleged effects on childbirth (as a useful relaxant) led us to examine it more closely. Stepwise logistic regression analysis revealed that the use of cannabis in the last month of pregnancy was independently predictive of a full-term pregnancy, and cannabis users were seven times more likely to carry a baby to full term than non-users. However, cannabis use was also associated with Neonatal Abstinence Syndrome (NAS) in the newborn baby, which might be expected in this group. Despite its controversial nature, it would be worthy of more detailed exploration through further research since it appears to be a part of the information available on the drug-using 'grapevine'.

Infant withdrawal: the Neonatal Abstinence Syndrome (NAS)

The difficulties associated with identifying the maternal risk factors for NAS became very clear when the infants were born. The unpredictability of the effects of drugs used by the mother during pregnancy is well known and there was no straightforward association between reported illicit drug use or methadone dose and the baby's health in these data. There are now guidelines on drug management and childcare (LGDF/SCODA, 1997; Mounteney, 1999; see also Chapters 14 and 17) which suggest that where there is a possibility of infant withdrawal, then delivery should occur in hospitals with a Special Care Baby Unit, and that medication should only be given to the neonate 'if needed'. The impact on mother–infant bonding of removal to Special Care is noted in most national and local guidelines. It is also observed that reassurance may be needed for mothers in order to alleviate the guilt that the majority of them experience.

While the short-term physical effects can be severe for the child, it seems that any long-term psychological and behavioural effects, if they exist at all, may stem from attachment problems that are then exacerbated over time. Among those claimed are poor self-confidence, hyperactivity, aggressiveness and learning disorders, but these are not substantiated since the co-occurrence of other influential factors such as malnourishment, poverty, poor access to health care and lifestyle can all be said to contribute. There may also be consequences that follow the labelling of a child that develops NAS as at high risk since the infant may be expected by the carers to suffer damage and lead to parenting that is overprotective and constraining.

The variability in the assessment and treatment of neonatal withdrawal has been described in several accounts (Morrison et al., 1995; Shaw and McIvor, 1994). Accurate diagnosis is difficult – for example, it is apparently easy to mistake the reactions to birth trauma for withdrawal symptoms. Not only their nature but also their timing is important, and beliefs about the time of onset of such symptoms tend to govern the procedures adopted. For example, they tend to determine the length of time that babies are retained for observation, a period that can vary from a few days to several weeks.

The majority of women had tried to reduce their methadone dose during pregnancy to avoid the baby's withdrawal in the belief that it offered the best chance of a normal delivery and postnatal treatment. Despite such attempts, it came as a shock to some when the baby was taken away. NAS was diagnosed in 26 (51 per cent) of the babies, and 25 were admitted to Special Care (not all of them for NAS). Seventeen were given medication:

> I was really shocked when he had to start on the morphine because I wasn't expecting it at all. I was surprised because the clinic and the hospital said he would be OK on only 20 ml a day. It could have been because he was premature. Betty [midwife] said she didn't think they needed to do it, but when the nurses in the Special Care Baby Unit get hold of the baby, they take over.

It was perceived as failure by the women and sometimes due to their own ignorance:

> *Was there an implication that the withdrawal could have been due to the methadone?* [The respondent had reduced her dose.]

I was smoking twenty cigarettes a day . . . they were more concerned about that. They also said it could have been due to drinking too much tea and coffee . . . well, I'd cut down on coffee but I didn't realise tea was just as bad. I used to have about ten cups of coffee a day but went down to two and had tea instead. I thought I was doing really well.

Although most respondents had been reassured by their experiences with staff on the labour ward and during the baby's birth, they were likely to fear censure at this point:

The midwife said, 'basically it's your fault . . . you did it'.

Understandably, the women felt that this was unfair:

One of them said, 'You've been taking methadone for seven months through your pregnancy, it has got to have affected it somehow.' I said, 'It doesn't, you don't know what you're talking about.' She said, 'I do, I've looked after babies who have had heroin. It's just the same, there's no difference really, in fact heroin comes out of your system quicker than methadone.' At first they said it would take three to four days [in the Special Care Unit], then they said five, then six, then seven, then ten and fourteen. I cracked up.

I bet it made you feel quite bad.

It did, that's why I'd got rid of my habit to prevent all that. My friend's baby didn't need nothing and she was taking 20–30 ml a day.

There were many signs of defensive reactions in mothers, particularly when they were overtly criticised in this way. With milder symptoms the response could take the form of challenging the diagnosis:

On the ward I was treated as a second class citizen basically. He was a little bit restless admittedly, but only for one day. They kept me in for six days and the minute he started crying it wasn't that he had a dirty nappy, it wasn't that he needed feeding, it wasn't that he needed winding or whatever, he was withdrawing straight away. All babies cry, there was other babies there crying from mothers who weren't using, but there wasn't anything wrong with them, you know, but because mine was crying mine was withdrawing. It was just a biased opinion. So they whipped him off to Special Care.

There were several claims that the staff were making such assumptions:

Yeh. Well, that's it, just because they knew that I had used methadone they automatically assumed that the minute he started crying he was withdrawing.

ADMISSION TO SPECIAL CARE BABY UNIT (SCBU)

Women who have a withdrawing baby no doubt feel guilty and may fear the reaction of staff in charge of the care of the child. Stories of parents' erratic visiting and sometimes anti-social behaviour were reported. Staff working on special care units reported being afraid of drug users when they came on the unit. The aggressive behaviour of some of the patients and particularly their visitors in these circumstances may be a way of deflecting overt censure, but it alienated the staff. This is unfortunate since the availability of expert care presents an ideal opportunity for professionals to offer support and practical guidance to the parents.

Predicting NAS

The monitoring of the infant for signs of withdrawal was part of normal procedures when the mother's drug use was known. In some cases removal to the Special Care Baby Unit was immediate, but for others the diagnosis was delayed:

> The only thing that upset me when she was born, she wasn't born withdrawing or anything like that and she wasn't put on Special Care, but when she was three days old she was taken down . . . I thought she was going to be all right. It shocked me because I thought she was safe and over it.

For this woman, the baby's removal was more immediate and she seemed to anticipate criticism in volunteering the information that she had chosen to stay:

> About an hour, well, near enough straight away really. I was really gutted about that because like they put him on me tits, you know so that I could feed him, but he didn't want any. So J [partner] went down with him [to Special Care]. I was down there all the time because you can go at any time. I could have come home if I'd wanted to.

The distress of the baby under these circumstances can give rise to complex emotions, some of which are difficult to acknowledge. A continuously crying infant that will not be pacified is not only stressful, but also makes the mother feel rejected and guilty:

> I thought he was withdrawing because he was screaming a lot when he was born. Whether that was normal I don't know because it's my first baby and I wasn't used to it. I was a bit tired and I just wanted

some quietness and a chance to be alone. I hated myself for thinking that. I said to Kitty, the midwife from the clinic, I said I felt like running away. I asked if he was withdrawing because he was screaming. She said no, he'd got a few snuffles. But I done good by coming down to 15 ml a day, if I hadn't come down to 15 ml he probably would have been withdrawing a bit stronger.

We found no significant relationship between withdrawal or removal to SCBU and the average maternal dose of methadone during pregnancy, which tends to confirm the unreliability of this as a measure of risk. Other than a diagnosis of NAS, the variables associated with the removal of the child to SCBU were largely those indicating heavy use of street heroin and included a lack of preparation for the baby.

In some hospitals there was automatic removal to the SCBU of infants known to be born to drug users. This practice persists despite its critics and recommendations that the infant should be retained on the postnatal ward with the mother (Hepburn, 1993; Morrison and Siney, 1996). Most respondents (72 per cent) had known of the policy in advance of their hospital confinement, which perhaps stimulated their efforts to reduce their drugs. However, it was then seen as a pointless sacrifice if the baby was removed and kept in the unit. An extended stay there posed many problems for the mothers who sometimes faced long journeys every day to see the baby. If there were other children at home their problems were magnified.

Problems with Special Care: staff attitudes

The occurrence of extreme and uncompromising attitudes towards the respondents by hospital staff was very rare. They were more likely from those with responsibility for the infant. However, some women made an effort to see the staff's point of view:

but when we went down to Special Care, the nurses were even worse than the other ones [on the postnatal ward]. It's a nurse to each child, he had two different nurses, and they were really funny with us, but then again they were the ones who sat with him and saw how much distress he was in, and I hated that, so I could understand why they were a bit funny. But it's still not right.

One Special Care Baby Unit (SCBU) nurse commented that the mothers did not stay long in the unit with the baby. Staff whose main focus was the child were, understandably, the most prone to fear for the baby and to adopt a protective attitude that assigned the role of aggressor to the mother. However, some obviously struggled to be fair:

We try not to be judgemental but it can be difficult at times. I mean, we've had families that have stolen from us . . . it's very difficult to be objective about these things.

The responses of staff working in paediatrics were driven by the view that the infant's distress was unnecessary:

One feels more for the babies who have problems which in theory could have been avoided.

However, the change in practice over recent years has been matched in some hospitals by a corresponding change in attitudes. The experience of Special Care was not always unrewarding. The quality of care for the infant was very high and often very reassuring for the anxious mother. It was an added bonus not to be openly blamed for the baby's presence in the unit:

Were any of the staff off with you about the methadone?

No . . . they said I wasn't the first one whose baby had turkeyed. She had sticky eyes and they were really good with her . . . they really cared for her.

The experiences of the women could be so markedly different that it seems likely that they are a product of an interaction between the attitudes of the participants – the overt or implied censure on the one hand and the defensiveness on the other. The major factors that reduced discord were the level of information among the staff about drug use and the degree of their co-operation with the drug team.

Over half of the women were unaware of the nature and extent of contact between drug and maternity services. However, the respondents who expressed most satisfaction with their treatment were those cared for in areas where service liaison was established, and particularly if this was mediated by a liaison midwife. Where this was lacking there were problems in interprofessional communication and co-operation. This arose mainly from the different perspectives of drug workers and maternity staff on a variety of issues. At times there was overt disagreement on policy.

Problems with Special Care: confidentiality

In addition to the emotional strain of the removal of the baby to Special Care and the interactions with staff, there was now an increased danger of exposure of their drug dependence. Visitors increased after the birth and the observance of confidentiality by SCBU nurses was uncertain and potentially disturbing for mothers who were likely to have difficulty in explaining to visitors why the baby was there. There was also a fear that a 'cover story' would not be confirmed by the staff. An even more obvious sign was a chart attached to the cot although this was comparatively rare.

> I told them that my parents didn't know I used drugs or methadone or anything and on his little cot they put 'Baby born to addicted mother'. I wasn't happy about that.
>
> *Did they move it?*
>
> No, I asked them but they said it had to stay there.

Paediatric staff were often conscious of the mothers' desires to maintain concealment of their drug use from relatives. It could be a sore point, however. There was at times only limited sympathy, and the effort needed to be fair was often apparent:

> We've had all sorts of problems on the confidentiality issue – no one knows the mother's on drugs . . . including the whole family. We've got into a sort of conspiracy with the mother – having to lie – she says 'will you tell them it's got a chest infection' . . . and so grandmother and grandad come in and you're expected to spin this yarn out to cover up for the mother wanting to keep it a secret. And it becomes clear that this kiddy is suffering from anything but a chest infection, and they can get quite aggressive to know why the baby's still here . . . and you find yourself saying 'ask your daughter about it'.

There was also resentment of the difficult position in which they were placed by the women whose drug use was unknown to the partner:

> The partner didn't know the mother was a drug addict and she'd been a heavy user for years . . . I don't think they should be lying to the father if there is a stable relationship . . . it's very difficult if you're asked by a father why the baby is ill.

The unthinking exposure feared by the women, and indeed that seemed to persist in some places, was confirmed by several of the older staff as a common part of history:

> When I first came [six years ago] one of the hospitals used to put the women in a side room and there were posters stuck all over the door 'Danger: risk of HIV'. They wanted them to wash themselves after they'd delivered, they were given a bowl and a sponge and the nurses wouldn't go anywhere near them because of the risk of HIV.

The arrangements in some hospitals were much appreciated if the infant's removal to SCBU was not open to enquiry from other mothers and access to the baby was encouraged:

> Anyway, they put me in a little room on me own, which I thought was good, and you can visit Special Care at any time you want, which I thought was lovely. And the father, although there's visiting times for me, he could have stayed at the hospital all day . . . if he wasn't with me he could have been in Special Care with the baby. There was no set times, he could be there all through the night if he wanted, he didn't have to go home or nothing like that.

Most (65 per cent) respondents found the treatment of the baby in Special Care good, a few (14 per cent) had mixed feelings and 22 per cent were not satisfied. This was largely influenced by their relationships with staff and sometimes involved challenges to hospital policy and diagnostic criteria.

TREATING NEONATAL ABSTINENCE SYNDROME

Taking the babies to Special Care was regarded as avoidable by ward nurses. They were faced with difficult decisions when beds were scarce. There were different views on this; those expressed by hospital staff were informed more by convenience than those of drug workers or liaison midwives.

> *Do you think that's the best way to go about it then, to take them to Special Care?*

> Well, let me put it this way, I don't think that we could cope with these babies on our wards the way things are now, because we're pretty busy. I think in an ideal world the babies should be roomed with their mothers, preferably in a special area within the maternity unit so that you can do the neonatal monitoring and look after the mothers, because putting babies on Special Care causes some separation and I think these people need separation like a hole in the head.

Part of the problem of decisions on infant care was the unpredictability of identifying the babies at risk and the variability in the delay before symptoms appeared. It was recognised that the NAS was likely to set up tensions between mother and child that could have serious implications for the bonding between them in addition to the direct health effects on the infant.

Various ideas were voiced about the best way to treat withdrawal and other drug-related symptoms in the newborn. One of the difficulties was predicting the nature of the damage in the face of their uncertainty about the range of drugs used by the mother and her patterns of use during pregnancy. The woman's account was not always accepted as valid:

> When we get the baby we do a urine sample to work out exactly what mum was on, because they don't always tell you the whole truth and we look for methadone, heroin, other narcotics, cocaine, amphetamines and benzodiazepines. That takes several days to come back. Now the methadone, from our point of view, is probably the worst because the withdrawal takes longer and is often a bit more severe. Heroin is actually better from our point of view, but obviously not from the mum's. And also we'll contemplate starting the mums on morphine syrup rather than methadone to see if it will actually reduce the severity of the withdrawal that the baby gets.

It was somewhat ironic that methadone was not always considered a good option and perhaps fortunate that a preference for morphine was not likely to be known to the opiate-dependent women. As a treatment for the infant, morphine was popular in some regions, but there were reservations about releasing the baby during treatment:

> I'm still undecided about which is the best treatment for the withdrawal in babies. At ———— [hospital] they have let a few of their babies go home with morphine, but what they actually do is get the Special Care nurses to go in and give the dose once a day – they're not usually on it for long once they're home and you can usually get them off within two to three weeks – which is faster sometimes than we do treating them in the usual way – and they do seem more settled.

Despite the problems of leaving an infant suspected of withdrawing on an understaffed ward, this was allowed in some hospitals. Disturbance caused by the child's crying was overcome by the mother taking the baby into a separate room. This was not an option in some hospitals, and there were also considerations of the mother's necessity to sleep. There was no doubt that most wanted the babies to stay with them and greatly appreciated this when it was allowed.

STAYING ON IN HOSPITAL

The average stay in hospital was five days, a median of four but a range up to 42 days. Eleven (22 per cent) stayed for over a week. Some mothers met with resistance in their efforts to be discharged. This seemed to be part of a cautious approach by staff to the possibility that symptoms of NAS might appear:

> She [liaison midwife] told them 'don't treat her different than anybody
> else because of the methadone'. And there was nothing wrong with
> him – some babies on the ward were going home and they'd never
> even started feeding, it was only because I was on the methadone that
> they didn't want to let me out. I said to the doctor, 'How come I'm
> not getting let out?' He said, 'Well your name's not on the list.' I
> said, 'What do you mean, I've been here five days and I'm going
> home whether you say so or not.' The nurse came up and said, 'Well,
> we think you should stay in another day.' I said, 'Why what's wrong
> with him?' She said, 'He's got a touch of jaundice.' I said, 'Well,
> there's a few babies on this ward who've got jaundice, there's only
> one that's not got it.' And there was nothing they could say about
> that, they had to let me out and they knew it. And when Sandra
> [liaison midwife] came in she said, 'All it is, is because of the
> methadone, I've told them but they won't listen, they just treat people
> different and they shouldn't really.'

Most babies (65 per cent) were discharged with their mothers. For those
discharged later the median number of days was ten with a range up to
77 days. The experience was not pleasant:

> It was dead weird coming out of hospital without a baby. I thought
> I'd be all right, but I weren't, I was just the same as what I was the
> first time I did it, you know coming out without them. And you see
> the other mums at the side of you, and they've got theirs with them.

Since most mothers with SCBU babies had been separated from them
since soon after birth, this delayed further the opportunity to care personally for the child and start the normal process of bonding. The chances
of a successful family life were thought to be questionable according to
this consultant paediatrician:

> the appropriate action even now is to see whether, having given the
> baby that bad start in life, the family continue the same way and don't
> cope terribly well . . . The next thing I hear is when a year or two
> down the line I'm suddenly asked to fill in adoption papers.

Following the birth, it was suggested by some staff that the mother's
interest in the baby could be low, the evidence coming from her behaviour while the baby was in Special Care:

> Whereas most parents of babies tend to be good reliable visitors, these
> tend to come up with an inordinate number of excuses why they can't
> come in to visit on Special Care.

In contrast, drug-using women have reported making great efforts to maintain contact with the baby when in Special Care. They also reported encountering hostile reactions from staff caring for the baby and feeling that their child was being singled out for attention unnecessarily. Given these circumstances perhaps it should come as no surprise that some parents visit their children infrequently or are wary of the hospital staff.

SUMMARY AND CONCLUSIONS

It seems that judgemental attitudes persist among certain health care professionals. When combined with anticipatory defensiveness on the part of the patient the result is mutual hostility – expectations are fulfilled on both sides and so consolidated and perpetuated. The views of drug-using mothers among maternity staff varied considerably, tending to become more negative with concentrated involvement with the infant. However, there were relatively few who were openly judgemental. Many were attempting to appreciate the women's difficulties. The more experienced were also realistic about their capacity for change.

In regions where drug and maternity services collaborated there was considerable success in ensuring that the women were not faced with hostility during their confinement. The liaison midwife played a key role in these developments. The resources available to her varied, however, which needs to be addressed in view of the importance of the functions they perform, one of which is to offer training to maternity staff. In clinics with drug liaison midwives the consultants and junior staff relied on them heavily, and were relieved to be able to do so. Those with a newly appointed liaison midwife had great hopes that the situation would improve since she would have access to the patient and better information. The most content women were those in contact with services with a policy that had been developed specifically to cater for them.

Understanding the women's complaints about their treatment in hospital should include an appreciation of their sensitivity to rejection. One or two negative staff members or encounters could lower the threshold of non-compliance and elicit a generally unco-operative response in return. Since the women were experiencing physical and psychological changes, it could be that these interactions assume disproportionate significance at this time.

The uncertain relationship between methadone use in pregnancy and NAS was not clarified by these data. All women had reduced their drugs but for some this was apparently to no avail, NAS was diagnosed and most of these babies were removed from the mother soon after birth. Removal of the baby has wide ranging effects on mother and child and the process of bonding. It seems that automatic removal of a baby born to a drug user can be a consequence of limited resources rather than for justifiable clinical reasons; a practice much resented by some paediatricians who felt the unit was being misused. Not only were the patients upset, the move put strain on Special Care facilities designed for more serious cases.

These accounts suggest that the disappointment of her infant's ill health reduces self-esteem and confidence in a woman who has tried to control her drug use. She believes that the baby's distress will be a signal to others that she is a bad mother, feels guilty that the baby is suffering and fears the consequences may be serious. Her low confidence will not help her reach the robust psychological state necessary to care competently for a new baby. If maternity services were consistently sensitive to these common reactions perhaps a less destructive relationship could be developed.

REFERENCES

Hepburn, M. (1993) Drug use in pregnancy. *British Journal of Hospital Medicine* 49(1), 51–55.

LGDF/SCODA (1997) *Drug Using Parents and their Children*. London: Local Government Drugs Forum and the Standing Conference on Drug Abuse.

Morrison, C. and Siney, C. (1996) A survey of the management of neonatal opiate withdrawal in England and Wales. *European Journal of Paediatrics* 155, 323–326.

Morrison, C., Siney, C., Ruben, S.M. and Worthington, M. (1995) Obstetric liaison in drug dependency. *Addiction Research* Vol 3, no 2, 93–101.

Mounteney, J. (1999) *Drugs, Pregnancy and Childcare: Drugs Work 6*. London: ISDD.

Shaw, N.J. and McIvor, L. (1994) Neonatal Abstinence Syndrome after maternal methadone treatment. *Archives of Disease in Childhood* 71, 203–205.

Chapter 10

Drugs and parenting

Hilary Klee

The social construction of motherhood that is apparently set up as the benchmark for all women yields an ideal of a virtuous, caring, self-denying woman that any relatively superficial empirical exercise will reveal belongs to early Hollywood films and TV soaps. It seems to transcend cultural and racial differences in being a universal baseline expectation. It is remarkable in contemporary society that it still retains such power in driving health and social service delivery and, more generally, the attitudes of the general public. Measured against this model, it is difficult to see how anyone can succeed. Such standards would produce feelings of inadequacy in many women, but among the more vulnerable of them who have little self-confidence and low self-esteem, they could induce feelings of guilt and anxiety at a stage when they are least likely to be able to handle them, which is the period soon after childbirth. It is at this point for a drug user, perhaps when coping with a fractious and sick baby as well as reduced drug consumption, that she can find herself the target of direct professional scrutiny about her ability to care for her child.

EARLY DEMANDS

The stress of a new baby was put in perspective by one drug worker:

> I think anyone that's had kids of their own knows what it's like trying to cope with a screaming baby when they've had no sleep. And if these girls have got the added problem of drugs on top of it maybe they haven't got the sense to put the baby on a blanket on the floor and go out of the room, have a cup of coffee and a ciggie and calm down for five minutes.

All mothers are under stress at some time and these women were no exception. However, given the women's belief in the dangers associated with the exposure of their drug taking, overt symptoms of stress could be signals that would attract unwelcome interventions. While in non-drug users the impact on the child would not normally be considered pathological unless severe, these symptoms could be seen as drug induced and therefore an indication of resumed dependence.

An account of her anxieties about the health of her baby provided by this new, young mother reflects the emotional strains experienced by most mothers. She had tried building her confidence as in the past by using amphetamine but feared it would get out of hand. She was a watchful mother and was aware of the effects of her own anxiety on the child:

How have you been finding it having him around?

He was really good at first, you know like when I first brought him home, and then he got colic, I mean I have actually been back to the doctor and got some Prozac, that was like last week. I was going a bit mad on the 'billy' (amphetamine) and I was scared. Like when I first come home I wanted to look after him when he cried, but with the colic you do your best and it doesn't get any better, you know, because they can have it for like three months. I probably make him worse because he knows I'm, you know, all wound up about it.

Some young women had difficulty in accepting the arrival of their baby and took time to come to terms with it. It seems unlikely that this was a feature specifically related to their dependency on drugs.

How did you feel when he was actually born?

I was just like overwhelmed. When he come out and she asked me did I want to hold him, I didn't have any feelings you know. I just said 'no'. And she cleaned him and because he was only small and that, she put him in a fan thing, you know to get him warm. And then because of the blood pressure they changed him and fed him all day and had him in the nursery. So I didn't see him really the first day anyway. I mean me boyfriend Pete come round and he was dead upset. He said to me mam, 'I think she's gonna ask the hospital to keep him.' But like I said, it was just too overwhelming. And then you get all the visitors there and I don't know what they expect you to do, but they was all holding him anyway. So no, I didn't really feel anything.

This may have been regarded as a failure to adapt to motherhood by the professionals in contact with her, but there is evidence that maternal ambivalence is prevalent even among mothers with relatively few problems (Featherstone, 1997).

For the mothers who had such severe doubts that they had considered abortion ($n = 20$; 40 per cent), the problems did not go away easily.

Analyses revealed that these were women with partners who were not emotionally or practically supportive. They were significantly less likely than other mothers to feel happy with the baby (52 per cent compared with 85 per cent) and more likely to get back early into the use of street drugs (60 per cent compared with 27 per cent) and injecting (45 per cent compared with 20 per cent).

There were several other variables significantly associated with negative responses to the baby, for example: admittance of the baby to SCBU while in hospital; the retention of the baby after the mother left; and the prematurity of the baby. The negativity could be due to poor opportunities for bonding or the occurrence of NAS, or both. There were babies whose attempts to communicate were perceived as too demanding and if the mother was depressed and anxious this seemed to be reflected in the baby too. According to Jeremy and Bernstein (1984) a destructive pattern of parenting under these circumstances could develop early from such interactions.

An infant with Neonatal Abstinence Syndrome can be a particular strain. Those caring for such babies faced acute problems immediately they were home and had to cope while experiencing the physical changes and psychological volatility following the birth. The withdrawing baby is harder to comfort and can seem rejecting and the mother often needs reassurance that her mothering skills are not at fault. For this mother, like many others, the need for support was critical:

You had a little bit of depression at first didn't you?

Oh, yeah. I still get that now. You know, like you're fed up sometimes when the baby's crying and crying. And like you check his nappy, you feed him and then when you look to see if everything's all right, nothing's wrong but he's still crying. I just crack up. And sometimes Michael [partner] goes out and he doesn't come in till all hours and I crack up. Sometimes you feel like it's a waste of time and I just feel like leaving. I wouldn't, but you just feel like walking out and shutting the door behind you.

A significant minority (18 per cent) of the women continued to find it difficult to cope with the new baby and in returning to street drugs some were additionally assailed with guilt. For this woman it did not decline:

Yeah. I felt a bit guilty an' all, I think that's why I've given her a lot, you know because like I'm using [drugs] and everything. She didn't withdraw or anything, but I felt dead guilty, I used to sit there and say 'sorry' to her and things like that, you know when I felt depressed and what have you . . . I wouldn't let go of her. I did the same with her (older daughter) and she's spoilt . . . and this one's going to end up the same way.

For some women, the stress experienced during pregnancy had not diminished over time; the stressors after the birth were different, but they could be just as acute, despite the return to home territory. The women were asked about their need for drugs now the child was born. There was a greater reluctance to commit to giving up street drugs completely; about a third (36 per cent) said they would continue with street drugs (cannabis and amphetamine, less commonly heroin) in contrast to the 10 per cent who would continue with methadone. Over a third (38 per cent) said they would try to give up methadone, which was regarded as chronically addictive, a common complaint among opiate dependents in treatment. It was very clear that the lure of street drugs was strong and that returning home was full of hazards. Strong craving was reported by 38 per cent at this time, 31 per cent described this as moderate and 31 per cent as weak. By the third interview those reporting weak craving earlier had diminished and there was a corresponding increase in those reporting moderate craving (34 per cent, 45 per cent and 21 per cent).

Talking of street drugs, do you ever feel tempted to go and score?

Loads of times. When I've seen people that I know and ask them where they're going and they tell me to score, I just want to go with them. I don't though.

One of the major concerns about using drugs with the children around, and often heard across all samples of parents, was that their children would take up drugs. There was an awareness of the example they might be setting and that this may lead to the child experimenting with them:

What makes me stop a lot of things is me kids . . . I just think 'I don't want them to grow up like that' . . . it would kill me if my kids ever went near drugs.

The concern is justified, there is much evidence that children of drug-using parents are likely to go on to use drugs themselves (e.g. Kumpfer, 1997; Tarter and Mezzich, 1992) and may be subject to mental health problems. The parents are subject to a considerable amount of guilt later. Nurco and his colleagues (1998) suggest that they are overwhelmed by the problems related to their dependence and cannot function well as parents. Their study revealed, in addition, that their children saw themselves as far more effective in their parenting practices than their parents.

Amphetamine users found it easier to contemplate using the drug in the future and there was less guilt, perhaps not surprising since they had found it functionally valuable in giving them energy and confidence (Klee, 1997):

Do you think once you stop breast feeding you might give up?

I can't say I'll never not have it again because I know I will, but it'll be when she's a lot older. I won't leave her with anybody and I won't have any of them into the house and stuff. And a lot of whizzheads smoke and I don't like anyone near them [the children] who smokes. But if I said I wouldn't use it again I'd be a liar.

THE POSITIVE ASPECTS OF MOTHERHOOD

Despite the stress, few women, even those whose babies were unplanned or unwanted, said they were unhappy with the baby, although for some the adaptation took a little time. There was a decline in numbers of those who reported pronounced positive interactions ('very high enjoyment') with the infant from 20 (40 per cent) soon after birth to 10 (20 per cent) at third interview. Perhaps this temporary 'honeymoon' could be expected. Notwithstanding the problems of bonding, the fractiousness of withdrawing babies and the struggle for equilibrium in drug use, the majority (94 per cent) continued to enjoy their babies throughout the period of study. Those who had healthy and happy babies felt particularly grateful, to the extent noted by Burns and Burns (1988) that the child was seen as a gift to them:

How do you feel about the fact you've had him then?

It was strange at first, I kept saying to myself, I wish I hadn't had another one. But you go with it, you know you get used to it. I wouldn't be without him now, you know it's like I said to me husband, he's like a 'Gift from God' sort of thing, you know because he's so much fun. He keeps you going.

The opportunity of being in an uncomplicated loving relationship was important to several mothers:

Don't get me wrong he does cry and all that, but he's someone to love isn't he? It's like, I don't know, I mean it's strange . . . he's always in your brain sort of thing. If you go out you know to go and check him and things like that. I love him to bits, I'm glad I've got him because I think he's just gorgeous.

It was clear that for others the baby was a catalyst for major change:

You sound like you're quite enjoying having her around. What sort of things are good about that?

I don't know. Just having somebody that I can look after and love. Before I got pregnant I was in a bit of a bad way anyway . . . so she actually sorted me head out in a way. I've always had my own freedom and, like, this was the chance to quieten down and settle down.

The baby inevitably made a significant impact on the women's lives. Mostly this was very positive. Despite a loss of freedom, this woman and her partner also benefited from their new baby:

Yeah, I can't just get up and do things that I've done before I had Kenny, you know the other two are grown up. But it does change your life. I mean before I had him I was bashing the drugs and everything, but since we've had him our whole life has changed, I mean we've really cut down, we don't do speed no more, we have gear (heroin) once a week. But it really has, he's done good more than anything I suppose, you know helping me get off the drugs, because I done everything for him.

There were some mothers whose previous children had been placed in care and who deeply regretted it. This woman admitted her neglect through heavy drug use and was determined to avoid her mistakes now she had a second chance:

I don't think I've been a good parent, not to Jess [first child]. I've lost her, she's gone to me mum and dad's. Dave [partner] was never here, she had no family, she got picked on at school, she never had nothing. I used to take her with me everywhere I went and they weren't nice places.

Most respondents did not think very highly of their mothering skills: 45 per cent thought they were 'good mums' and 16 per cent felt they were adequate and not worried about it, the rest (39 per cent) felt guilty or had problems. Such views seemed to be part of a more general lack of confidence in many cases and suggest a need for reassurance and encouragement, and interventions that would endow them with skills that would increase their confidence.

COPING

An operational definition of coping satisfaction was computed comprising the data from three related variables: self-reported level of coping, feeling happy about the baby and enjoyment of the baby. Analyses revealed other variables that were significantly associated with this measure which were largely about opportunities for bonding during hospital confinement, for example: the baby being kept on the ward or returning home with the mother. Predictably, relatively poor coping satisfaction was associated with sick babies and the feelings of guilt about the baby's problems. However, there were accounts of fears that would affect most mothers of new babies:

> It's most probably just me, I worry and that . . . at one stage I was dead paranoid over him, I had this thing about cot deaths and I used to be all the time thinking it was gonna happen to me. I was terrible, checking him all the time and that. But there was loads of things on the telly then about them cot mattresses and it just got on me mind.

Although the majority ($n = 36$; 72 per cent) reported that they were coping fairly easily, it is important to be able to identify and offer support to the sizeable number of women who do have difficulties. The main problems were the demands of the child, the child's health, and having no break. Multivariate tests showed that coping well was strongly associated with a full-term baby, illustrating perhaps the problems that premature birth can bring.

Much indirect 'evidence' for poor parenting has accumulated among practitioners and has been widely accepted partly because it could be predicted from what is known about the psychoactive states induced by drugs. It seems quite logical to suppose that a child will suffer if cared for by a person in a state of inebriation. However, few service providers are able to base their assumptions on first-hand experience of the homes of drug-using families, and equally they would be unable to compare them with non-drug users of similar background, income, education and informal, social support. Fortunately, the determinants of child neglect or abuse are increasingly recognised by practitioners and policy makers (LGDF: SCODA, 1997; National Children's Bureau, 1994) as a product of a number of inter-related factors that include substance misuse but also include others, primarily poverty, deprivation and psychiatric disorders.

Eleven women (22 per cent) had been in care as children and this variable was significantly associated with a number of variables that together indicated their perceptions of lack of support, for example the need for more help, and irregular contact or poor relationships with their natural mothers. They were also more likely to report a criminal record. Finkelstein (1996) points out that such women may never have been exposed to healthy or appropriate models of parenting.

A range of views were expressed by service providers about the parenting capacity of drug users. Even the most sympathetic and insightful among them acknowledged that problems of dependence and an established drug-oriented lifestyle meant that extraordinary efforts would be needed by mothers, many of them involving major change. Women returning home with a new child may feel fulfilled and happy but are also likely to face unfamiliar problems. The rest of this chapter examines the challenges of parenting and how these were met.

RISK FACTORS AND PARENTS' PREVENTION STRATEGIES

The data in this section are supplemented by the accounts of other groups of drug-using parents from studies carried out in the same geographical regions and using the same research methods (Klee *et al.*, 1998). The observations are organised in terms of the categories of risk for the child that were derived from thematic analyses of qualitative data in these studies and the pregnancy research, and reports the strategies used to remove or minimise them. The interview data were informed by direct observations of the women's interactions with the child(ren) and other members of the household. These provided many insights. Three broad categories of risk were identified:

- risks associated with the mental state and behaviour of the parent;
- risks in the social environment;
- risks in the physical environment.

1 Risks associated with the mental state and behaviour of the parent

Depression

Chronic and severe depression was the most common complaint reported by 33 women (66 per cent) at first interview. This was often linked to drug withdrawal but is likely to have been a persistent feature in many cases. Observations of depression, social isolation and low self-esteem have been made repeatedly in the literature on substance-dependent women (Finkelstein, 1996). Logistic regression analyses of changes in methadone doses used during pregnancy revealed depression as an independent predictor. A higher proportion (87 per cent) of those not achieving a reduction reported depression compared with 53 per cent of those reducing. After the birth of the child nearly half of the women (46 per cent) were still reporting depression, although this time it could have been confounded with postnatal symptoms. The manifest forms of depression often include immobility, insensitivity and unavailability, which are frustrating and potentially provocative for the child according to Reder and Lucey (1995). Such effects impact on many aspects of the child's life: providing the food, shelter and warmth that ensure his or her physical well-being; and the support, guidance and consistency in behaviour which are critical for cognitive, emotional and psychological development.

Heroin reduces emotional responsiveness and at high levels has a sedating effect. Withdrawal can lead to a level of craving that allocates further administration of the drug a high priority. With resources depleted by high financial costs, other aspects of family life can get neglected. This was acknowledged by some opiate users who paid more for their drugs than amphetamine users:

> No it doesn't make you a better mum, it makes you worse, I think. I think you're a good mum in the sense that like everybody else, you look after them an' everything, but you're still wondering like all the money you're spending on that, you're thinking what you could have for the kids an' that.

Irritability

The majority of parents recognised the dangers when inebriated or withdrawing and attempted to avoid harm by removing themselves or by using other drugs to improve their mental state. This was a standard protection strategy for both opiate users and primary amphetamine users. With frequent dosing of amphetamine, however, there could be a loss of control in which such considerations were not maintained and led to irritable behaviour:

> If I didn't have Gary [son] I'd probably take it a lot more through the week, but I don't in case I get a bad comedown or because you don't sleep you're gonna feel tired in the afternoon, aren't you? And like when I'm tired I get ratty an' it's not his fault, an' I know I'd take it out on him because he's the nearest person to me.

Seriously aggressive acts tend to be associated with paranoid delusions and, more rarely, amphetamine psychosis among problem users (Klee, 1992).

Among primary amphetamine users the symptoms appeared during periods of hyperactivity too (when 'speeding'). Some of the irritation was through impatience. For a person who is 'speeding' other people can appear to be very slow:

> Yes. You want people to hurry up and do things – kids can't. And you can't be bothered sitting down talking to them like you're supposed to. You want to go out, you don't want to be sat in the house so you'd leave them with anybody. I never left them on their own, I really didn't, but I left them with people who weren't suitable really.

Irritability that takes the form of harsh criticism, emotional and verbal abuse can damage not only the parent–child relationship but also undermines the self-esteem of the child (see Rutter, 1990).

A common way of tempering the irritability was to use cannabis. In the parenting study this appeared to be more common among women than men probably because few had the option of detaching themselves physically from the child and leaving, and unless they could call on family or peer support there was little they could do:

I can get pretty bad-tempered when I'm coming down, that's why I try an' have a smoke [cannabis] or get someone to take the kids out.

The consequences of impatience and aggression directed at children were usually soon regretted but not always remedied in an appropriate way.

I shouted at me son . . . you know what I mean. I shouted at him when I was coming down and I felt dead guilty. I went into the other room and started crying . . . it's not his fault I haven't got any speed. So now I let him do what he likes . . . wreck me house or whatever. I give in to him too much . . . but it's not his fault . . . why should I take it out on me son?

(Single mother)

Neglect

Instances of neglect arose largely through failure to monitor effectively the child's whereabouts and actions:

He fell and hurt his head today so he's getting spoiled today. He's had presents an' that. All his face was a mess an' I was really frightened. I was stoned at the time an' I felt really guilty.

(Single mother)

The children of women with little support in the home could be at greater risk. This woman had the co-operation of her own mother:

I usually take my little girl to me mum's, you know, get out of me head for about an hour or summat, get myself straight and then go and pick her up.

Primary amphetamine users liked to draw a distinction between themselves and heroin users, the women placing particular emphasis on their housekeeping standards:

I keep the kids warm and fed and the house tidy . . . I play with the kids. With junkies like, the kids are out on the street with no clothes in the middle of winter . . . I'm not going to get like that.

However, the attitude of amphetamine users towards heroin users, and the statutory drug services associated with them, effectively removed the possibility of seeking professional help, which could have implications for the future welfare of their children:

Sometimes I think she should go.

(Partner)

I don't see myself as having a problem on whizz. I probably have, but I don't think I have. Because no one would look at me and say 'oh, you're on drugs'.

The difference is, like, if she has £10 in her pocket and we needed electric, she'd go out and buy the electric card, whereas junkies would rather buy the drugs rather than buy the electric, and that's the difference.

(Partner)

The kids come before anything.

I know they'd do that, empty fridges, but they're all smack heads, not whizzheads.

(Partner)

They're all junkies not users. There's a big difference between a junkie and a user.

While field observations tended to support this distinction between primary heroin and amphetamine users, it was not as absolute as claimed (see Taylor 1989, 1993). There were heroin users, in particular those stabilised by methadone treatment, whose standards in self-care and care of their home and children were high. On the other hand there were the more chaotic users for whom the craving for heroin took precedence over most other aspects of life, including the monitoring and care of the child (see Nurco *et al.*, 1998).

The drug-using mother is likely to meet fairly comprehensive hostility from the non drug-using community. It will not matter that she may aspire to give up drugs but fail because of lack of support or environmental or psychiatric forces; nothing less than total abstinence is acceptable. However, like amphetamine users, opiates and other 'downers' fulfilled a positive function that users were unwilling to forgo and often perceived as beneficial to the child:

You just have a bit to help you get through the day and that's it . . . that's all I want, just to be OK so I don't be horrible, otherwise the kids would cop it then, wouldn't they?

They're expecting me to get off it [heroin], but it's really hard though, being at home and coping with the kids . . . keeping the place tidy . . . it's a hassle without anything.

Attending to personal needs was a first requirement for most opiate-based polydrug users, and this was a regular feature of everyday life:

If you've got a habit – when you get up in a morning before you can even think about the children you've got to think about getting yourself better.

Summary

Observers of the drug scene place much emphasis on the dangers inherent in the inebriated state of the parents. These data suggest that drug users themselves pay most attention to this form of risk and attempt to protect the child. However, they are not the only risks and the social environment and lifestyle present dangers of a rather different kind that are much less easily identified and controlled. Parents may wish to change this by moving away but frequently are caught, not only in a poverty trap, but also through fear of change. Entering 'straight' society is not easy for a long-term member of a drug subculture and requires much determination and confidence.

2 Risks in the social environment

Some potential hazards for the child were identified that were a part of the social environment. This was mostly in the form of interpersonal inter-actions, and protective actions were aimed at preventing the child from seeing drugs being used and people in a drug-induced psychoactive state.

Concealment

At a very basic level there were rules about not administering drugs in front of the child. When both parents used drugs there was usually an agreement about the degree of concealment and the age at which this would be necessary. No respondent reported injecting in front of children. It seemed to be their major concern, even prior to the child's birth:

> We're saying that nothing is to be done in front of it. If we're still both using it then we'll go into the kitchen and do it, but we're not going to be cooking it on the spoon in front of it.

Drugs were being used at home by 33 (66 per cent) of the women, the majority having resumed their use of street drugs within a few weeks of arriving home. All respondents had some procedures worked out to try to protect the child from witnessing parental drug administration but they tended to vary in terms of what was considered safe. They were asked about their drug administration practices:

> We always go upstairs.

> We don't always go upstairs! Be truthful.
>
> (Friend)

> To inject we do.

I don't. We put the kids in the kitchen and I turn me back in case
they walk in . . . it's done that quick.

(Friend)

We set it up in the kitchen because it's easier to put away in there.
But I do it upstairs, and if the kids are in bed or whatever I just do
it down here, or if they're in here playing we'll just close the door.
But most of the time I go upstairs.

No one in their right mind would do it in front of the kids anyway.

(Friend)

Role modelling

The influence of more subtle drug-related harms, such as overheard conversations and attitudes, were often overlooked. These were frequently
recorded in the observational field notes of interview settings and seemed
more insidious and pervasive and therefore potentially more dangerous.
The majority had drug-using friends and some only had drug-using friends.
Since most were unemployed, the typical pattern of day-to-day living
involved visiting or visits from friends. The risks associated with the social
environment were, in the short term, not life threatening, but they were
more likely to shape the behaviour and attitudes of the growing child
(Loeber and Stouthamer-Loeber, 1986). This was through mechanisms of
role modelling and social learning of the norms and values of the reference culture.

There were many ways that these were transmitted – through direct
observation of drug-related behaviour by parents and their associates, by
their conversation – the content and vocabulary used in verbal interactions, by inferences made of repeated patterns of behaviour associated
with drug administration, by their attitudes towards non-drug-using society
and the societal norms that governed behaviour outside the home – which
could be very different from those within it. It is these continuous and
very powerful mechanisms that establish a child's identity and role within
the group, but which could conflict with the norms and values that would
be encountered outside at school and perhaps in the local neighbourhood.
The conflict between them could itself be damaging in terms of social
integration and psychological health if these were so opposed that the
child was forced into compliance with them on the one hand and labelled
as deviant by authority figures on the other. These were factors that were
recognised by some parents as potentially damaging but ways of avoiding
them were much more complex and effortful than simply hiding drugs.

Some parents became aware eventually of the impact on their children,
like this man who saw the difference only after he had entered treatment,
but was still struggling in his efforts to give up the drugs:

What's your relationship like with your children at the moment?

Great, no problems. Me daughter's growing up and I worry about her a lot, you know picking up on things, the atmosphere . . . cos it affects them, doesn't it? And she's seen us arguing a lot. I think it's affected her, made her a lot quieter, you know – withdrawn. I find that hard to deal with. Like I say, I know the reasons why I shouldn't do it [use drugs] but I still do . . . just because I do that doesn't mean I don't care about me kids, because I do.

Some parents were vigorous in their efforts to ensure the child did not become submerged in the lifestyle and would be accepted in the outside world. They were aware that the children had to be integrated if they were not to suffer at school and in the neighbourhood:

Mandy goes to Sunday school and she goes to the Brownies on a Monday. I thought 'If I get her in with the right crowd, doing the right things' . . . because the worst fear in my life is the kids coming across drugs. I try me best to keep it from me kids, that they don't hear anything and they don't see anything at all . . . but she's so advanced it's hard. I never lock the bathroom door but all of a sudden it's 'Mum, why is the bathroom door locked?' . . . 'Go away . . . I'll be down in a minute.'

Role reversal

The parenting of respondents at times appeared dysfunctional, but their emotional attachment to their children was mostly very high. If women feel lonely and isolated from family and other social support, they may turn to the infant for human comfort. The emotional investment in the child was a prominent feature among several mothers, and some of their partners too. It seemed to be intense and exclusive and there were signs of role reversal (Glaser, 1995) with the parental need for emotional support being met by the child. From a psychoanalytic perspective, parents who have been emotionally deprived as children may try to conceive in the hope that they will provide the affection they never received (Pines, 1993; Steele, 1980). Such relationships can be potentially problematic for the child at a later stage when forming adult relationships.

There are other negative consequences, for example if it interferes with the child's school attendance and educational development. The most disturbing example was an older single parent with a large family. This woman's eldest daughter avoided school if possible and her mother colluded with her truanting:

How many kids have you got?

Four.

You've got your hands full!

I haven't, the older one has. I've had to keep her off school today because I've had to do all the bedding and everything, you know, to get rid of the lice [infestation found among pupils at school]. But they're trying to take me to court, that's how bad it is . . . but she doesn't care.

So have you had the education welfare officer around and everything?

Yeah. They 'want a word with me' . . . they're 'there to help me'.

And what do you think of that?

Bollocks!

Termed the 'Cinderella syndrome' (Burnett, 1993), this is emotionally abusive if carried to an extreme, and normalisation of family relations might ultimately need more intensive interventions than advice and education.

Children who know

Some children knew of their parents' drug use, often revealed accidentally or by gradual accumulation of information. The impact of this type of revelation is unknown but is likely to affect the parent–child relationship, the child's self-image and social integration. Those with other older children were more aware of the impact on them and had few illusions that it went unnoticed.

Do you think it has affected the kids in any way?

Oh yeah . . . like when you're withdrawing and poorly they know. Like she [daughter] said to me, 'I don't like seeing you poorly.' Oh, it definitely affects them.

The interviewer had witnessed occasions when respondents had injected with babies or very young children in the room and had observed their interest in what was happening. It seems that some mothers believe that children cannot understand what they are seeing while they are so young. Similarly when talking about drugs to the interviewer some were unaware that an older child was listening. The age at which such information will affect the child is not predictable and the point at which this is occurring may not be noticed for some time. This highlights the importance of education and awareness raising about these issues.

Summary

Undoubtedly there is much evidence that confirms the drug-using home as a high risk area for a child. Comparisons between developmental outcomes of children born to drug-using mothers who were adopted and those who remained with the mother have indicated poorer development and more behavioural disorders among those who stayed (Ornoy *et al.*, 1996). This was the case even when both groups were diagnosed with NAS at birth. These authors believe that *in utero* exposure to drugs is less important than the home environment. While most concern among the medical fraternity focuses on the physiological impact of NAS on the child, the evidence suggests that the drug-oriented home and lifestyle is the more important factor in the child's cognitive, emotional and social development.

3 Risk from the physical environment

In addition to possible damage caused through neglect, if not direct abuse, by parents who use drugs, many health and social welfare professionals believe that there may also be the detritus from communal drug taking and injecting as well as the drugs that are not securely out of reach.

The risk of children consuming the parents' drugs is a prominent part of public concern for their safety. Most households use pharmaceutical preparations and other substances that are potentially lethal if consumed by a child – bleach and cleaning fluids, for example. As with any dangerous substance there is a risk, if it is unconcealed, within reach and not child-proof, that the child's curiosity will prevail, particularly if their role models are seen to consume it. There were very few respondents who did not try to keep drugs out of the way although the security of the hiding place was not always adequate:

> *Have you used any street drugs since the baby?*

> No. Just some methadone, but I don't let him see me doing it. I take it to the toilet upstairs. I don't like the others [children] seeing me do it as well because if they see me they might think they can do it. I keep the Calpol in the fridge and I wouldn't want them taking that.

Not allowing the child to observe access and administration of drugs was a part of the strategy for many people:

> I have to do it early on in the day when I get up. I get them out of the cupboard and it's a bit of a pain taking ten at a time [methadone tablets]. I keep them well away from him, I don't want him to get used to seeing them at all.

The safeguarding of injecting equipment, given the association with HIV transmission, has been the subject of close attention by health professionals and the message thoroughly disseminated. The consequent raising of awareness seemed to have resulted in extra care by some parents:

> There's people that use them [needles] here. My boyfriend will take them off them and put them in a box so he knows where they are, because of the kids and that. He doesn't like the idea of the kids getting hold of them.

However, another mother believed that her warnings were sufficient:

> I'm on diazepam in the mornings and Angie [3-year-old daughter] will get me tablets and give them me before I get up. But she doesn't touch them or open them, she'll just get me the bottle. She knows not to touch them, she knows they're mine and they'll do her harm. I've told her if she ever touched my medicine it'll kill her.

Summary

There were many instances of ignorance of child development and miscalculation of the capacities of the child's comprehension of danger and risk that indicate the need for intervention in the form of training in parenting skills. Since many drug users have poor models of parenting, it is particularly important to offer them opportunities to safeguard and nurture their children which is something most of them want. In this they are no different from non-drug users.

CONCLUSIONS

According to Dore and her colleagues (1995) sickness in the newborn makes them more difficult to care for, hence parenting skills are particularly important for the drug-using mother. However, if she is still using psychoactive drugs there may be a number of direct as well as indirect effects of her inebriation on the child's cognitive and psychosocial development. Various researchers (Johnson and Montgomery, 1989: see Kumpfer, 1998 and Reid et al., 1999 for an overview) have found evidence of impaired intellectual functioning, conduct disorders, anxiety, low self-esteem and, ultimately, the later use of illicit drugs. The nature of the physical and social environment adds more subtle influences to the hazards and makes the burden on the mother's parenting capacity more difficult. There is strong evidence that informal support from those close to her is essential at this time if she is to succeed in avoiding such harm. The potential for her relapse back into street drugs increases and, if it occurs, will bring in its wake anxiety and depression, loss of self-esteem, hopelessness and greater fear of welfare services.

Some protective strategies used by parents were simply aimed at separating the child from the source of the hazard, for example access to dangerous drugs, or someone (including themselves) in an inebriated state. The time to take real action was seen by them as a series of thresholds: the child's active unrestrained movement; comprehension of adult actions and words; playing with children outside the family: and, in particular, going to school. The more subtle influences that could affect older children – overheard conversations, attitudes and interactions with drug-using visitors – tended to go unrecognised. However, mothers with older children were less likely to accept that the child could be kept in a perpetual state of safe ignorance, presumably through having failed to achieve it previously. As a matter of priority there is a real need for professional interventions that educate and inform parents about the range of such dangers to their children, their time scale, and how to avoid them.

An aspect of parenting that was consistent across all research samples was that of good intentions. Drug-using parents have a high emotional investment in their children that should provide the motivation for adequate childcare within the range provided by non-drug users. In a controlled study, Sowder and Burt (1980) compared the families of 160 drug users with 160 non-drug users and found no difference between the groups in terms of child rearing practices, methods of discipline and their expectations of their children. The roots of the differences may lie, hypothetically, not only in the drugs but also the social factors associated with drug taking. Suchman and Luther (2000) examined three parenting dimensions: involvement, autonomy and limit setting, and three potential determinants of parenting behaviour: maternal drug dependence, socio-economic status and children's maladaptive behaviour, with the aim of identifying those aspects of parenting attributable to these factors. Using matched groups they found a significant negative association between maternal addiction and involvement with the child, which was congruent with other studies; but equally strong were the socio-demographic factors. They concluded that these could contribute as much if not more to parenting behaviour than maternal addiction.

It seems that what is needed is informed and non-judgemental guidance for drug-using parents, which raises issues about remedial and educational interventions. For example, realistically, what actions can be implemented by the mother, assuming that her drug use could continue; what type of strategy will effectively safeguard the child; how can co-operation be achieved that will ensure a constructive dialogue with mothers about their problems; how are secrecy and deception to be avoided? To develop effective interventions is a major challenge that could be met more easily if the use of drugs is well controlled. After the birth of the child much of a drug user's ability to cope will depend critically on preventing a return to the use of illicit drugs and the associated lifestyle. A skilled and sympathetic professional who provides a 'listening ear' would be valuable in sustaining her attempts to avoid relapse by reassuring her that the negative feelings, doubts and confusion are normal. Where informal support is lacking and confidence is low, such formal support is essential. The focus in the next chapter is on the roles of both formal and informal support systems in preventing relapse and helping to reduce the strains of parenting.

REFERENCES

Burnett, B.B. (1993) The psychological abuse of latency age children: a survey. *Child Abuse and Neglect* 17, 441–454.

Burns, W.J. and Burns, K.A. (1988) Parenting dysfunction in chemically dependent women. Chapter 12, in: I.J. Chasnoff (ed.) *Drugs, Alcohol, Pregnancy and Parenting*. The Netherlands: Kluwer Academic Publishers.

Dore, M.M., Doris, J.M. and Wright, P. (1995) Identifying substance abuse in maltreating families: a child welfare challenge. *Child Abuse and Neglect* 19(5), 531–543.

Featherstone, B. (1997) Crisis in the western family, in: W. Hollway and B. Featherstone (eds) *Mothering and Ambivalence*. London: Routledge, 1–16.

Finkelstein, N. (1996) Using the relational model as a context for treating pregnant and parenting chemically dependent women, in: B. Underhill and D.G. Finnegan (eds) *Chemical Dependency: women at risk*, 23–44.

Glaser, D. (1995) Emotionally abusive experiences, in: P. Reder and C. Lucey (eds) *Assessment of Parenting: psychiatric and psychological contributions*. London: Routledge.

Jeremy, R.J. and Bernstein, V.J. (1984) Dyads at risk: methadone maintained women and their four month old infants. *Child Development* 55, 1141–1154.

Johnson, R.J. and Montgomery, M. (1989) Children at multiple risk: treatment and prevention. *Journal of Chemical Dependence and Treatment* 3(1), 145–163.

Klee, H. (1992) A new target in behavioural research: amphetamine misuse. *British Journal of Addiction* 87, 439–446.

Klee, H. (1997) A typology of amphetamine misuse in the United Kingdom. Chapter 3, in: H. Klee (ed.) *Amphetamine Misuse: international perspectives on current trends*. The Netherlands: Harwood Academic Publishers.

Klee, H., Wright, S. and Rothwell, J. (1998) *Drug Using Parents and their Children: risk and protective factors*. The Manchester Metropolitan University, Manchester: SRHSA.

Kumpfer, K.L. (1997) Special populations: etiology and prevention of vulnerability to chemical dependency in children of substance abusers, in: B.S. Brown and A.C. Mills (eds) *Youth at High Risk from Substance Abuse*. No. (ADM) 87–1537 National Institute on Drug Abuse (NIDA), Department of Health and Human Services. Washington DC: US Government Printing Office.

Kumpfer, K.L. (1998) Links between prevention and treatment for drug-abusing women and their children, in: C.L. Wetherington and A.B. Roman (eds) *Drug Addiction Research and the Health of Women*. National Institute on Drug Abuse (NIDA), Rockville, MD: US Department of Health and Human Services.

LGDF/SCODA (1997) *Drug Using Parents and their Children*. London: Local Government Drugs Forum and the Standing Conference on Drug Abuse.

Loeber, R. and Stouthamer-Loeber, M. (1986) Family factors as correlates of juvenile conduct problems and delinquency, in: *Crime and Justice, an Annual Review of Research Volume 7*. Chicago, Ill: University of Chicago Press.

National Children's Bureau (1994) *Drug Misuse*. Highlight series 7. London: NCB.

Nurco, D.N., Blatchley, R.J., Hanlon, T.E., O'Grady, K.E. and McCarren, M. (1998) The family experiences of narcotic addicts and their subsequent parenting practices. *American Journal of Drug and Alcohol Abuse* 24(1), 37–59.

Ornoy, A., Michailevskaya, V. and Lukaslov, I. (1996) The developmental outcome of children born to heroin-dependent mothers, raised at home or adopted. *Child Abuse and Neglect* 20(5), 385–396.

Pines, D. (1993) *A Woman's Unconscious Use of Her Body: a psychoanalytic perspective*. London: Virago.

Reder, P. and Lucey, C. (1995) Significant issues in the assessment of parenting, in: P. Reder and C. Lucey (eds) *Assessment of Parenting: psychiatric and psychological contributions*. London: Routledge.

Reid, J., Macchetto, P. and Foster, S. (1999) *No Safe Haven*. New York: (National Center on Addiction and Substance Abuse at Columbia University) CASA Publications.

Rutter, M. (1990) Psychosocial resilience and protective mechanisms, in: J. Rolf, A.S. Masters, D. Ciccieth, K.H. Nuechterlein and S. Weintraub (eds) *Risk and Protection Factors in the Development of Psychopathology*. Cambridge: Cambridge University Press.

Sowder, B. and Burt, M. (1980) Children of addicts and non-addicts: a comparative investigation in five urban sites, in: *Heroin addicted parents and their children: Two reports*. National Institute on Drug Abuse (NIDA) Research Report, Department of Health and Human Services. Washington DC: US Government Printing Office.

Steele, B. (1980) Psychodynamic factors in child abuse, in: C.H. Kempe and R.E. Helfer (eds) *The Battered Child*, 3rd edition. Chicago: University of Chicago Press.

Suchman, N.E. and Luther, S.S. (2000) Maternal addiction, child maladjustment and socio-demographic risks: implications for parenting behaviours. *Addiction* 95(9), 1417–1428.

Tarter, R. and Mezzich, A. (1992) Ontogeny of substance abuse: perspectives and findings, in: M. Glantz and R. Pickens (eds) *Vulnerability to Drug Abuse*. Washington DC: American Psychological Association.

Taylor, A. (1989) Post natal depression. What can a health visitor do? *Journal of Advanced Nursing* 14, 877–886.

Taylor, A. (1993) *Women Drug Users*. Oxford: Clarendon Press.

Tyler, R., Howard, J., Espinosa, M. and Doaks, S. (1997) Placement with substance abusing mothers vs placement with other relatives: infant outcomes. *Child Abuse and Neglect* 21(4), 337–349.

Chapter 11

Relapse

Missing the window of opportunity

Hilary Klee

Pregnancy is widely regarded as an opportunity for a drug-using woman to give up drugs and become rehabilitated into society. Drug dependence is, however, a chronically relapsing condition and progress is easily disrupted. The motivational forces need to be strong to withstand the challenges presented by a new baby. From earlier chapters we have learned that drug-dependent women tend to come from deprived backgrounds in which they may have been subjected to neglect, abuse and a variety of other stressors that leave them low in self-esteem and prone to anxiety and depression. As their dependence increases they may become detached from the usual support systems of family and stable friendships. Their need for support increases when they become pregnant. The frequency of premature births and NAS among the children creates the potential for additional strain. There is evidence that babies that are premature or have feeding problems are more at risk of neglect and abuse (Browne and Saqi, 1988). A crying child can be perceived as a rejecting child, the rejection is regarded as unnatural and the mother is confirmed in her belief that she is a failure, the tensions increase and their interactions become unrewarding. This is a pattern seen in non-drug-using mothers and is linked to symptoms of anxiety and depression. It is likely that the impact on the drug-using mother is much greater. If she is also without informal support from partner, family or friends she is particularly vulnerable to self-medication at this time with her own form of therapy and may resume using the drugs that have worked for her in the past.

COPING WITH DEMANDS

Adapting

The reality of motherhood is one of multiple roles, high levels of responsibility and long hours of work. Mothers are criticised if they fail in their duties and if they are punished publicly they are stigmatised. The stigma can persist long after the original charges are over and circumstances have changed (Glenn, 1994). We witnessed widespread and convincing evidence of good intent among the respondents about drug control and abstinence during pregnancy. In some women it appeared to be unrealistic given their degree of dependence and their home circumstances.

The return home with a new baby required adaptation to a lifestyle that would need to be different from the one that had existed when she left. Now back in familiar territory replete with drug-related cues, a battle commenced to establish control of consumption and it was one that most of the women eventually lost. Nonetheless, drug use during pregnancy had declined as the women responded to a desire to avoid damage to their children. According to Rosenbaum and Murphy (1987), they would find further adaptation to be slow and full of disappointments.

A losing battle

Between the birth of the child and two or three months later, three-quarters of the women showed changes in the pattern of their drug consumption. Among the opiate users, managing without methadone after the birth of the child was difficult and only achieved by a few women. Seventy-eight per cent ($n = 39$) were being prescribed methadone at the start of their pregnancy and at the end of the study period the number was little reduced at 66 per cent ($n = 33$). There were also changes in the amounts prescribed, with a significant increase over time, the mean value rising from 28.8 ml per day (range 5 to 75 ml) in the last month of pregnancy up to 40 ml (range 10 to 90 ml) after six months. It appears that while slightly fewer women were requiring methadone at this stage, those that did needed higher doses. This could be predicted on the basis of a model that assumed a heightened degree of stress at this time, a state that might previously have been medicated by some with illicit drugs as a matter of course.

There was also a tendency for the use of street drugs to decline, and in some cases stop, during pregnancy, which persisted for the first month after childbirth. A steady climb in the numbers using then occurred. From 54 per cent of women using heroin early in pregnancy this reduced to 22 per cent in the final month then rose to 26 per cent in the first month post-partum and 40 per cent after six months. Eventually all the opiate-dependent women relapsed. The figures for primary amphetamine users were 38 per cent, 12 per cent, 20 per cent and 28 per cent. These trends were highly significant <0.01. There was also an interesting switch during pregnancy by a small number of women who replaced the heroin with amphetamine, believing this to be a safer drug for the foetus. There was a marked curvilinear trend in cannabis use: 94 per cent, 64 per cent, 74 per cent and 86 per cent. The numbers injecting showed the same pattern: 36 per cent, 16 per cent, 18 per cent and 30 per cent. However, some caution is needed in interpreting the severity of these relapses since the quantities consumed of the various illicit drugs were not recorded because of the potential unreliability of the respondents' estimates. Anecdotal evidence strongly suggested that the quantities consumed decreased and remained fairly low for some women during this period, not least because of the expense and the associated diversion of money away from the child. An analysis of a composite variable comprising all illicit drugs illustrates this depressing picture: 94 per cent, 64 per cent, 74 per cent and 86 per cent.

Contributing to success

We need to ask why good intentions ended in failure for so many. A number of variables were found to be associated with reported abstaining from illicit drugs (not including cannabis) after six months. These were: a partner not using hard drugs (<0.001); support from partner and mother (0.006); being prescribed methadone (0.034); a highly supportive partner (0.041); and a partner committing himself to abstinence (0.051). Logistic regression analyses identified high informal support (partner/mother), a methadone prescription and partner's drug use as independent predictors of a woman's abstinence. Of these the most powerful was a non-drug/cannabis-only partner, and abstinence was six times more likely for a woman living with such a partner (0.005). The important role for practical and emotional support during pregnancy that has been revealed in other research (e.g. Cameron *et al.*, 1996; Collins *et al.*, 1993; Cowan and Cowan, 1995), and described in earlier chapters, was shown to be equally important in the early months of the child's life.

Partners' involvement

There is a widespread belief that emotional and practical support should come mainly from the partner, but in fact there is evidence that mothers tend to have fairly low expectations and hence are satisfied with relatively little input (Mauthner, 1995). Six months after the birth, nearly half (48 per cent) of the respondents with partners ($n = 44$) reported that the level of support from them was high and two-thirds (66 per cent) said they were completely satisfied. Those complaining that support was low and not satisfactory were rare. Partners' involvement changed over time with 36 (82 per cent) described as providing both emotional and practical help during pregnancy, 32 (76 per cent) at one month after birth and 43 (95 per cent) six months later. Their involvement was much appreciated by the women:

> He feeds him, he doesn't have to get up in the night cos he [baby] just sleeps right through the night. So he does all the cleaning up an' all that for me, he feeds them for me, he'll see to the kids an' that if I'm seeing to the baby. He does half of everything.

He's better at being a father than the other [previous partner]. He's brilliant with them . . . he gets up and takes them to school, especially when I was first pregnant. I was really sick . . . he was brilliant.

Partner support tended to decrease when the mother returned from hospital but increased again later. It may be important to find ways of encouraging the partners of drug-using women to be involved during pregnancy in planning for parenthood to alert them to the additional strains that may occur in the early months.

Changing relationships

Men's low contribution to household and childcare tasks is regarded as a major factor in the decline in marital satisfaction (Cowan and Cowan, 1992; O'Hara, 1986). However, despite generally good support for these respondents, their relationships with partners were subject to some change. Postnatally, about a third (35 per cent) of the women said the relationship was better, 24 per cent said it was worse, for the rest there was no change.

There were several factors significantly associated with change. The most serious was the woman's reported psychological problems of depression and anxiety, which was associated with deterioration. It is difficult to determine cause and effect here, the problems may have caused the breakdown or been a consequence of it. Other factors were the respondent's injecting of drugs with associated censure by the partner, and contact with the social worker. A rather weaker factor was the baby's health; the healthier the baby the stronger the relationship with the partner.

THE RELATIVE IMPORTANCE OF SUPPORT AND CONTINUING DRUG USE BY THE PARTNER

The causes of a mother's relapse do not seem to be associated wholly or directly with partner support in child rearing and practical help. For drug-using couples there were strong indications that the partner's use of drugs emerged as a critical issue even when his investment in the relationship was maintained. The state of this man had made him incapable of helping at first but he did eventually change, though this was more in terms of increasing involvement, not changing his use of drugs:

So when did that start changing? When I last saw you about six months ago he was still using gear [heroin].

It's been in the last four to five months. It was when I was going into a depression and that and I had a heart to heart with him and told him that he was probably the cause of the depression because I was just stressed out. I don't like to let things get the better of me and I can't go to bed if there's dirty pots and things in the sink. He'd be sat there falling asleep and I'm running about – I was ironing at one and two in the morning trying to get everything ready for the next day, while he's sat there watching the telly, you know it just used to piss me off. But he's really started helping a lot, so that's all right now.

While the intention to abstain was expressed as a firm conviction by most partners in the early days, unfortunately it was not sustained. One man had delegated the responsibility for control of his drugs:

Is he reducing?

He wants to get off it. He wants me to keep hold of it and start reducing him. If he's got it he won't. We both want to get off it . . . we don't want to be like this for the rest of our lives.

None of the drug-using partners of the women succeeded in giving up their illicit drugs completely, though there were modifications made, mostly by reducing the amount, or changing to drugs perceived as less harmful, usually cannabis. Some switched from injecting to oral administration but this was not reliably maintained: 30 per cent of partners were injecting during the woman's pregnancy, this fell to 14 per cent in the first month post-partum but rose again to 26 per cent at third interview. The impact of the partner's failure on the woman was predictable. This woman spoke about her return to street drugs with regret and resignation:

I stay in most of the day and when I do go out it's to me mum's or downtown or whatever. So it's him who goes out and gets it [drug], otherwise I wouldn't really bother. But with it being there in front of me I can't knock it back.

The psychological health of the women was strongly influenced by their partners' support. If the partner was a drug user this was undermined by a failure to change his use of drugs since it affected his capacity to help with chores and with the care of the child. Obtaining street drugs took up time in each day and the expense, in addition to diverting money away from domestic items, usually meant criminal activity. His activities were a constant reminder of what could be a reliable and easy way of easing the strain. Thus the comparative fallibility of the two groups of partners, users and non-users, lay not in their wish to support or even in their efforts to provide that support, but in their priorities. For drug-using partners their dependence was too strong to sustain abstinence for a period longer than a month or so from her returning home.

The partners' use of drugs and the influence this has on the women are not necessarily straightforward. During pregnancy many women expressed doubts about their capacity to avoid street drugs once they had returned home. Relapse is unlikely to have been due solely to the partner's use but due to multiple and complex interactions between factors such as: the demands of the child; confidence in meeting the child's needs; doubts about coping; bouts of depression; a sense of guilt; the partner's struggle to abstain or reduce drugs, and the friction this induced. However, the partner's use of drugs, and the implications this has for the lifestyle they share, is a prime determinant of her ability to avoid relapse.

Familiar drugs are particularly attractive choices for self-medication if known as effective therapy for past problems. Oakley (1992) drew attention to the self-medicating and functional use of nicotine. Cigarettes are not only effective, they are easy to get and legal. An alternative strategy to dealing with problems may not be so easy, quick or reliable. The resumption of previous methadone dose levels can be seen as part of this pattern and as safer and more productive in the context of treatment and the reassurance that this brings.

A ROLE FOR GRANDMOTHERS

Support from the extended family is also important, with a positive relationship with the mother a predictor of maternal well-being in the early months after the birth (Cutrona and Suhr, 1990). Over a quarter (27 per cent) of the respondents had no help from their own mothers early in their child's life. However, half the women saw their mothers regularly and 50 per cent of those reported support from them. This woman's mother regularly cared for her granddaughter:

> I think like with being on the methadone, there are times when I don't feel up to doing things. I might wake up in a morning and I feel rough . . . when I go to me mum's I dress her, I do everything for her, and me mum does the washing. Me mum's just dropped her off now and she's brought a tin of spaghetti for her dinner.

Grandparents were frequently involved in the upbringing of the children, whether formally through fostering or through providing informal support (see Tyler et al., 1997). They are investigated as first choice for the care of children by social services. However, the relationships were not without strain:

> When I had our Jenny I got kicked out of me mam's, an' me mam was trying to get custody of our Jenny. That's what drove me back into drugs because I was all uptight an' that.

Is she with your mum now?

Yeah, just for the time being. As soon as I get off drugs I'm going to get me head together . . . with me an' me mam . . . get it all sorted out an' get me daughter back. Me mam doesn't know I'm on drugs, she's no idea whatsoever. She's no idea that I was taking them at 16. I do wanna come off desperately, not just for my sake, but for me daughter's sake.

The grandmother's ignorance of the daughter's drug use was regarded as a necessity by many women, but it was difficult to sustain the conceal-ment, and meant that the potential for support was not realised. The mother of another respondent was aware of her daughter's history but unaware of her relapse:

Me mum doesn't know that we still dabble, if she did all hell would break loose again. Like me brother still has a smoke and he walks in and she susses him out straight away, and she's shoving him back through the door.

Grandmothers were seen as a valuable resource by those women in regular contact with them. If their help was complemented with that of a supportive partner, the prospects were improved not only for coping with the child but also in avoiding relapse.

FRIENDS

Opiate dependence tends to lead to a form of social isolation that is set in a context of a large network of other drug users, but few friends. Thus, although heroin is often used in the company of associates, the peer group becomes increasingly restricted and mutual trust is rare, reliance upon partners is enhanced as a result. The use of amphetamine is different in that it is a social drug and rarely used alone – it generates high activity, sociability and talkativeness (Klee, 1992, 1997). However, prolonged use gives rise eventually to some paradoxical effects and patterns change – company is no longer sought and the user can become reflective and more isolated (Morgan and Beck, 1997). Excessive use of opiates or stimulants therefore is not conducive to maintaining supportive and trustworthy friends:

Have you got any friends you're close to?

No, not any more. I have a few who come round here like, but you don't have friends when you're on drugs.

Close relationships with friends were comparatively rare, for many of these respondents their partner was their only real friend. Other drug users did not seem to count. As a part of the total system of support to the woman the contribution made by friends may be limited.

The support of other mothers is critically important according to Mauthner (1995) and if the use of drugs cuts women off from other mothers this should be a cause for concern. Most of the women (71 per cent) were in contact with mothers of their own age, but only 24 per cent said that this was important to them. For many of them other relation-ships seemed sufficient. Those with extended families had sisters, for those in treatment there were possible contacts when attending the drug agency. Some mothers simply wanted relief from the constant focus on the child rather than a get-together with mums:

> I know some people go to mother and toddler groups and stuff like that for a break. I can't be bothered . . . all they do is sit there talking about kids. You know 'mine's doing this, mine's doing that'. It's not a break.

SEEKING PROFESSIONAL SUPPORT

Two-thirds (67 per cent) of the women sought professional advice in the early months, mostly about child health and they chose to go to their GP or to the hospital. Most (72 per cent) of the respondents were also in contact with their health visitor at this time. Of those who were in contact, 75 per cent reported good relationships with them.

Thirty-six (72 per cent) of the women had a 'key' worker assigned to them by a drug agency and 46 per cent saw their worker regularly. Seventy per cent of them said their relationships were good or excellent. Only three were in regular contact with a social worker and nine occasionally in contact because of the baby, 29 (62 per cent) reported that they had contact pre-viously as an adult. Of the 12 currently in contact, seven reported good or excellent relationships with them. The women's concerns about social work intervention did not always result in an attempt to conceal their troubles. This woman believed that being open about drugs was the best approach:

> I've told me social worker, the health visitor and the doctors [about her drug use], so you know, if anything did go wrong at least they'd all know. And I'll tell you what – I get more respect off them all now for telling them.
>
> *So the fact that you're using speed isn't a problem?*
>
> No. As long as the kids are all right. They check up just to make sure, I mean me health visitor she doesn't come because she knows

> I can look after the kids and she knows they're okay. But I do get a lot more respect for telling them the truth . . . definitely.

Other women had made the same observation. This woman went further, despite her fears, and demanded help, with some support from her friend:

> It's like if you tell them the truth and you're straight with them they're all right with you. She respected me a lot more as well for asking her for help. Because I phoned her up and I said, 'If I don't get some help then I'm gonna put me kids in care.' Not because I couldn't cope with them.

> You were frightened of telling them weren't you?
>
> (Friend)

> Yeah. I needed to see somebody just to talk to me. I said if I don't I'm gonna end up putting them in care because I felt that guilty. They weren't suffering but I felt so guilty I couldn't cope.

> Now she comes and asks you if you've had anything and you don't have to lie to her.
>
> (Friend)

> It's brilliant.

Support from social workers and health visitors was available to the women but their experiences with them were very variable. Relationships with professionals could be supportive and appreciated, but there was also evidence that traditional fears concerning the removal of children persisted that could lead to deception and concealment. The majority of respondents (88 per cent) felt they had no need of help. More important, two-thirds (66 per cent) would not seek advice from a social worker. The well-established finding that women avoid becoming involved with social workers because their children might be taken into care was confirmed in this study. Multivariate analyses showed, however, that there were certain individuals who were more likely to fear such interventions, for example those with a family environment heavily into drugs, who were using heroin throughout pregnancy, and who were finding it difficult to cope with the baby.

There were many women who were pleasantly surprised at the service they received from a social worker and were keen to dispel their image on their behalf. Qualitative analyses of the experiences of those who had been in contact with them revealed more positive than negative comments. It seems that a bad reputation precedes social workers, and hearsay about specific cases fuels this in drug-using networks. There were several who had benefited from their help and said so:

I've got a social worker, yes, she comes round, she's all right, with me being on the drugs and that. People are under the impression that the social workers will take your kids off you when you take drugs and that's just not true, you've got more chance of it if you're drinking than taking drugs . . . they're all right.

Practical help was much appreciated, particularly in an emergency:

I just see them when I want them . . . I had no milk and no electric so he give me £10 towards some electric, you know, and little things like that. And he said I can smoke cannabis and do what I want so long as the children are all right. He said, 'My sole concern is the children and if I see you spending money' . . . like if there's no food in the cupboard and I'm going buying drugs with the money, he'll step in. And he has a right to do so. He says he just wants to keep an eye on the children to make sure they're all right.

Another woman had caused concern to her health visitor by the severity of her postnatal depression and contact with a social worker had been suggested:

I think they're supersensitive, they've got to be, haven't they? That's what I said to the health visitor before Christmas. She said, 'I can refer you to the doctor or we can get you somebody to talk to.' And I said, 'No, they read too much into it.' If I'd seen them then they could have taken Ben off me, and that was really what was at the back of my mind, . . . I couldn't have coped with that, it would've been a real kick in the teeth. But I think with the way he's [baby] turned out I think I'm not that bad. I am capable of looking after him right.

Another woman had been full of anxiety but similarly was not keen on inviting an interaction:

If I want to see her I just ring and she'll come round and see me. But I've never bothered. You see you have this thing about them don't you? Before I'd ever spoken to one . . . 'they're dead nosy, they wanna take your kids off you' and all that. But when I spoke to her I thought, 'Oh my God, all that for nothing.'

There were several accounts that were positively enthusiastic:

So do you think social workers need to change in any way at all?

Well, like I say, I used to think they were just there to take your kids away, but they weren't. I've seen a couple of social workers since I've grown up and they've both really helped me. One took me to town, she took me all over in the car, she took me to playgroup and everything. She was really great. And the other one phoned up the housing where I was staying, she wrote letters to them and everything, contacted the solicitor. And I didn't know they could do all that, I just thought they were there to take your kids off you. But they were really great.

Respondents were asked if they thought social workers needed to change in some way in order to be more approachable 66 per cent said yes, and those that offered an opinion on the type of change necessary ($n = 19$) mentioned less interference, a less judgemental attitude towards drug users and improved communication with drug and other services.

SUMMARY AND CONCLUSIONS

Heavy and prolonged use of drugs increases the risk of damage to a child, and continued control over drug use would be a vital first step in child protection. Whether opiates or amphetamines, many mothers had been self-medicating by using illicit drugs to treat their problems of depression and anxiety for many years. It seems that this pattern of use was re-established in response to an inability to cope with the arrival of the new baby.

Sustained support from partners and/or mothers was critical to the well-being of the mother. The lack of secure support, according to Rutter and his colleagues (Rutter *et al.*, 1983) makes parents more vulnerable to external stressors, mental health problems and parenting breakdown. For these mothers, the continued use of drugs by the partner was particularly destructive to their hopes of rehabilitation.

The presence of a supportive partner who is a non-drug user or a user who is willing and capable of joining with her in her efforts to abandon the use of illicit drugs seems to be the single most important determinant of a woman's capacity to avoid relapse in this 'window of opportunity'. The absence of such support has to be remedied. The mental health of mothers who are struggling to cope with their child is at risk. Returning to an environment that facilitates a return to previous habits increases the strain and the probability of relapse. Comprehensive, sustained professional help is needed if this is to be avoided and the health and integrity of the family is to be preserved.

REFERENCES

Browne, K. and Saqi, S. (1988) Approaches to screening for child abuse and neglect, in: K. Browne, C. Davies and P. Stratton (eds) *Early Prediction and Prevention of Child Abuse*. Chichester: Wiley.

Cameron, R.P., Wells, J.D. and Hobfoll, S.E. (1996) Stress, social support and coping in pregnancy. *Journal of Health Psychology* 1(2), 195–208.

Collins, N.L., Dunkel-Schetter, C., Lobel, M. and Scrimshaw, S.C. (1993) Social support in pregnancy: psychosocial correlates of birth outcomes and postpartum depression. *Journal of Personality and Social Psychology* 65, 1243–1258.

Cowan, C. and Cowan, P. (1992) *When Partners Become Parents. The Big Life Change for Couples.* New York: Basic Books.

Cowan, C. and Cowan, P. (1995) Interventions to ease the transition to parenthood. *Family Relations* 44(4), 412–423.

Cutrona, C. and Suhr, J. (1990) The transition to parenthood and the importance of social support, in: S. Fisher and C. Cooper (eds) *On the Move: the psychology of change and transition.* Chichester: Wiley.

Glenn, E. (1994) Social construction of mothering: a thematic overview, in: E. Glenn, G. Chang and L. Forcey (eds) *Mothering: ideology, experience and agency.* New York: Routledge.

Klee, H. (1992) A new target in behavioural research: amphetamine misuse. *British Journal of Addiction* 87, 439–446.

Klee, H. (1997) A typology of amphetamine misuse in the United Kingdom. Chapter 3, in: H. Klee (ed.) *Amphetamine Misuse: international perspectives on current trends.* The Netherlands: Harwood Academic Publishers.

Mauthner, N. (1995) Postnatal depression. The significance of social contacts between mothers. *Women's Studies International Forum* 18(3), 311–323.

Morgan, P. and Beck, J. (1997) The legacy and the paradox: hidden contexts of methamphetamine use in the United States. Chapter 7, in: H. Klee (ed.) *Amphetamine Misuse: international perspectives on current trends.* The Netherlands: Harwood Academic Publishers.

Oakley, A. (1992) *Social Support and Motherhood.* Oxford: Blackwell.

O'Hara, M. (1986) Social support, life events and depression during pregnancy and the puerperum. *Archives of General Psychiatry* 42, 801–806.

Rosenbaum, M. and Murphy, S. (1987) Not the picture of health: women on methadone. *Journal of Psychoactive Drugs* 19(2), 217–226.

Rutter, M., Quintin, D. and Liddle, C. (1983) Parenting in two generations: looking backwards and looking forwards, in: N. Madge (ed.) *Families at Risk.* London: Heinemann Educational.

Tyler, R., Howard, J., Espinosa, M. and Doaks, S. (1997) Placement with substance abusing mothers vs placement with other relatives: infant outcomes. *Child Abuse and Neglect* 21(4), 337–349.

Chapter 12

Mothering and drugs

Four case studies

Marcia Jackson

The case studies presented in this chapter were selected from the sample of women who were interviewed as part of the study of drug use and motherhood that was funded by the UK Department of Health. Drug-using women are not a homogeneous group and the variety of lifestyles and circumstances identified in this research illustrate the necessity for services to be flexible when planning for the needs of women seeking help. The choice of cases was difficult. The criteria for choice included the extent of their engagement in the study, which lasted over several years, and the depth of knowledge acquired. This offered opportunities for greater insights into each individual that would be lost with a comparatively superficial coverage of more cases. At the same time an attempt was made to reflect the diversity found across the larger sample. The women who were chosen are very different in a variety of ways but, when combined, the events in their lives illustrate most of the major themes to emerge from this research. The names of the women have been changed to protect their identity.

CASE 1: MANDY

Background

Mandy was 18 years old at the beginning of the study. She and her husband, Jason, lived on a council estate on the outskirts of a small town in the north-west of England. They had been married a year. Mandy spent her formative years in care, and from the age of 10 to 16 was moved from one home to another. Her use of drugs began while she was in care. She had tried a variety of drugs including temazepam (a benzodiazepine), amphetamine and heroin.

Mandy had been physically abused by her stepfather as a child and her parents were now separated. She had little contact with her mother during the pregnancy, a situation which had developed over several years and one which she accepted. This was her first pregnancy, despite having rarely used any contraception, and she and her husband had planned the baby.

However, it seemed to be a surprise when the pregnancy was confirmed and Mandy was now *worried* about how they would manage financially.

Drug use

Mandy was in treatment and had been put on a reducing course of methadone, nitrazepam and diazepam when she became pregnant. She aimed to be drug free by the birth and succeeded in reducing the methadone from 50 ml to 10 ml per day. She felt guilty about the potential effect of her own drug use on the developing foetus and saw the pregnancy as an incentive to address her drug problems. By the birth she was taking no street drugs except cannabis and aimed to abstain from illicit drugs once the baby was born. Her primary concern was to maintain custody of her child:

> *You've not been using any street drugs [during the pregnancy], so do you think that having the baby will keep you from using street drugs?*
>
> I won't touch them again.
>
> *Will it be difficult for you?*
>
> It's hard but if you've got something to do it for, you will, or it'll be taken into care.

Despite her successful efforts at drug reduction, Mandy and her baby remained in hospital for several weeks postnatally while the baby was screened for signs of withdrawal and medicated accordingly. She had hoped to avoid drug withdrawal in the baby and her inability to do so may have adversely affected her efforts at controlling her drug use after the birth. She lost the incentive to reduce her methadone once the baby was born, was diagnosed by her GP as suffering from postnatal depression and, by the time the baby was five months old, her methadone prescription had been increased to 40 ml daily. However, she had stopped taking benzodiazepines and was still free from street drugs, with the exception of cannabis:

> *Was that your decision [to increase the methadone]?*
>
> I would have gone back on heroin if I hadn't.

The partner

Mandy's husband was a supportive father and showed concern for the welfare of the baby. Both of them intended to become drug free in the near future, and Mandy was determined that her child would not end up in care as she had herself. She felt that social workers and other professionals were interested in her solely because of her drug use and was wary of their interventions:

> The social worker came, the family outworker comes, the doctor comes, the drug worker comes, about eight people come, it pisses me off.

What do they come down for?

> To be nosy, I think. They had a meeting after I had him to see if I could keep him and whether he should be put on an at risk register, but he wasn't . . . they had no grounds to put him on it.

Resenting professional 'interference', Mandy found the support of her partner had been important in coping with the early months of motherhood. However, her circumstances changed when the baby was around five months old when her partner was put on remand. She was unsure how long he was likely to be away and was finding single parenthood increasingly difficult. Her depression worsened. When the baby was ten months old she was interviewed, and reported that there was little help offered by any other members of the family or friends:

Has there been anyone to help you out?

> No. His family is just starting to come round now. My mum says, 'don't have none of it', and Jason's saying, 'don't have none of it'. But they're still his grandma and his aunty at the end of the day.

At this time Mandy wanted to maintain regular contact with Jason, not least for the baby's sake, and despite limited finances would visit him in prison every week. However, his absence exacerbated her postnatal depression. Her use of street methadone increased to compensate for a reduction in prescription drugs:

Have you changed your dose of valium?

> I've come down [on valium], but I've gone right up on my methadone. I get prescribed 80 ml a day but really I'm on like 100/150 a day. It's a lot of money extra, it's a lot of methadone as well. I hate it, I just want to get off it.

Mandy did not feel that her increasingly chaotic drug use affected her parenting skills but was desperate for help to control her drug use for fear of inviting an intervention from social services. The child always appeared clean and cared for during interview visits. She had made sure that he had all the necessary health checks and immunisations and had taken advice from a dietician regarding the introduction of solid foods into the baby's diet. She was generally enjoying motherhood and could not foresee any difficulties arising as the baby got older. However, on occasions the drugs visibly affected her ability to concentrate and stay alert. It could be argued that this has implications for childcare. Despite her escalating drug use, she was still determined to maintain custody of her child. As well as concern for the welfare of herself and the baby, Mandy was also worried that her continued drug use would increase the chances of her husband using again when he came home from prison:

> He wants me off it otherwise when he comes out he'll be dabbling in it again.
>
> *So you want to be off it by the time he comes home?*
>
> Yes, but I want to be off it for myself and the baby.

As her drug use became less controlled and single parenthood proved more demanding, Mandy acknowledged that she needed professional support. With the offer of appropriate practical help, her attitude to her social worker began to change:

> They've offered me respite care, a night nurse so I can have a rest. I haven't taken them up on it, but they've offered.
>
> *A lot of people say they don't like social workers.*
>
> Well, I get on with her.

By the time the baby was two and half years old, there had been major changes in Mandy's life. Her trust of social workers continued, and she felt confident to admit to them that she was not coping. Continued chaotic drug use combined with another pregnancy had made life increasingly difficult. She had voluntarily given up custody of her child who had been living with his aunt, Jason's sister, for the past seven months:

> I got really bad on the methadone and I told social services myself that I just couldn't cope with him. So I put him in voluntary . . . so if I wanted him back now I could just go and take him.
>
> *So do you actually get a chance to see him?*
>
> Oh yeah, I see him every morning.

The relationship with her husband, Jason, had also ended. Having been released from a period on remand he continued to commit crime and was subsequently imprisoned. Mandy now had a new partner and at the last visit they had an 11-week-old baby together. It emerged that in the preceding months the relationship with Jason had deteriorated. His support in caring for their child had diminished; he had been drinking and had subjected Mandy to physical violence. His imprisonment helped to accelerate an end to their relationship. She stopped allowing the child to visit his father in prison, and she herself had no contact with him. Although the child was not living with her she still showed considerable concern for his welfare:

> Jason's mum got caught taking gear [heroin] up [to prison]. His mum used to take him [their son] but I've had it stopped now because if she gets caught taking gear up with my son I'll go off my head.

Loss of control

During this period Mandy was taking benzodiazepines and increased amounts of methadone; as a result her tolerance had become very high:

> I can take about 300 ml a day but I'm just like I am now, I just cannot get stoned on it anymore no matter how much I take. Like the other week I took 600 ml to try and get stoned but it didn't get me stoned it just made me go over [overdose].

Her prescribed drugs were stopped some months earlier because she had been caught 'double scripting' (that is, getting more than one GP to supply prescriptions). Now she was pregnant again it was interesting to note the difference in her attitude to her drug use within the two pregnancies. We did not discuss this difference, but it seems likely that her relationship problems, depression and childcare difficulties during the first increased the chances of Mandy self-medicating to help her cope during the second pregnancy. In order to fund this habit she had started shoplifting again. She had been caught, charged and threatened with a custodial sentence. On appeal, she was put on probation because she was eight months pregnant.

Increasing support

Mandy was aware that she had lost control of her drug use and was hoping to stabilise once she had re-established contact with the drug team, something she planned to do the following week after we spoke. She was also well aware that this would be difficult, and was relying on her new partner to take some of the responsibility for childcare while she readjusted. Mandy had also become accepting of the input from social services. Both of her children were registered as 'at risk' and she saw her social worker at least twice a week. This professional relationship had developed over the months and she had come to find reassurance in the contact with him:

Some people have said that when they've got a social worker they worry about them taking the kids away?

Oh, I have worries, yeah. But I know he's trying his best to keep them with me, and I know he's not just saying that to me, I know he is. He does a lot for me. But it's like he said, if he just banged Lee back with me now, he'd be setting me up to fail. He would, because I wouldn't be able to cope.

Mandy found her relationship with her new partner more stable than the previous one and felt she could rely on him for help and support. Although he himself was prescribed methadone he tended not to use it and was keen for Mandy to reduce her drug intake.

They were planning to move to a new address and hoped to have the two-year-old living back with them once they were settled. Her new circumstances had brought about an improvement in the depression she had experienced over the previous months:

it's getting better these last few months.

Has anything changed, I mean, why has it got better?

I think it's better because Jason's gone, and he was making me worse anyway with his drinking, because I was getting leathered [beaten] all the time. Since he's been in prison it's just got better, I suppose.

How do you think you'll manage?

I'll be all right because I've got him now [new partner]. Before I was just on me own.

The relationship with her mother also improved over the study period. Mandy attributed the change in her mother's attitude to a change in her own marital situation since her mother and stepfather had divorced. She was now benefiting from the practical and emotional support that was available from her mother.

Comment

This case study illustrates the importance of a supportive partner and the effects on the woman when such relationships fail. It was all the more important for Mandy as she had little support initially from other members of her family or friends. As with many drug-using women, Mandy found pregnancy an opportunity to address her drug use, but subsequently returned to her established pattern. She had been using drugs from a young age and it could be argued that her deteriorating circumstances induced a reliance on medication as a way of dealing with the stresses of life. Mandy ultimately benefited from professional support but it took some time for a trusting relationship to develop. Indeed, Mandy's circumstances demonstrate how an untrusting relationship with social workers and other professionals can be improved once the value of their support is accepted. It seems that service providers may need to persist in their efforts to reassure drug-using mothers that they really are working to keep the family together.

CASE 2: DIANE

Background

When Diane was first interviewed for the study she was 25 years old, this was her first pregnancy and very much unplanned. Although she had her own flat, she was staying with her mother in the family home. They lived on the outskirts of Manchester in a somewhat isolated area of council housing. It was a stable background and she had a close relationship with her mother and other family members. However, the relationship with the baby's father, Phil, who was also a drug user, was going through a difficult period. They had been together for eight years but had separated some months earlier. The discovery of the pregnancy had led Diane (after some persuasion by her mother) to re-establish contact with him. The drug of choice for both Phil and Diane was and always had been orally administered amphetamine.

Diane had not planned to have children and was over five months pregnant when the pregnancy was discovered. She had been using regular contraception (pill) and, although she occasionally forgot to take the pill, had assumed (with some reassurance from her drug worker) that missed periods could be due to the use of amphetamine:

> I'd missed a couple of periods . . . she [drug worker] said, 'don't worry if your periods aren't regular because it's due to the speed.' So I didn't bother when they weren't . . . but I got this bad stomach ache so I gave her a sample and I was pregnant.

The late discovery of the pregnancy limited Diane's choice as to how to proceed and seemed to affect how she responded to the baby once he was born:

> I didn't know how I'd feel when I had him because I don't like babies. I mean I was buying things but it was like it didn't register, and then when I had him it was a shock. I didn't bother with him for the first day, but I'm all right now.

Diane was fortunate in that she had a very supportive family, particularly her sister and mother. She was very grateful for the sensitive way in which they helped her through the pregnancy and early months of motherhood. She had also been pleasantly surprised at the involvement of the baby's father who gave both emotional and practical help with the child.

Drug use

Since Diane had been unaware of the pregnancy she had carried on taking oral amphetamine daily. Despite her apparent ambivalence to the pregnancy, she made her first conscious effort to limit her consumption once it was confirmed:

> *When you found out did you make any changes to your drug use?*
>
> Yeah, because I didn't know what it would do. I did have the odd one [dose] but it wasn't half as much, you know, it was to sorta like satisfy the craving thing.

A few weeks after the baby was born Diane was finding motherhood extremely difficult. She was relieved initially that she had bonded with the baby but was concerned that her difficulty in coping would result in her rejecting the child. Some of Diane's fear seemed to stem from a need to prove to everyone, including herself, that she could be a good parent. By the time the baby was seven weeks old she was feeling depressed and had started to take amphetamine on a more regular basis. She approached her GP for help and he prescribed Prozac.

Although her sister was giving her advice, Diane said she would have liked more professional help and information regarding the care of the baby in the early weeks. However, the people who would have been appropriate to offer this advice were the very ones in whom Diane felt she could not trust or confide. She had chosen not to discuss her drug use with anyone other than her drug worker and her GP. She had assumed that the staff on the maternity ward would be aware of her history through her hospital notes. Interestingly when she did realise that they did not know about her use of drugs, she chose to keep it to herself because she was worried about how she would then be treated by the staff:

> I didn't realise, I just thought they'd know automatically, you know you go in hospital and they've got your files.
>
> *So you assumed it would be on your records?*
>
> Yeah. But I wasn't gonna tell the midwives anyway, you know I don't think I would've done because I know how funny they're going to be.

A changed lifestyle

Diane was interviewed for the last time when the baby was around eight months old. Her life had changed dramatically. She had moved out of her mother's house and was living alone with her son in a flat after an argument with her mother. Her relationship with the baby's father had also deteriorated. However, she was finding it easier to cope alone than she had anticipated and was finding parenthood increasingly fun, although difficult at times. She was using Prozac and illicit amphetamine to give her more energy and to help her cope with the stress, particularly through persistent periods of colic in the baby.

It is interesting to note that the increase in amphetamine use coincided not only with the baby's disturbed sleep, but also with a breakdown in the relationship with her mother and having to deal with the baby alone. The baby's father was still involved with their son's upbringing, but Diane was becoming unhappy with this. To some extent she blamed him for the increase in her use of amphetamine, since it was he who brought it into the flat.

Despite a clinical diagnosis of depression and periods of chaotic amphetamine use there were no professional concerns about Diane's ability to cope with the child. It was Diane herself who feared rejecting the baby and neglecting his needs. As with Mandy, she did not feel that her drug use per se had any detrimental effects on her son, rather she saw it as a way of dealing with the demands that motherhood imposed. Nonetheless, she felt guilty at using drugs. Despite Diane's initial fears about motherhood and the stresses she faced in the early months of motherhood, by the end of the research period she was identifying many positive aspects to having a child:

> he makes me laugh and that now so it's better and it's easier.

Comment

Although Diane did not find motherhood easy she felt that having the responsibility for her son had helped her to improve her own health and self-care. With the help of her drugs worker she had also begun to take more control over her drug use. Before she had the baby she did not eat or sleep, but she now felt that unless she cared for herself, she would be unable to care for her child. She now put the needs of her child before her own need for drugs. Although she could not foresee a time when she would be drug free, having a child had given her an incentive to think about her future and how she could provide for him. Diane's case demonstrates that continued drug use does not inevitably lead to neglectful parenting; she sought and obtained support from a number of people, both family and professionals, when she felt she needed it. Her use of amphetamine was her way of coping with the day-to-day pressures of motherhood.

There may be differences due to the type of drug used; the energising effects of amphetamine contrasting with the more calming effects of opioids. Her able parenting shows that drug use should not immediately be linked with problematic behaviour that is damaging to the child.

CASE 3: LINDA

Background

Linda was 23 years old at the beginning of the study and was pregnant with her third child. This was her first pregnancy since becoming a drug user, which caused her some concern. Her marriage to the father of her previous children had ended in divorce. She was a recreational ecstasy and intravenous amphetamine user when she became pregnant, living with her children in a two-bedroom council flat.

Linda was not currently in a stable relationship and had not planned this pregnancy. She had considered termination, primarily because she was concerned that her use of drugs in the early months may have harmed the developing foetus. However, she decided that this may be her last chance to have another child and cancelled the appointment for termination.

Drug use

Fairly early in her pregnancy Linda stopped using ecstasy and stopped going to raves. However, her concern regarding the effects of her drug use did not prevent her from increasing the frequency with which she took amphetamine, and also taking cocaine occasionally. This was precipitated by the changed pattern of use. Amphetamine increasingly became part of her normal daily routine rather than used in her social life. She also chose to ignore professional advice to stop injecting the drug because she preferred the immediate effect. She had mixed feelings about the possible effects on the foetus. Linda believed that she had used amphetamine in the past as a way of coping with stress. It is possible that she was finding the reality of a third child difficult to cope with in prospect, although she denied it would affect her lifestyle to any great extent:

Has anyone said there'd be any problems?

No, they said there'd be no side effects to harm the baby . . . but they don't really know until it's born.

After the birth, Linda found that her use of drugs altered in a way she would never have anticipated. She started to take both amphetamine and cocaine intravenously and the additional cost led to crime:

Now I'm getting to the stage where I'm going out stealing, and that's not like me. I've never done anything like that before. I've been to people's houses before and they've left money lying around and it's never bothered me, but this time it did.

Is there any reason you've done this?

Because I needed money for drugs. I was so run down and I wanted some.

Like many drug-using mothers, Linda identified her living circumstances as major contributors to her increased need for drugs. The family was living in a first floor flat with few local facilities for the children. She had applied for rehousing but was becoming disillusioned at the length of time she had to wait. Her growing frustration had a negative effect on her emotional state and illustrates well how the inability to cope with the practicalities of motherhood can be a catalyst for drug use. However, she thought there would be a simple solution:

If I get a house I just won't want to touch the drug, I'll get off it totally.

Loss of control

Linda had begun a new relationship with a man she had known for some years. She described him as both emotionally and practically supportive. She was impressed that he treated the children as his own. Bob was also taking amphetamine, but despite Linda's increasing dependence on the drug, at this stage drugs did not seem to be a major part of their relationship.

When interviewed a third time Linda's baby was 15 months old. The family circumstances had dramatically deteriorated. They were living in temporary accommodation because of a fire in their flat, and Linda and her partner were under investigation for child abuse (the baby had been identified as having a non-accidental injury). All three children had been registered as at risk and put into foster care. Linda had been granted limited supervised access. The allegations were later dropped due to lack of evidence but the children remained registered and subject to regular visits and reviews by social services.

The stress of dealing with the investigation seemed to precipitate further complications. The removal of the children shocked her into action and she had successfully obtained a reducing prescription for dexamphetamine. However, she continued to take street amphetamine, which effectively increased her overall consumption. Her use of illicit drugs meant that her criminal activity continued and led to a deterioration in her relationship with Bob. Disagreement over the sharing of childcare responsibilities and, to a greater extent, the sharing of their drugs and funding activities, created conflict within the relationship which eventually culminated in physical violence.

It is hard to speculate about the direct role of drugs on her parenting skills, but the indirect result of her use, the involvement of social services and the removal of the children to foster care appeared to have had an impact on her relationship with the children. Linda herself felt that the resulting police and social work involvement affected the children more than the witnessing of physical violence:

> like my little girl, every time she sees a police car or a social services van or a council van, she wets her knickers because she thinks the police are coming to take her away or to take me or Bob away. You know she's only four years old and that is distressing.

Surprisingly, Linda maintained that her own drug use had no effect on the children. Perhaps laying blame with the professionals was a way of distancing herself from the idea of personal responsibility.

Steps towards rehabilitation

Linda was interviewed for the final time around a year later. The baby was now two and a half years old. There had been further police and social work involvement regarding the care of the children and they remained registered as at risk. There had been a change in Linda's choice of drug use. She and Bob had both successfully detoxified from amphetamine some months earlier, mostly because Bob had been experiencing severe mental health problems:

> We stopped the amphetamine because they were going to section him . . . he was getting paranoid and was like getting dead protective of me . . . and then he started getting psychotic and we had a lot of problems with social services, you know, that side of it.

It is unclear to what extent Bob's state of mind had affected his relationship with Linda and her children other than Linda's comment that it improved once Bob stopped taking amphetamine. Their amphetamine habit was soon replaced by daily heroin use. Linda's change in attitude is worthy of note, since, when we first met, Linda was very much against heroin. One cannot help but question the influence of Bob on her life. She was impressed with the support she received from him and his self-imposed role as a father, given that none of the children were his. However, until he entered her life it had been comparatively stable, her drug use was controlled and she had never had any criminal involvement. Linda hinted that Bob had been a heavy heroin user before she met him, although she would not be explicit about his past. One must wonder to what extent he influenced her choice of what was effectively self-medication, to cope with the pressures of motherhood.

Linda felt that even though she was still taking drugs, her relationship with her children had improved since she had started taking heroin, which she was now funding from money she earned from work rather than crime:

> I talk to the kids, we have a very close relationship . . . We do communicate, I'm a lot closer to them than I was before, you know I make more time for them now.

What do you think has changed?

> I think rather than running around after drugs and all that, now, you know, I spend most of my time in here with them, I always seem to be with them.

Linda continued to blame the authorities for problems in her life but did little to improve the situation herself. She complained that the children were unnecessarily registered as at risk simply because she had failed to attend meetings where their current assessment could be discussed:

> they reckon because I'm not going to enough appointments and don't seem to be communicating with them they're not quite satisfied about the children . . . they don't see enough of them. They don't see me with the kids so they don't think the children's names should be taken off the list. That's just because of appointments, not of the way I am with them. It's a bit stupid, isn't it? Their names don't need to be on there.

She did not acknowledge the impact that her lack of co-operation may have had on the situation:

> I've got to let them know where I'm going. You've got no privacy at the end of the day when you think about it. They're your children and you've got no say in the matter, it's down to them if you can't come and go.

However, her more recent opinion of her social worker was positive:

> If I have a problem I'll go in and see her in the office. She trusts me a hundred per cent now. I've come a long way.

One possible explanation for these changes could be the depressing effect of heroin. Her personality changed over the later interviews from open and honest disclosures to a closed and monosyllabic style. Furthermore her main concern, that of being rehoused, had still not progressed from our first meeting some three years earlier. This situation continued to have a negative effect and may have added to her feeling of powerlessness to effect a change in her life, resulting in a high degree of inertia.

Comment

Despite her many problems, Linda remained a very proud mother. She enjoyed talking about the children and how well they were progressing and indeed, perhaps paradoxically, the children always appeared to be well cared for and very much loved. The case illustrates how a young mother can progress from recreational, controlled drug use to daily dosing that involves criminal activity. Through a series of stressful life events Linda's drug use changed from being a fun way to socialise to a way of dealing with the increasing pressures of motherhood that started when she was a single mother. Although she had felt that her drug-using lifestyle had not affected the children, by the end of our interviews she admitted that, since her family life had regained what she saw as increased stability, her relationship with the children had improved. Her story demonstrates the rapidity with which involvement with drugs can spiral in and out of control. Linda had received help from drug and social workers but her problems were by no means resolved by the end of the study. She was in need of long-term and sustained support in order to deal not only with drug use, but also the practical issues that users often consider to be more of a problem than drug use itself.

CASE 4: BRENDA

Background

Brenda was 21 years old when she was first interviewed for the study. She had been a difficult child who had played truant from school and was in trouble with the police from an early age. By 13 years she was taking intravenous heroin. Her mother put her into voluntary care when she was 14 when she could no longer control her behaviour. Within two years she was dealing drugs and using heroin and crack cocaine intravenously, interspersed with periods of intravenous amphetamine use. However, Brenda's life had become more stable by the time she became pregnant. She and her partner of a year and a half, Steve, were living in a two-bedroom flat in inner city Liverpool.

Drug use

Brenda had been through drug rehabilitation in the year before becoming pregnant and, although she had recently relapsed, had again taken control of her habit. She was receiving a reducing methadone prescription from the local drug agency. This was her first pregnancy and the baby had been planned. Brenda was very pleased that she was pregnant and was well prepared for the baby's homecoming. Like the great majority of the women in the research sample, she showed concern for the welfare of the developing foetus. She hoped to be drug free by the birth but she was advised not to make any further changes to her drug use through the pregnancy:

> I wanted to come off it by the time I had Joe but they said, 'wait till afterwards now, because it's not safe to come down while you're having a baby.' I was pretty upset about that because I didn't want to be on it while I was carrying.

Once the baby was born Brenda immediately tried to reduce her drug use to the extent that she asked the midwives on the ward to dispense just half her usual daily dose. She soon realised that this was an unrealistic aim, which caused some problems for her during her hospital stay. However, by the time the baby was ten weeks old she had gradually reduced her daily dose of methadone by half. Brenda always appeared a confident parent and the responsibility of caring for the baby increased her determination to become free from hard drugs:

> because I've got Joe now . . . that's another reason why I'd never go back on it. I wouldn't have gone back on it anyway, but because I've got Joe I definitely wouldn't go back on it, not now I've got the baby.

The partner

Brenda's partner, Steve, was very supportive. From the very beginning of the pregnancy he showed great concern for Brenda's welfare. Unusually, they discussed the best way to control their drug use during the pregnancy. He too was on methadone and was also reducing the amount. Steve's support was particularly welcome since Brenda did not have any other close friends.

Unlike the previous case studies, she did not expect to use drugs as a means of coping with her role as a mother:

> *Some people worry that when they've got a child and it's demanding all the time, they worry that they'll be tempted to go out and score [buy drugs].*

> No. Joe makes me want not to go out, I wouldn't leave him . . . I'd never go out and score.

Brenda's mother lived about 30 miles away in Manchester. She was pleased at Brenda's pregnancy, but was unaware that her daughter was currently using drugs. Brenda felt unable to confide in her mother because of this, but did discuss the pregnancy and asked for advice from her on childcare.

Once the baby was born, Brenda and Steve shared in the child's care. Brenda had not anticipated the input Steve would have and while on the whole she appreciated sharing the responsibility, she also felt her role as a mother had been somehow hijacked:

> Before I had Joe I honestly thought that I'd be doing the stuff, but it's not like that. He won't let me do it, he wants to do it. He does all the feeds and that. I don't like that, I want to do it!

By the time the baby was ten months old Brenda was drug free apart from smoking cannabis in the evenings. She had now taken over more of the parenting but found she was becoming bored with her lifestyle. Given her background it would have been very easy for Brenda to choose to return to drugs to help relieve her boredom. She still knew a number of drug users locally and had a bottle of methadone in the flat. Her determination to remain drug free prevented her contacting her old drug-using friends:

> It was just because there was nothing to do during the day and I had no friends and that. I don't want to get involved with anyone who's near drugs and I don't know anyone in Liverpool who doesn't.

Considering her youth, Brenda behaved in a very mature and confident way. Rather than return to her old routine she decided to contact the nearby Family Support Unit to enquire about local activities in which she and Joe could participate. She used the information and made friends with other young, non-drug-using mothers. Brenda did continue to smoke cannabis and had no desire to stop this. She saw it as a means of relaxing:

> I just have a weed [cannabis] of a night time, once he's in bed because that's my time . . . I have a joint then because I know he won't wake up.

She believed that being opiate free had helped her in her role as a mother:

> He wants to play all the time, and now I'm not on methadone I can get up and play with him . . . but then I couldn't.

As well as a supportive partner, Brenda also enjoyed a good relationship with her mother. The child stayed with his grandmother in Manchester over a long weekend every couple of weeks. Steve felt this was excessive, but Brenda felt it was right that her mother had the opportunity to spend time with her grandchild. In view of the complaints from other mothers who felt they needed a break, she did not seem to appreciate how fortunate she was to have an arrangement which gave her and Steve the chance to spend time together.

Brenda's relationship with her mother had evidently improved from her teenage years and it is interesting to note Brenda's attitude to her own upbringing:

So do you think you will bring up Joe in the same way that you were brought up?

In some ways like, but not in others. Like my mum never hit me, an' that's something I'd never do to Joe. I'll just keep him in if he needs to be punished . . . but with school I'm gonna be much stricter than me mam was. I used to say, 'I don't want to go to school today' and she said, 'all right then, go back to bed'. But I'm not going to be like that with Joe, he's going to school and that's it.

The responsible nature with which she approached Joe's future was impressive, particularly given her own early experiences. Her acknowledgement of mistakes she had made in her own adolescence may have reinforced her desire to provide her son with a better opportunity for his future.

Comment

Brenda's case demonstrates how a young and heavily chaotic drug user can rehabilitate. The last time Brenda was interviewed, her mood was very optimistic. She was proud to announce that this was the first time in seven years that she had not been on probation. She and Steve had secured a tenancy on a house in what they described as a good part of the city. They were both drug free (apart from cannabis) and determined to stay that way. Although Brenda had made a relatively successful attempt to become drug free before she became pregnant, the birth of her son increased her determination to lead a drug-free life. She is an example of a woman who was able to take advantage of the pregnancy as a 'window of opportunity' in providing the catalyst for a change in lifestyle, and illustrates the responsibility that women with previously chaotic lives can show in raising their children.

SUMMARY

These four cases illustrate the diversity of issues that present themselves to drug-using mothers. There are the obvious differences such as drug type and mode of administration, and the nature of the informal support available to them, but there are also similarities in the concerns of the women reviewed here. These include the feelings of guilt at using drugs during pregnancy; a desire to do what is best for the child; and the fear of professionals who could separate them from the child.

To varying degrees each woman was the subject of an intervention from professional services. Mandy and Linda had input from a variety of professions. Their initial suspicion and resentment changed over time as the relationship with workers improved and trust developed. Ultimately Mandy came to rely on their help. Coping alone with a young child is very difficult and it is worth noting that it was this situation that motivated her to seek extra support. Linda, although not entirely trusting the help available, realised that there could be practical benefits to social work intervention. Diane chose to have little formal support from her drug worker but was grateful for an understanding GP. Brenda on the other hand sought very little professional help. However, she had a very supportive partner and mother. It is worth noting that for the other three women the relationship with the baby's father had failed, and the support from family was limited.

All four women made changes to their lifestyle for the benefit of their child. Mandy reduced her intake of prescribed and illicit drugs during pregnancy; Diane drastically reduced her intake of amphetamine, even though she had never considered doing so before; Linda chose to stop going to raves and consequently reduced her drug use in the early stages of pregnancy. Her subsequent acceleration in drug taking made her feel guilty and concerned about the effects of drug use on the developing foetus. Brenda sought to change her network of friends because she was concerned that she would be vulnerable to relapse if she resumed contact with her drug-using associates.

By the end of the study each woman had experienced a major life change and was facing a very different future. For Mandy, Diane and Brenda this appeared to be mostly positive. Linda's problems were not over and seemed to be worsening. They had arrived at this point with differing degrees of optimism and perceptions of control and illustrate the variety that can be expected among drug-using women in pregnancy and early motherhood. The cases highlight their need for support at this time and the responsibility of services to respond to this by offering help that takes account of individual circumstances.

Chapter 13

Child protection

Social workers' views

Julian Buchanan and Lee Young

Professionals working in the area of drug use will know that parents experiencing uncontrolled and chaotic drug use can pose potentially serious risks with regard to the safety and/or care of children and standards can fall below what social workers used to call '*adequate parenting*'. However, we would contend that serious 'at risk' situations constitute only a minority of cases overall with the majority of drug-using parents providing – in the wider context of their lives – adequate care for their children. For many of these parents, however, should they be brought to the attention of social services, it is likely that they will face a lottery in terms of how they will be responded to. Research shows (Bates *et al.*, 1999) that this is because social workers (and other professionals) are at best confused about the issue of parental drug use and at worst moralistic and punitive.

This chapter is an attempt to gain some understanding into why many social workers – and other childcare professionals – respond in this way. In doing so, it is hoped that policy and practice might be informed in such a way so as to improve working relationships between parents who use drugs and those professionals charged with safeguarding the welfare of children – particularly social workers. Moreover, it is also hoped that this chapter will act as a challenge to those childcare professionals who hold judgemental attitudes towards such parents.

A recurring theme running through a number of chapters is the fear, mistrust and at times outright condemnation of social workers by drug-using parents. There are, admittedly, a number of positive comments as well, but on the whole service users tend to be overwhelmingly anti-social work, fearing that intervention will inevitably lead to removal of their children. Indeed, research shows that non-drug-using parents are also critical and fearful of contact with social services (Corby *et al.*, 1996). Whilst accepting that it is perhaps unrealistic, given their child protection remit, for social workers to be welcomed, the potentially serious consequences for such parents begs the question – why has this perception become so deeply embedded in the psyche of parents and – in the context of this chapter – parents who use drugs? It is all the more surprising when one considers that social work values promote the ideals of respect, partnership and empowerment. Indeed, qualifying social workers are required to demonstrate their commitment to a practice model based on anti-oppressive and anti-discriminatory values (CCETSW, 1995). What then has gone wrong to cause parents who use illicit drugs such fear and apprehension of social work intervention?

To make sense of social work in the area of child protection, it is necessary to look beyond the confines of the profession itself and the specific issue of drug use and parenting. Indeed, it is necessary to locate social work in the changing social, economic and political context of the late 1970s and 1980s in Britain. This is not to say that social workers were any better thought of and/or received prior to this, but it is unlikely that public or political consciousness (or indeed the profession itself) was so aware of the perceived shortcomings, failures and criticisms of social work as in the period post-1979. One of the consequences of the changing nature of childcare social work since then is that it has become a narrowly focused and defensive activity, highly sensitive and extremely concerned with public and political disapproval. Under siege on many fronts, the profession, in its work with children and families, has been forced to surrender its core values and turn the focus of its attention on surveillance and policing families who are defined in some way as problematic. This chapter will show that this role is not without its tensions and/or conflicts, resulting in confusion and uncertainty for many social workers.

THE IDEOLOGY OF CHILD PROTECTION: FROM 'CARE' TO 'CONTROL'

> The policies and professional practices previously designated as childcare, which formed the basis of the Children's Departments and formed a central plank of the Seebohm reforms of local authority social work in the early 1970s, have not just been redesignated, but have been reconstructed around the axis of child protection.
>
> (Parton, 1991: 203)

Many professions can point to events and/or defining moments that have influenced and shaped their development. This is certainly the case with social work. The profession had barely come together as a unified occupation in the early 1970s, when events impacted profoundly to begin a process that redefined its role, responsibilities and future direction (Clarke, 1993). This is what Parton is referring to when he talks of the 'reconstruction' from childcare to child protection.

The events and defining moments for the social work profession are the many high profile public inquiries (in excess of 40) following the tragic deaths of a number of children at the hands of their parents or step-parents in the 1970s and 1980s (Maria Colwell 1974; Darryn Clarke 1979; Jasmine Beckford 1985; Tyra Henry 1987; Kimberley Carlile 1987; Doreen Ashton 1989). The situation was further compounded by the events surrounding Cleveland, Rochdale and the Orkneys in the late 1980s and early 1990s. Because of the public nature of the inquiries, over more than a 20-year period, these events became a watershed for the social work profession (Corby, 1993). This is not the time or place to examine in detail the short-comings or otherwise of either the child protection system generally or indeed of social work practice in relation to these specific cases. However, an important point that should not be lost from this period of intense public, political and media scrutiny is that:

> The resulting [inquiry report] is something of a view of what happened, and who was to blame – rather than why.
>
> (Cochrane, 1993 in Clarke, 1993: 85)

This quotation, referring to the Beckford Inquiry, encapsulates the public, political and legal response to the death of children under the supervision of social services. The need to apportion blame took precedence over many other important factors. For example, whilst acknowledging the major problems that social workers faced in dealing with the multiple roles with which they were charged, and the limited resources available to undertake this difficult area of work, inquiry reports consistently failed to take these issues into account when making recommendations. Indeed, what is clear is the increasing emphasis towards a more child protection focus:

> rather than indulge in a massive reinvestment of resources, which at the optimum can minimize marginally the risk of injury, fatal or serious, to the child at home . . . society should sanction in high risk cases the removal from home of such children for appreciable time . . . It is on those children who are at risk – but where the risk is problematical – that Social Services should concentrate their efforts.
>
> (Jasmine Beckford Inquiry, 1985: 288–289 in Clarke et al., 1993: 88)

Social workers were consistently criticised as 'naïve', 'gullible', 'incompetent (and negligent)', 'barely trained (and training misguided any way)', and 'powerful, heartless bureaucrats' (Wroe, 1988 referring to the Jasmine Beckford Inquiry, in Parton, 1991: 64) and on the basis of acts of commission or omission, were held responsible for the tragic deaths of a number of children under their supervision:

> The Beckford Inquiry Report argued that the tragedy occurred not because the child abuse system was particularly misplaced or lacking, but because the professionals' attitudes were inappropriate.
>
> (Parton, 1991: 57)

We turn now to examine how social work responded to these critiques of its competency to protect children. In doing so, we begin to make some sense of why drug-using parents might be fearful of coming under the gaze of social services. Drug use in British society is an illegal activity. More than this, for some categories of drug users, particularly women, it transgresses societal norms and becomes both a moral and an illegal activity (Ettore and Riska, 1995). Whatever the nature of their drug use, society defines them as 'problem families' and their children self-evidently in need of protection. In disclosing or having their drug use discovered parents make themselves easy targets for intervention. Moreover, social workers are compelled to intervene as much out of societal expectations and the fear of not being seen to do something, as for any concerns about child protection.

Many professionals will know that drug use does not necessarily equate to harm or neglect of children. However, societal discourse creates its own reality. How then are social workers to make sense of societal expectations about childcare concerns when in the majority of cases there are no such concerns? Drawing on research that examines the operation of child protection systems in Australia and Wales (UK), Thorpe comes to the conclusion that:

> Investigations, judgements, assessments and interventions appear to fit more into the activity [social work], which could be described as the regulation of parenthood, the enforcement of standards and the imposition of norms rather than the protection of children. It is not entirely clear in many cases precisely what 'protection' actually consists of since the focus of the observation and intervention is on parents who are responsible for looking after children and in the case of the very few vulnerable, minimising as far as possible actual and potential environmental hazards. Why do accounts of child protection workers dwell so readily on the moral character of parents, which is used to qualify other observations about actual child rearing practices? It is probably because the category of competent 'parent' carries with it, has embedded within it assumptions about moral character. It is one thing to speak of someone being 'drunk' but quite another to speak of a 'drunken mother' or a 'drunken father'. Even if the drunkenness does not in any obvious way affect the care of children, 'drunken parents' are in some sense worse than 'drunks'.
>
> (Thorpe, 1994: 197)

If as Thorpe argues it is moral character and child rearing practices that are being judged and not any actual 'risk' of harm or neglect to children, it is clear then why drug-using parents (and parents more generally) might feel so threatened by social work intervention. Thorpe continues:

> By presenting information (or misinformation) on allegations and using the word 'abuse' as a decontextualised and highly emotive signifier, the new ideology appears to have succeeded in changing the role of child welfare agencies from predominately one of service provision, to one of policing and 'normalising' [parenting]. It can be construed as a switch from a view of the child in a context where caregivers are encouraged and supported by the state to look after and protect children, to one where the state 'intervenes' to 'protect'. It sees parents not as nurturing and supporting agents whose difficulties and structural disadvantage require compensation, but as potential threats from which children require protection.
>
> (Thorpe, 1994: 199)

This is an important point. The switch from 'service provision' to 'policing and "normalising" [parenting]' acts as the ideological frame of reference for social workers. An 'ideology of child protection' will inform not only observations and interpretations of events, which can be crucial in determining outcomes, but will also frame the workers' perceptions of themselves, their role and responsibilities. If the social work role is perceived only in terms of child protection, how meaningful are the concepts of working in partnership with families to achieve this end? What support systems can or will be provided to enable parents to meet required standards? Indeed can socially and economically excluded families ever hope to meet such standards? If as Thorpe states this ideology is about policing and normalising parenting, can a parent who uses illicit drugs ever be considered acceptable as a parent? How does the concept of 'Care' fit with societal expectations of 'Control' of problem families? These questions raise significant dilemmas for social work as a profession.

Another important consequence of the 'ideology of child protection', is that drug-using parents will come into contact with social workers only at times of crises in their lives or at the point of investigation and/or assessment about childcare concerns. This acts to confirm and perpetuate the idea that social workers are not an agency to turn to when requiring support or assistance during times of difficulty. In spite of the multi-agency and multi-disciplinary nature of decision making in child protection cases, for parents who use drugs, social workers more than anything else represent the *public face of child protection*, to be avoided if at all possible. Moreover, social services and social workers have done little if anything to dispel this perception with many workers fully engaging with the ideology of child protection and actually referring to themselves not as social workers but '*child protection workers*'. This shift in ideology cannot be overemphasised in that it frames a worker's understanding, approach and, most importantly, response to parental drug use.

THE RESTRUCTURING OF THE WELFARE STATE AND ITS IMPACT ON SOCIAL WORK

The discussion so far has provided some context of the situation in which social work found itself during the late 1970s and 1980s. A lack of public confidence left the profession wounded and lacking in confidence. As a consequence of this the profession was pushed into adopting an ideology of child protection, becoming more of an agency of 'control' than 'care'. However, this is not the whole story with another and equally significant and defining moment for the profession – the election of the Conservative Party in 1979. One of the major planks of Tory social policy was a commitment to 'reform' the welfare state. The rhetoric used to legitimise the reforms was that the state could no longer afford the increasing costs of the so-called burgeoning welfare budget. The extent, success or otherwise of the reforms have been widely debated (Hutton, 1996; Marsh and Rhodes, 1992; Report of the Commission for Social Justice, 1994; Savage and Robins, 1990) with little consensus being reached between protagonists. However, what is clear is that the Conservative Government, led by Margaret Thatcher, had a clear ideological agenda that was intent on sweeping away the collectivist ideals of the welfare state. The vision for the future was one of individual choice and responsibility free from an overpowering and interfering 'nanny state' (Thatcher, 1993).

One of the main targets for change was reform of welfare benefits. It was claimed that welfare – particularly benefits – undermined the will of benefit recipients to take responsibility for themselves and their families. Indeed, some commentators held the welfare state responsible for the creation of an 'underclass' (Dennis, 1997; Murray, 1996). Social problems were blamed on an overgenerous benefits system acting as a disincentive for people to look for work. The way to resolve the problem, it was argued, was to tighten eligibility thresholds and reduce benefit rates. Legitimacy for such measures was gained through the construction of the stereotypical benefits claimant – work shy, scrounger, dishonest.

This is the social, economic and political context in which many young people found themselves in the mid-1980s (Buchanan and Young, 1995). Manufacturing in the major industrial conurbations had collapsed with 1.7 million jobs lost in manufacturing industry between June 1979 and January 1981 (Jackson, 1993 in Marsh and Rhodes, 1992: 16). Unemployment reached post-war records and averaged 2.7 million throughout the

1980s (Report of the Commission for Social Justice, 1994: 34). Levels of poverty also rocketed in the period post-1979 (Hills, 1995) with many working-class communities experiencing harsh social and economic conditions not of their making.

One of the major social problems resulting from these high levels of unemployment and poverty during the 1980s was widespread drug addiction. And although the concept did not exist in the mid-1980s, a whole generation was being subjected to a process of social and economic exclusion. The Commission on Social Justice commented:

> The most disturbing evidence of social disintegration is the rise in drug addiction and drug-related crime. The number of deaths from solvent abuse increased at least four fold during the 1980s, while the number of notified new addicts in 1993 was five times higher than in 1981 and fourteen higher than in 1973.
>
> (Ibid.: 50)

Many young people, families and poor communities suffered severe social and economic hardship. What part did social work play throughout this period of intense social and economic change? Unfortunately at a time when the social work profession might have been expected to have provided some ameliorating services or at least been advocating on behalf of communities under stress, it was unable to respond in any positive way. Social work – already under attack for its apparent failure to protect children – found itself, along with the trade union movement and local authorities, being held responsible for the creation of the so-called 'culture of dependency' that was said to be responsible for the social and economic ills of the United Kingdom (Seldon, 1982: 8).

In the new mixed economy of welfare, social workers and others of their ilk were seen to be part of the problem with few supporters. As part of the wider reconstruction of the welfare state, social work also underwent considerable reconstruction losing much of its professional autonomy. The Children Act 1989 and the NHS and Community Care Act 1990 created new frameworks for practice in which social workers would work more closely with health professionals, the police and legal services. Their new role was more clearly and closely proscribed. The fragile nature of the profession at this time can be seen in the words of John Patten, the then Minister of State at the Home Office:

> Is it really necessary for some of our big cities to have approaching 10,000 or so social work and related staff on their pay role? Are such large groups of people appropriate, any more than it is for one local authority to own vast holdings of council houses and flats?
>
> (*The Times*, 3 January 1991)

Implicit in this statement is not just a question about the organisation and role of social services departments, but also a question about the future of social work itself.

This then was the social, economic and political context in the post-1979 period. A profession under siege, used as a political scapegoat for social ills and a failed profession based around outdated collectivist ideals. Unlike the teaching profession, which found some public and political support in its resistance to central government initiatives, social work was unable to defend its humanistic values in the face of wider social acceptance of self-interest and raw individualism. No longer able to advocate on behalf of the poor and dispossessed, social workers in the area of childcare were remodelled into child protection workers.

Within this context, parents who used drugs could expect little support from social services. Any pretensions to preventative social work were long gone, replaced by an ideology of child protection. The primary role of social workers in the restructured welfare state was to carry out surveillance on problem families. Moreover, in adopting an ideology of child protection with regard to *all* families where drugs are used, social workers succeed only in alienating already fearful parents. The likely outcome of this scenario was not a more, but a less effective model of protection. This assessment is based on the premise that, the most effective model of protection is through working with and supporting parents. Ultimately it is not social workers that protect children but their parents and carers.

CHILD PROTECTION: SOCIAL WORKERS' VIEWS

Although the '1989 Children Act' and the '1991 Working Together' guidelines promote a multi-disciplinary and multi-agency response to child protection concerns and decision making, social workers still represent the *public face of child protection.* Indeed, on the basis of our own experience as practitioners, we would argue that this is not only the case for the public at large but also other childcare professionals who look to social services as the lead agency in child protection. This places social workers in a very powerful position at the very centre of the child protection system. However, this also means that they carry a disproportionate degree of responsibility vis-à-vis other childcare professionals, and are likely to be held publicly and politically accountable if things should go wrong.

Because of issues surrounding confidentiality, social workers rarely have an opportunity to respond to criticisms of their practice and/or the operation/effectiveness of the child protection system more generally.

This section now draws on empirical material taken from a study that set out systematically to explore, compare and contrast the attitudes, values and practices that exist between some of the main agencies that are involved with drug-using parents and their children (Bates *et al.*, 1999). The three groups of professionals – social workers, health visitors and drug workers – were chosen because they represent key workers in the child protection system. It is the professional judgements of these workers that heavily influence the decision-making process and 'outcomes' for parents who use drugs. Views of professional workers with regard to drug use more generally have been discussed earlier (Chapter 10); however, in this section the intention is to focus attention specifically on the views of social workers.

What this section will show more than anything else are the tensions that exist for social workers. Public and political discourse has been for social work to move towards an ideology of child protection. Some workers have embraced this role and see no conflict between the professional values of social work and this explicitly controlling function. However, the situation is not as clear-cut for all social workers. Mindful of societal and political expectations, they continually find themselves having to balance rights and responsibilities with regard to their mandate to protect children. A selection of data from the study will show how complex these dilemmas can be.

Child protection registration

The majority of social workers in the study questioned the effectiveness of child protection registration as a means of protecting children, with some feeling that the decision to register a child was more about protecting the professionals involved than the children. Indeed, some workers were also concerned about the infringement of parental rights simply because of a parent being a drug user. These thoughts and feelings are illustrated in the following comments:

> Registration does not prevent risk. Only removal of children would do this. Registration is a waste of time.

> The child protection register only protects the professionals.

> I sometimes question the use of the register because I am not sure how much having a child's name on the register actually protects a child . . . I do not see how you can anticipate every risk.

The responses of this sample of social workers raises serious questions about the use of the child protection register and whether it contributes anything towards actually protecting children. Implicit within the responses is the issue of how registration is perceived by professionals, that is, whether registration is understood as the beginning of a process of child protection or indeed the end of the process. Research undertaken by Corby and colleagues (1996) shows that, for many professionals, child protection registration constitutes the culmination and end of the process with very little else happening following the decision to register. These responses support the arguments discussed earlier (Parton, 1991; Thorpe, 1994) that child protection might not actually be about child protection at all but more about 'normalising' parental behaviour.

It is interesting to note that within all three professional groups only a very small minority was in favour of a policy of blanket registration for all children of drug-using parents. However, whether this positive attitude is translated into practice remains questionable.

Issues of confidentiality

The issue of confidentiality has always proved a difficult area for professionals in the social care field and never more so than in the area of drug use and parenting. In addition, there are of course legal considerations, which only further compound the problem of information sharing. Within the study, the inherent difficulty of information sharing across agencies was a major area of concern expressed by a number of professionals. Asked whether there are times when information is ever withheld from other agencies, the comments of this social worker make explicit the tensions faced by workers not wanting to stigmatise or disadvantage either children or parents:

> Sometimes [information is withheld from] health visitors and schools. It is hard to say what is collusion and what is not. There have been times when I have been working with families [who use drugs] and have made particular note not to tell the school. I have waited for the school to feed back to me any concerns they have before informing them. I am pretty sure that had I initially said that these parents use drugs their response would be different.

This is a clear example of a social worker taking risks in withholding information. Should anything go wrong, there is no defence for the worker in claiming they are protecting parental rights to privacy. This is an example of the conflict that exists between the requirements of the child protection system and the workers faced with having to do the job.

Parental drug use

Social workers were asked whether some agencies adopt a heightened sense of concern about childcare issues when they become aware of parental drug use. All social workers and drug workers felt this to be the case either always or sometimes, with the majority of health visitors agreeing that this was the case. Health visitors and, to a lesser extent, teachers featured significantly in response to this question:

Yes, health visitors are anxious. It would be helpful to share these concerns and anxieties. They get anxious because it is illegal and want to check with other agencies because they are not sure whether to report it. It is as much to do with the anxiety of the professionals as it is drug use.

Yes, the medical profession – GPs, hospital staff and health visitors in particular. They have a set model of what good parenting is supposed to be and this is divorced from the real world, in which we live and work.

The responses to this question raise some important issues vis-à-vis drug-using parents and childcare professionals. The idea of a model of normative parenting is raised once more. The responses also indicate that social workers feel themselves to be more 'grounded' in relation to issues of illegality, models of parenting and drug use. This view is challenged, however, by both health visitors and drug workers:

Social workers – they are laid back about it [drug use and parenting]
(Health visitor)

Some agencies overreact – it causes a lot of problems. Drug-using parents feel everyone is against them and social workers are scared of the repercussions.

(Drug worker)

The notion that professionals have a different perception of what constitutes social reality (Howe, 1992) gives some indication of why practice both within, and across, professional groups can be so variable. This raises serious questions with regard to the idea that all that is required to prevent 'bad' practice is multi-agency training. This issue will be discussed further in the recommendations section of the chapter.

Inter-agency 'working together'

A small number of professionals felt that inter-agency working was improving. However, the majority amongst all three groups expressed significant levels of dissatisfaction. Moreover, responses to this question, more than any other, showed the extent of the differences in perspective held between – and within – professional groups about parental drug use and the child protection system more generally. The comments of this social worker show rich insights into the problems associated with inter-agency working:

It needs improving. There is a façade that we are working together but in reality everyone is doing their own thing. It is about professional values and protecting your own back. Different professions view drug use differently with most condemning it. This makes working together difficult. Some joint training would help bring down these barriers but only to a certain extent. If individuals think drug use is wrong then there is always room for conflict.

Many drug workers felt ambivalent about the involvement with other agencies with several expressing concerns about individual workers:

It depends upon the individual worker. Some are prejudicial against drug users.

Of the health visitors that felt inter-agency working was poor, one commented that:

No one seems to understand each other's role. There's a long way to go.

The issue of inter-agency working appears problematic and not to be working effectively for many of the professionals questioned. This is in spite of more than 20 years of policies consistently emphasising the importance of working together to safeguard the welfare of children. Of concern also is the issue that problems are not solely confined to difficult working relationships between agencies. Indeed, there are also serious critiques of the attitudes held by some workers within the same agency.
    This is clearly demonstrated in the following comments by social workers:

Yes, it's a dependency. Their [parent's] needs will come before the child's needs every time.

Yes, because of their lifestyle. Drug use prevents a normal existence for the children.

On the other hand, some social workers seem more attuned to the wider social and economic context within which the majority of drug-using parents live:

It depends on their resources to an extent. The drug use combined with poverty that we have [in the area] tend to cause problems. A lot of their money goes on drugs. If they had a good job and reasonable income they could afford to spend a certain amount on their drugs, and it may not present in the same way. It does not mean that they are bad at looking after their children but that money is in short supply.

To conclude this section, it is refreshing to note that only a small minority of professionals from all three groups supported a blanket policy of child protection registration for children of drug-using parents. However, that aside, what this section shows more than anything else is a serious lack of working together not only between agencies but also surprisingly within agencies. The beginning of this chapter referred to the 'lottery' that drug-using parents are subject to when brought to the attention of social services. Some of the reasons for this appear to be because there is little agreement between or indeed within professions about the acceptance of drug use per se. Some professionals are concerned about the illegality of the issue; others take a moral stance on the basis that drug use is simply not acceptable in any circumstances. A number of professionals, on the other hand, see controlled drug use as relatively unproblematic. A confused and seriously worrying state indeed.

CONCLUSION

The main aim of this chapter was to address the question of why drug-using parents are so fearful of social work intervention. Whilst appreciating the obvious point that social workers represent the public face of child protection, the question still remains of why an agency with values so firmly embedded in anti-discriminatory practice should be so over-whelmingly feared. Moreover, this is not simply an academic question but one that raises fundamental issues with regard to social work practice.

It has been shown how the social work profession has been subject to a prolonged onslaught of public and political criticism resulting in the profession adopting a defensive strategy in order to adapt and survive in a hostile political environment. This has meant that at a structural level the profession has been reconstructed around an ideology of child protection. Thus social work has been forced to compromise its core values as an agency of care and become focused on control. It has been argued that the issue of child protection is the Trojan horse that legitimises intervention into private family lives and unacceptable models of parenting. On another level of analysis, however, it can be seen how many social workers, whilst required to operate within this context, struggle to balance the rights and responsibilities of drug-using parents. Their role is an unenviable and thankless task with little support and/or acknowledgement of the very real tensions and dilemmas inherent within such complex areas of work.

Having surveyed the recent history of social work one final but crucial question remains: can anything be done to improve the situation? Many writers have argued that it is indeed possible to work more constructively with parents (Bates et al., 1999; Cannan and Warren, 1997; Corby et al., 1996; Klee and Jackson, 1998; Klee et al., 1998; Mounteney and Shapiro, 1997; Parton, 1997; Parton, et al., 1997; Taylor, 1993). Ultimately, however, the basis on which any improvement is founded is to work with parents, not against them. Parents who use drugs can be defensive, hostile and secretive but given the attitude of many professionals and society generally, this is only to be expected. Social workers, moreover, must be prepared to resist the structural pressures to collude in an ideology of child protection.

The following recommendations drawn from the study by Bates and colleagues (1999) represent a number of tangible actions that can go some way towards improving responses to parental drug use and child protection concerns. They are not meant to be exhaustive – more the beginning of a process. Moreover, they are not confined only to social work professionals but involve all workers in the childcare/protection/parental drug use field.

RECOMMENDATIONS

Training

It is clear that this is an important issue that needs addressing urgently. It is also clear that all professionals involved in the field of drug use and childcare/protection should be involved together in such training. There is a caveat to this, however. Understanding of different roles and responsibilities will not come simply from multi-agency and multi-disciplinary training. Working relationships may be significantly improved from such a process and this is to be welcomed. However, there are fundamental differences between professional groups in terms of theoretical perspective. What we mean by this is that different professional groups hold fundamentally different views about people, the nature of social problems and how they might be resolved (Howe, 1992). These are quite profound issues that basic training in itself will not address.

Area Child Protection Committees (ACPCs)[1]

No agreement exists between workers about whether it is possible to provide adequate parenting when using drugs. There is a need then for a clear statement on the part of the ACPC about professional attitudes towards parental drug use and childcare. Clearer policy and practice guidelines, that is, inter-agency protocols, are required to develop greater consistency between agencies. This is no easy task, given the illegal nature of the activity, but without such policy, workers are lacking in confidence and the variability of response is unacceptable.

The views of parents

Whilst the views of parents are not the sole criteria for organising and developing services and/or professional practice, they do nevertheless raise important issues for intervention. Their views should be further researched and utilised to inform inter-agency training.

Resources

The issue of ensuring adequate and appropriate resources are available to support parents where drug use is a concern that should not be overlooked, especially the need for day care and nursery provision for young babies and children. Too many workers and families see the child protection system as a gateway to such services. This is clearly wrong.

Specialist inter-agency teams

ACPCs should consider seconding staff to form specialist inter-agency teams to improve expertise, consistency and overall standards of practice. Such teams could be used to develop inter-professional policy and best practice in respect of working effectively with drug-using parents and their children. Such teams could do much to challenge and improve inter-agency understanding and co-operation.

Finally, it is with some optimism that we conclude this chapter. Recent publications from the Department of Health: *Working Together to Support Children: New Government Guidance on Inter-Agency Co-operation* (1999), and the consultation document, *Framework For The Assessment Of Children In Need And Their Families* (1999), indicate a shift in political thinking towards the concept of children and families in 'need'. If this is indeed the case, then social work will find itself once more providing services on a proactive and preventative basis. If this is the case, it is good news for both the profession and – more importantly – parents who use drugs.

REFERENCES

Bates, T., Buchanan, J., Corby, B. and Young, L. (1999) *Drug Use Parenting and Child Protection: towards an effective interagency response*. University of Central Lancashire.

Buchanan, J. and Young, L. (1995) *Drugs Relapse Prevention: giving users a voice*. Bootle Maritime City Challenge.

Cannan, C. and Warren, C. (1997) *Social Action with Children and Families*. London: Routledge.

Central Council for Education and Training in Social Work (1995) *The Rules and Requirements for the Diploma in Social Work*. London: CCETSW.

Clarke, J. (ed.) (1993) *A Crisis in Care? Challenges to Social Work*. London: Sage.

Corby, B. (1993) *Child Abuse: towards a knowledge base*. Buckingham, UK: Open University Press.

Corby, B., Millar, M. and Young, L. (1996) Parental participation in child protection work: rethinking the rhetoric. *British Journal of Social Work* 26, 475–492.

Dennis, N. (1997) *The Invention of Permanent Poverty*. London: Institute of Economic Affairs.

Ettorre, E. and Riska, E. (1995) *Gendered Moods: psychotropics and society*. London: Macmillan.

Hills, J. (1995) *Joseph Rowntree Foundation Inquiry into Income and Wealth, vol. 2*. York: Joseph Rowntree Foundation.

Howe, D. (1992) *An Introduction to Social Work* (2nd edition). Aldershot, UK: Arena.

Hutton, W. (1996) *The State We're In*. London: Vintage.

Klee, H. and Jackson, M. (1998) *Illicit Drug Use, Pregnancy and Early Motherhood*. Manchester Metropolitan University, UK: SRHSA.

Klee, H., Wright, S. and Rothwell, J. (1998) *Drug Using Parents and Their Children: risk and protective factors*. Manchester Metropolitan University, UK: SRHSA.

Marsh, D. and Rhodes, R.A.W. (eds) (1992) *Implementing Thatcherite Policies: an audit of an era*. Buckingham, UK: Open University Press.

Mounteney, J. and Shapiro, H. (1997) *Drugs, Children and Families*. Birmingham: Venture Press.

Murray, C. (1996) *Charles Murray and the Underclass: the developing debate*. London: Institute of Economic Affairs.

Parton, N. (1991) *Governing The Family: childcare, child protection and the state*. London: Macmillan.

Parton, N. (ed.) (1997) *Child Protection and Family Support: tensions, contradictions and possibilities*. London: Routledge.

Parton, N., Thorpe, D. and Wattam, C. (1997) *Child Protection, Risk and the Moral Order*. London: Macmillan.

Report of the Commission for Social Justice (1994) *Social Justice: Strategies for National Renewal*. Institute for Public Policy Research, London: Vintage Press.

Savage, S. and Robbins, L. (eds) (1990) *Public Policy Under Thatcher*. London: Macmillan.

Seldon, A. (1982) 'Introduction', in: H. Parker (ed.) *The Moral Hazard of Social Insurance*. Research Monograph 37, London: Institute for Economic Affairs.

Taylor, A. (1993) *Women Drugs Users: an ethnography of a female injecting community*. Oxford: Clarendon Press.

Thatcher, M. (1993) *Margaret Thatcher: the Downing Street years*. London: Harper Collins.

Thorpe, D. (1994) *Evaluating Child Protection*. Buckingham, UK: Open University Press.

Part IV

Service delivery and development

The whole of this part is devoted to contributions from health professionals working with pregnant drug users. The main issue of concern to the opioid-using respondents in our research was the effects of the substitute drug methadone on the foetus and the predictability of the baby withdrawing (the Neonatal Abstinence Syndrome: NAS). This was the driving force behind their efforts to control their use of drugs during pregnancy. The part opens with an account of the NAS by Stephen Walkinshaw, a consultant in maternal and foetal medicine, Benjamin Shaw, a neonatologist and Catherine Siney, a drugs liaison midwife. Most maternity services in the UK are currently examining their procedures and practices with respect to drug use and attempting to improve them. These authors are key members of a Pregnancy Support Group for drug-using women. This group provides the framework within which the Specialist Drug Service in Liverpool works. It is an innovative model based in a drug dependency clinic and is the subject of the next chapter written by Susan Ruben, the consultant psychiatrist in charge of that clinic, and the specialist health visitor, Frances Fitzgerald.

Subsequently, Faye Macrory gives an account of the development of the service she provides in Manchester, from the conceptualisation of the idea to the eventual delivery of the service. Mary Hepburn, an obstetrician and gynaecologist internationally known for her pioneering work among socially deprived women in Glasgow, ends the section by describing the model that has been so influential in the UK and abroad.

The chapters in this part illustrate the ways that services can respond to their patients' needs, for guidance and reassurance as well as appropriate health care. The hard work involved in developing these models does not come across in these accounts. The initial organisation of such enterprises has required many months, if not years, of networking, fund seeking and struggling with intransigent bureaucratic procedures. On the back of this work will rise other variations to be used to meet the challenge of caring for pregnant drug users in other regions. It is a privilege for us to have their contributions.

Chapter 14

Neonatal Abstinence Syndrome

Stephen Walkinshaw, Benjamin Shaw and Catherine Siney

Opiate dependency carries many adverse effects in pregnancy, though many may be related to the confounding social variables (Siney *et al.*, 1995). The one constant and specific problem of concern to pregnant women dependent on opiates or other drugs is that of drug withdrawal in their babies.

The majority of opiate-dependent women in the Liverpool area are entered in methadone replacement programmes within specific pregnancy drug clinics (Siney *et al.*, 1995) and attempts are made to reduce both polydrug use and total opiate dose using a stepwise approach in the second and early third trimester (Medical Working Group on Drug Dependence, 1992).

Neonatal Abstinence Syndrome (NAS) is common though dependent on definition. Up to 80 per cent of pregnancies have been claimed to have this complication for both heroin and methadone (Kandall *et al.*, 1977) although rates of 40 per cent for heroin and 60 per cent for methadone have been reported (Bell and Lau, 1995). Severe withdrawal, requiring treatment, is less common, with half to three-quarters of infants showing signs of abstinence needing an intervention treatment (Fulroth *et al.*, 1989; Kandall *et al.*, 1977; Madden *et al.*, 1977). The incidence of NAS may be less in those infants whose mothers have smoked heroin (Gregg *et al.*, 1988).

Pregnancy may be a driving force in encouraging women to reduce their drug use (see Chapters 6 and 11), and a potent tool in this struggle would be the knowledge that reduction in drug use would directly help the baby. One of the commonest questions asked by new patients is, if they can reduce their methadone or heroin, will it stop the baby withdrawing? Because of this, there has been long-standing interest among health professionals and researchers in predicting neonatal opiate withdrawal, in addition to its recognition and treatment.

PREDICTION OF NEONATAL OPIATE WITHDRAWAL

Measurement

The two most commonly used outcome measures for prediction of withdrawal are the neonatal abstinence score of Finnegan (Finnegan *et al.*, 1975), and the need for therapy in the neonatal period. A number of factors have been considered as antenatal predictors. These include: the main drug used; other drugs used; duration of drug use; dose prescribed; gestation at delivery; size of infant; timing of last dose; labour; delivery; and analgesia in labour.

The earliest work suggested that doses of methadone less than 20 mg per day were associated with either no symptoms or mild symptoms (Ostrea *et al.*, 1976; Ramer and Lodge, 1975) and that polydrug combinations were linked with the most severe withdrawal. Strauss and colleagues (Strauss *et al.*, 1976) showed that infants of mothers on the higher doses were more likely to have symptoms of withdrawal, more likely to have severe symptoms and more likely to have these symptoms longer. This was particularly true of tremulousness (shakiness) and hypertonicity (stiffness). As a consequence the higher dose group were twice as likely to need treatment. However, the findings were confounded by a higher rate of polydrug use in the higher dose group. In a detailed analysis of a small group of 'pure' opiate users, Harper and colleagues (Harper *et al.*, 1977) found a relationship between total dose in final 12 weeks of pregnancy and daily dose and severity of withdrawal. Again there was a twofold likelihood of the need for treatment.

Other early workers were unable to confirm a dosage phenomenon (Blinick *et al.*, 1975; Kandall *et al.*, 1977). Although more recent studies have tended to confirm a dosage relationship, they have found this relationship to be weaker (Doberczak *et al.*, 1991; Mayes and Carroll, 1996). Others have challenged arbitrary divisions on dosage (Brown *et al.*, 1998) emphasising that severe withdrawal can occur with very low doses (Kempley, 1995). In local studies using self-reporting of drug use, a twofold difference in severe symptoms was confirmed between those on less or greater than 20 mg (Shaw and McIvor, 1994).

Polydrug use

The most complex and difficult task is in determining the effects of other drugs, largely other opiates, cocaine and benzodiazepines. In population screening, about one-third of drug screen positives had more than one drug detected (Ostrea *et al.*, 1992). For opiate use, only one-third of patients used the prescribed opiate alone, compared with half for cocaine use.

In Ramer and Lodge's early work (Ramer and Lodge, 1975), the six worst scores were in infants born to women on both methadone and heroin. However, others could find no difference in the proportion of infants with abstinence, its time of onset, duration or severity between women on methadone alone and those taking both methadone and heroin. This lack of a difference has been confirmed by several researchers (Doberczak et al., 1991; Doberczak et al., 1993).

Cocaine use is common in women receiving prescribed methadone or heroin (Brown et al., 1998). Combined use has been said to worsen neonatal abstinence (Fulroth et al., 1989). These workers found that almost two-thirds of infants born to women on either drug alone had Finnegan scores less than 9, but where both drugs were used, only one-fifth had low scores. As a consequence both the need for treatment and the duration of treatment were substantially increased. Using a different scoring system (Brazelton) Chasnoff (Chasnoff et al., 1985) also showed differences in the combined drug group. Doberczak, however, could find no difference either in mean score or need for treatment between infants born to mothers using methadone alone or methadone and cocaine (Doberczak et al., 1991). In a recent study (Mayes and Carroll, 1996), the only difference found was an increase in the first neonatal abstinence score after delivery. No differences were found in the maximum score, or in treatment. Our own local data supports a view that polydrug use has less effect on neonatal abstinence than predicted, and that knowledge of such use is not particularly valuable in predicting the neonatal outcome (McCarthy et al., 1999).

Other factors

Obstetric factors may also influence neonatal abstinence symptoms. Infants who are small for gestational age may be more likely to have withdrawal symptoms (Wagner et al., 1998). It has been suggested that infants less than 35 weeks gestation may be at less risk (American Academy of Pediatrics Committee on Drugs, 1998). This could be as a consequence of neurological immaturity or reduced drug exposure. However, most scoring systems have been developed for term infants, and it is equally possible that the screening tool is not appropriate. Certainly, mean scores were reduced in one study (Doberczak et al., 1991) and severe clinical symptoms including seizures were rare in the preterm.

It is clear that there are substantial difficulties in predicting neonatal abstinence in the antenatal period. There may be a dose effect, but this is not as clear-cut as one would like to allow directive counselling of patients. Similarly it is uncertain if additional use of cocaine increases the risk. At present, management is still reliant on observation of the infant, identification of symptoms, and appropriate treatment.

IDENTIFICATION AND RECOGNITION OF NEONATAL ABSTINENCE SYNDROME

In Liverpool, mothers and babies are cared for together within the post-natal area. There is no 'routine' admission of infants of known drug users to the neonatal intensive care unit. Symptoms of neonatal abstinence are outlined to the mother during the antenatal period, so that mothers are involved in the observation of their babies. The likely duration of their hospital stay is also described.

Encouraging a system whereby women are happy to volunteer infor-mation about their drug habit to health care providers is clearly the key to early recognition of NAS. Reassurance of the normality of their post-natal care goes a considerable way towards this. All professionals involved in postnatal care need to be aware of the issues of prediction outlined above, the features of withdrawal for each of the main drugs of misuse in their area, and the time course of these symptoms. It is important for staff to understand that withdrawal from opiates may occur early (under 24 hours), withdrawal from opioids may occur three to four days after birth and that polydrug use may delay or distort withdrawal signs.

The syndrome: how it is assessed

Features of NAS *arising* from maternal opiate use have been extensively described in the literature and consist of hyperactivity, irritability, tremors, hypertonicity, dehydration, seizures, weight loss and aspiration (American Academy of Pediatrics Committee on Drugs, 1983; Finnegan *et al.*, 1975).

A number of early assessment regimes of drug withdrawing infants cate-gorised signs into mild (infant tremulous), moderate (tremulous with exces-sive salivation, yawning, sneezing and loose stools) and severe (diarrhoea and vomiting and seizures in addition to moderate signs) (Nathenson *et al.*, 1971). Others graded withdrawal depending on the degree of irritability from mild (grade 1) to marked irritability when disturbed (grade 2) to marked fre-quent irritability when undisturbed (grade 3) (Kahn *et al.*, 1977). A major disadvantage of both these approaches was their subjectivity. In an attempt to minimise observer bias, Finnegan and colleagues assessed twenty signs most commonly found in neonatal withdrawal, scoring them when present according to their severity (Finnegan *et al.*, 1975). A total score was allocated to each infant. This system had a low inter-observer variability. Treatment for withdrawal was only prescribed when an infant reached a score of eight or more. The authors found that, using this system, infants received less drug treatment and had a shorter hospital stay. It has also been suggested that the Finnegan score enables an estimation of progression, and response to treatment. As a consequence, the 'Finnegan chart' is commonly used for assessing an infant with NAS in the UK (Morrison and Siney, 1996).

However, once members of staff have had experience in assessing infants with NAS it is still possible that a large subjective element comes into play. In addition there is a lack of clarity over which signs of NAS are predictive of later adverse outcome in these infants.

At Liverpool Women's Hospital we have developed a simplified chart and assessment strategy, which aims to treat signs of NAS that either cause distress or are potentially dangerous to the infant. This strategy depends on the recognition of fairly objective clinical symptoms such as profuse watery stools, profuse vomiting or a need for tube feeding due to inco-ordinate sucking. It also recognises distress in the infant as a sign of significant NAS. This is defined as not settling after comforting and swaddling or use of a pacifier following two consecutive feeds. The threshold for a decision rests on the need for treatment, rather than the results of 'scoring' the infant. This clinical approach simplifies observation procedures on the postnatal ward.

Time course of NAS

Signs of opiate withdrawal are clinically obvious at a mean age of 13 hours (range: 5–48 hours). The incidence of NAS requiring treatment in infants of mothers taking methadone is approximately 40 per cent and generally presents within 72 hours of birth. The signs of NAS may persist for longer in infants exposed to methadone compared with other opiates. There have been anecdotal reports of a later withdrawal occurring at one to two weeks of age (Challis and Scopes, 1977), although local data from a controlled study could not demonstrate an increased risk of signs in the methadone exposed group compared to a control group (Shaw and McIvor, 1994).

Infants born to mothers using cocaine are more likely to be born prematurely or growth retarded (Calhoun and Watson, 1991; Fulroth et al., 1989). Behavioural abnormalities in the newborn period, usually excitability, are more likely than in non-exposed infants, although these are probably due to a direct neurotoxic effect of cocaine metabolites rather than true NAS (Zabaleta et al., 1995). Whatever the cause, neurobehavioural abnormalities in the newborn, usually presenting as tremor and hypertonia or occasionally depressed activity, are more likely with cocaine exposure compared to other drug exposure in utero (Chiriboga et al., 1993). As a result infants born to cocaine-using mothers are more likely to be admitted to the Neonatal Intensive Care Unit and to stay in hospital for longer. Infants born to mothers using benzodiazepines, a common drug of abuse on Merseyside, may be floppy at birth or exhibit NAS. Care needs to be given to identifying those mothers with a significant benzodiazepine use as withdrawal may occur later than with opiates, starting often at 7 to 14 days (Sutton et al., 1990) after discharge from hospital postnatal care. This may persist for up to a month following its presentation and usually means an increased need for treatment. Community midwifery staff play an important role in these situations, and must be aware not only of the symptoms but also the temporal variations in their arrival.

Chronic alcohol abuse can cause foetal alcohol syndrome and result in NAS with similar signs to that seen in infants who have been exposed to other drugs *in utero*. Infants born to mothers who have used marijuana may exhibit mild withdrawal.

Treatment of drug withdrawal

Drug-using women and their infants in Liverpool are managed in the standard postnatal areas of maternity wards. Mothers are encouraged to participate in the recognition of withdrawal signs and symptoms in the child. Staff are trained, with regular updating, in the recognition and treatment of NAS, and the simplified Liverpool chart is used as a recording tool and guide. The aims of managing an infant at risk of Neonatal Abstinence Syndrome are: to maintain a normal temperature; to ensure adequate sleep between feeds; to reduce hyperactivity and excessive crying; to reduce motor instability; and to ensure adequate weight gain. Simple measures that can be undertaken by the mother such as cuddling, swaddling and using a pacifier may be effective. It is equally important to avoid excessive sedation. There is some evidence that nursing the infant on a waterbed reduces both the risk of NAS and the need for treatment (Oro and Dixon, 1988).

Using our chart (Figure 14.1), treatment should be considered if the baby has profuse watery stools or profuse vomiting or requires tube feeding due to inco-ordinate sucking. The only other indication for commencing treatment is if the infant has not settled after comforting, swaddling or use of a pacifier following two consecutive feeds. We do not advocate prescribing treatment for individual minor signs of drug withdrawal. Using this approach, approximately 35 per cent of infants born to known opiate users in this region receive treatment.

Drug treatment for NAS

A survey of Neonatal Units in England and Wales revealed great diversity with regard to the different drugs used for treating NAS (Morrison and Siney, 1996). There is little objective evidence to support the use of a particular drug for the treatment of NAS. A recent systematic review identified 14 randomised trials of drug treatment for NAS (Theis *et al.*, 1997). The quality of the trials reviewed in this paper was poor, with only a minority objectively verifying drug use, and none employing any kind of blinding procedure. The outcome measures assessed were mainly NAS scores.

ASSESSMENT CHART FOR NEONATAL DRUG WITHDRAWAL

Name:_____ Number:_____ Date of Birth:_____ Gestation:_____

Please ensure early feeding post-delivery. Commence 4 hourly monitoring after the first feed.
Note: if the baby has profuse watery stools or profuse vomiting or requires tube feeding due to
inco-ordinate sucking – consider commencing treatment.

Please tick the relevant box. Has the baby settled at all since last feed?
Note: if the baby has not settled following two feeds – consider commencing treatment.

Date:						
Time:						
YES:						
NO:						

Date:						
Time:						
YES:						
NO:						

Date:						
Time:						
YES:						
NO:						

Date:						
Time:						
YES:						
NO:						

Figure 14.1 Liverpool neonatal drug withdrawal chart

The majority of these trials assessed the use of Paregoric, a mixture of morphine, alcohol, camphor, tincture of opium and benzoic acid. The use of diazepam was assessed in nine of the trials and chlorpromazine, morphine and methadone were assessed in one each. Given the range of drugs used to treat the NAS, a meta-analysis was not undertaken.

Firm conclusions are difficult to draw from this review, but it appeared that treatment with morphine reduced symptom scores more than pheno-barbitone or diazepam. No differences were found between methadone and phenobarbitone or diazepam or chlorpromazine and diazepam. When an opiate was the main drug used in pregnancy, Paregoric was more effective at controlling symptoms than phenobarbitone or diazepam. When there was polydrug usage in pregnancy, phenobarbitone appeared better at controlling signs. Paregoric also improved co-ordination of the infants' suck whereas diazepam may have impaired this. This has to be balanced against concern that the use of diazepam or phenobarbitone can result in an increased risk of seizures either during their use or after stopping them. Although some useful information can be obtained from the randomised controlled trials reviewed, none of them took into account the important effects of variable antenatal care, maternal smoking, poverty, neglect and ill health.

In Liverpool, NAS is initially treated with morphine sulphate (Figure 14.2). Paediatric staff review the infant daily and the level of treatment is reduced every 24 hours provided the baby is feeding well and settling better between feeds. If improvement does not occur, the infant's condition is discussed with a senior paediatrician. Additional therapy may be indicated at this stage. We generally treat the effects of benzodiazepine usage, which often shows up later as withdrawal, with diazepam, however clonazepam is used by practitioners elsewhere. Where there is known polydrug use and a biphasic withdrawal pattern appears that is consistent with

GUIDELINES FOR MANAGEMENT OF DRUG WITHDRAWAL

Minor signs do not require treatment.
Withdrawal from opiates may occur in less than 24 hours (e.g. heroin).
Withdrawal from opioids may occur 3–4 days after birth (e.g. methadone).
Polydrug use may delay or skew withdrawal signs.

Aim of treatment is comfort not sedation.
Baby is reviewed daily by paediatric staff.

Treatment plan: *Level 4*
                      0.04 mg/kg morphine sulphate; oral preparation given 4 hourly
                      Level 3
                      0.03 mg/kg morphine sulphate; oral preparation given 4 hourly
                      Level 2
                      0.02 mg/kg morphine sulphate; oral preparation given 4 hourly
                      Level 1
                      0.01 mg/kg morphine sulphate; oral preparation given 4 hourly
Level reduced every 24 hours if the baby is feeding well and settling better between feeds.

If the feeding and settling does not improve or profuse watery stools and profuse vomiting continue – discuss with senior paediatrician.

Other medication may be required, e.g. diazepam for benzodiazepine use or chloral hydrate for cocaine/crack use.

If pharmaceutical treatment not required – the mother will still require support to help her comfort the baby – cuddling and swaddling is helpful. An infant soother 'dummy' may be necessary.

Figure 14.2 Liverpool guidelines for management of drug withdrawal

this, we use phenobarbitone or chloral hydrate to ease the baby's distress over the withdrawal period.

The majority of infants receiving treatment can be nursed on the postnatal wards. We keep known drug users and their infants in the hospital post-natal ward for at least 72 hours if there is no evidence of significant symptoms of withdrawal. In our experience, late opiate withdrawal has not been a clinical problem. Where treatment is required, infants and mothers are kept in hospital until the child is off all medication. Rarely, as a result of either prolonged withdrawal or difficult social circumstances, is there a need for the infant to be admitted to the neonatal unit.

When benzodiazepine use is a substantial part of the mother's drug use, she and the community midwifery staff are made aware of the continuing risk of later withdrawal, and similar observations are made at home.

SUMMARY

Neonatal Abstinence Syndrome is common in infants born to opiate-using mothers. It is generally unpredictable, though there is some tentative evidence linking extent of drug use with the frequency and severity of withdrawal symptoms. Polydrug use appears to have less influence on NAS than initially thought.

The majority of such infants should be managed on the normal post-natal areas. Simple clinical observation is sufficient to determine the need for medical therapy for the symptoms of NAS. Unless symptoms are severe, or there are other confounding medical or social factors, treatment should also take place on the postnatal ward. The best treatment appears to be morphine if the main drug used has been an opiate or opioid. If other drugs have been used alone or in combination, therapy may be individually tailored towards a longer or biphasic pattern of withdrawal. After many years of research and clinical observation there still remains a need for simple objective measures of assessing drug withdrawal in the infant. Better quality clinical trials are still needed to determine the best therapy for drug withdrawal.

REFERENCES

American Academy of Pediatrics Committee on Drugs (1983) Neonatal drug withdrawal. *Pediatrics* 72, 895–902.
American Academy of Pediatrics Committee on Drugs (1998) Neonatal drug withdrawal. *Pediatrics* 101, 1079–1085.
Bell, G.L. and Lau, K. (1995) Perinatal and neonatal issues in substance abuse. *Pediatric Clinics of North America* 42, 261–281.

Blinick, G., Inturrisi, C.E., Jerez, E. and Wallach, R.C. (1975) Methadone assays in pregnant women and their progeny. *American Journal of Obstetrics and Gynaecology* 121, 617–621.

Brown, H.L., Britton, K.A., Mahaffey, D., Brizendine, E., Hiett, K. and Turnquest, M.A. (1998) Methadone maintenance in pregnancy: a reappraisal. *American Journal of Obstetrics and Gynaecology* 179, 459–463.

Calhoun, B.C. and Watson, P.T. (1991) The cost of maternal cocaine abuse: 1 Perinatal cost. *Obstetrics and Gynaecology* 78, 731–734.

Challis, R.E. and Scopes, J.W. (1977) Late withdrawal symptoms in babies born to methadone addicts. *Lancet* 2, 230.

Chasnoff, I., Burns, W.J., Schnoll, S.H. and Burns, K.A. (1985) Cocaine use in pregnancy. *New England Journal of Medicine* 313, 666–669.

Chiriboga, C.A., Bateman, D.A., Brust, J.C. and Hauser, W.A. (1993) Neurologic findings in neonates with intrauterine cocaine exposure. *Pediatric Neurology* 9, 115–119.

Doberczak, T.M., Kandall, S.R. and Friedmann, P. (1993) Relationship between maternal methadone dosage, maternal-neonatal methadone levels and neonatal withdrawal. *Obstetrics and Gynaecology* 81, 936–940.

Doberczak, T.M., Kandall, S.R. and Wilets, I. (1991) Neonatal opiate abstinence syndrome in term and preterm infants. *The Journal of Pediatrics* 118, 933–937.

Finnegan, L.P., Kron, R.E., Connaughton, J.F. and Emich, J.P. (1975) Assessment and treatment of abstinence in the infant of the drug dependent mother. *International Journal of Clinical Pharmacology* 12, 19–32.

Fulroth, R., Phillips, B. and Durand, D.J. (1989) Perinatal outcome of infants exposed to cocaine and/or heroin in utero. *American Journal of Diseases of Childhood* 143, 905–910.

Gregg, J.E.M., Davidson, D.C. and Weindling, A.M. (1988) Inhaling heroin during pregnancy: effects on the baby. *British Medical Journal* 296, 754.

Harper, R.G., Solish, G., Feingold, E., Gersten-Woolf, N.B. and Sokal, M.M. (1977) Maternal injected methadone, body fluid methadone, and the neonatal withdrawal syndrome. *American Journal of Obstetrics and Gynaecology* 129, 417–427.

Kahn, E., Neumann L. and Polk, G.A. (1977) The course of heroin withdrawal syndrome in newborn infants treated with phenobarbital or chlorpromazine. *The Journal of Pediatrics* 75, 495–500.

Kandall, S., Albin, S., Gartner, L.M., Lee, Kwang-Sun, Eidelman, A. and Lowinson, J. (1977) The narcotic dependent mother: fetal and neonatal consequences. *Early Human Development* 1, 159–169.

Kempley, S. (1995) Pregnant women taking methadone should be warned about withdrawal symptoms in babies. *British Medical Journal* 310, 464.

McCarthy, J.E., Siney, C., Shaw, N.J. and Ruben, S.M. (1999) Outcome predictors in pregnant opiate and polydrug users. *European Journal of Pediatrics* 158, 748–749.

Madden, J.D., Chappel, J.N., Zuspan, F., Gumpel, J., Mejia, A. and Davis, R. (1977) Observation and treatment of neonatal narcotic withdrawal. *American Journal of Obstetrics and Gynaecology* 127, 199–201.

Mayes, L.C. and Carroll, K.M. (1996) Neonatal withdrawal syndrome in infants exposed to cocaine and methadone. *Substance Use and Misuse* 31, 241–253.

Medical Working Group on Drug Dependence (1992) *Guidelines for good clinical practices for the treatment of drug misuse.* London: DHSS.

Morrison, C.L. and Siney, C. (1996) A survey of the management of neonatal opiate withdrawal in England and Wales. *European Journal of Paediatrics* 155, 323–326.

Nathenson, G., Golden, G.S. and Litt, I.F. (1971) Diazepam in neonatal narcotic withdrawal syndrome. *Pediatrics* 48, 523–527.

Oro, A.S. and Dixon, S.D. (1988) Water bed care of narcotic exposed neonates. A useful adjunct to supportive care. *American Journal of Diseases of Childhood* 142, 186–188.

Ostrea, E.M., Brady, M., Gause, S., Raymundo, A.L. and Stevens, M. (1992) Drug screening of newborns by meconium analysis: a large scale, prospective, population study. *Pediatrics* 89, 107–113.

Ostrea, E.M., Chavez, C.J. and Strauss, M.E. (1976) A study of factors that influence the severity of neonatal narcotic withdrawal. *The Journal of Pediatrics* 88, 642–645.

Ramer, C.M. and Lodge, A. (1975) Clinical and developmental characteristics of infants of mothers on methadone maintenance. *Addictive Diseases* 2, 227–234.

Shaw, N.J. and McIvor, L. (1994) Neonatal Abstinence Syndrome after maternal methadone treatment. *Archives of Disease of Childhood* 71, F203–F205.

Siney, C., Kidd, G.M., Walkinshaw, S., Morrison, C. and Manasse, P. (1995) Opiate dependency in pregnancy. *British Journal of Midwifery* 3, 69–73.

Strauss, M.E., Andresko, M., Stryker, J.C. and Wardell, J.N. (1976) Relationship of neonatal withdrawal to maternal methadone dose. *American Journal of Drug and Alcohol Abuse* 3, 339–345.

Sutton, L.R. and Hinderliter, S.A. (1990) Diazepam abuse in pregnant women on methadone maintenance. Implications for the neonate. *Clinical Pediatrics Philadelphia* 29, 108–111.

Theis, J.G.W., Selby, P., Ikizler, Y. and Koren, G. (1997) Current management of the Neonatal Abstinence Syndrome: a critical analysis of the evidence. *Biology of the Neonate* 71, 345–356.

Wagner, C.L., Katikanemi, L., Cox, T.H. and Ryan, R.M. (1998) The impact of prenatal drug exposure on the neonate. *Obstetric and Gynaecology Clinics of North America* 25, 169–186.

Zabaleta, I., Jhaveri, R.C., Rosenfeld, W., Sahdev, S. and Vohra, K. (1995) Maternal use of cocaine, methadone, heroin and alcohol. *Neonatal Intensive Care* 3, 40–43.

Chapter 15

The role of drug services for pregnant drug users

The Liverpool approach

Susan Ruben and Frances Fitzgerald

Drug dependency is more common in men than women but the prevalence seems now to be increasing in women. It is well recognised that women may be reluctant to access treatment, often because of fear of the consequences for their children and a general mistrust of services. Pregnancy is one of many life events for a drug-misusing woman and we consider that services should be provided for this vulnerable group in a flexible, accessible way with the objective of providing support and care to minimise the potential harm of dependent drug use for the pregnant woman and her developing foetus. Multi-agency co-operative working practices seem to us to be the best approach to meet the multiple needs of this general group.

This chapter describes in detail the role of the Specialist Drug Service for pregnant drug users in Liverpool, with its emphasis on multi-agency and multi-disciplinary working. The outcomes described here met the service's objectives and have assisted in identifying the cases with more complex problems, some of which have included child protection issues. This demonstrates that it is possible to provide treatment and health care for this vulnerable and traditionally marginalised group, with positive outcomes in the majority of cases.

Research evidence indicates that regular antenatal care, methadone treatment programmes and social support improves outcomes for both the mother and the child. In an attempt to address the particular needs of pregnant drug users in Liverpool, the Specialist Drug Service works within the framework of a Pregnancy Support Group (PSG) comprising representatives from the drug services, the local Women's Hospital and the Social Services Drug and Alcohol Team. All the members of this team work directly with the client group, as well as liaising with other agencies if appropriate.

AIMS AND OBJECTIVES OF THE PREGNANCY SUPPORT GROUP

The PSG aims to:

- identify pregnant women within the city for whom illicit drug use is a problem;
- co-ordinate referrals from any source;
- collect and share relevant information on an inter-agency basis;
- oversee the pregnancy using a holistic approach and identifying health, childcare, child protection and social problems in order to form an individual care plan. This is agreed with the client and attempts are made to address the problems in a proactive way.

The PSG is a forum for multi-agency information sharing for pregnant drug users that can facilitate the best possible care and planning for this client group. Regular, fortnightly meetings of all members are held.

Core members

- Specialist health visitor (representing the Liverpool Drug Dependency Unit: DDU).
- Specialist midwife (representing the Women's Hospital).
- Social worker (representing the Social Services Drug and Alcohol Team).
- Deputy clinic administrator (representing Drug Dependency Unit Admin. Support).

Other individuals may be invited to attend this group on an ad hoc basis.

AGREED PROTOCOL FOR THE PREGNANCY SUPPORT GROUP

Information provided by the PSG

- Personal circumstances of the client plus general practitioner, health visitor and social worker reports if these are involved.
- The client's pattern of attendance at the Drug Dependency Unit and Antenatal Services.
- Contraceptive advice given and the client's practice.
- Information on drug use includes:
  - Level of substitute prescription if any, and compliance with it. Monitoring of illicit drug use and the impact of illicit use on the client's lifestyle.
  - Social issues, for example welfare, benefits, debts, housing, relationship problems.
  - The other agencies involved with the client especially probation, and district social services, if relevant.

Process

Any problems are identified during meetings and, if appropriate, the necessary action agreed upon, along with the name of a professional who would take responsibility for that action. For example, if a client was not attending drug dependency appointments, this would be followed up by the relevant worker at the clinic who would alert other agencies and if necessary undertake a home visit. The new referrals from any source are discussed at the end of the meeting.

THE PREGNANCY CLINIC

Pregnancy testing

The Clinic and local Syringe Exchange Scheme offers free pregnancy testing on site to any drug user for the following reasons:

• To encourage early confirmation of pregnancy.
• To allow the woman to consider termination of pregnancy, if appropriate.
• To give women more opportunity to access antenatal care.

We believe that this also encourages women to make initial contact with staff in a non-confrontational manner and be more likely to engage fully with the service.

Referrals to the pregnancy clinic

Referrals for pregnancy assessment come from:

• GPs and health visitors
• Maternity services
• Clinic attendees who become pregnant
• Social services
• Outreach workers, voluntary drug projects, probation
• Self-referrals

All referrals are deemed a priority and offered an assessment within one week of presenting.

Non-attendees for assessment are given a further series of appointments and may even be seen at home initially to encourage attendance. Some women fail to attend because they fear automatic Social Services referral, and reassurance can help to allay their fears. We ensure that the family health visitor, general practitioner and maternity services are all aware of non-attendance and that another referral can be made later in the pregnancy. We have observed that women who have lost touch with the drug clinic often return later in their pregnancy even when previous children have been removed from their care.

All pregnant drug users in Liverpool should have access to:

- antenatal care;
- drug treatment services if appropriate, including substitute prescribing, detoxification and drug counselling;
- social support, including advice around welfare rights, housing, budgeting, childcare support and other social issues;

that result in a healthy mother and baby living together in the community with appropriate support.

Clients of the clinic

The nature of the clientele can best be described through brief case descriptions:

- A 20-year-old single woman told antenatal services at 12 weeks that she was smoking heroin but adamantly refused to be referred to the drug clinic saying that she would be able to wean herself off. At 28 weeks she accepted a referral and was seen the next day, having realised that she needed help and support and having been unable to stop heroin use unaided.
- A 28-year-old sex trade worker whose previous child is now six years old and is in care of the local authority. She had not been seen for three years following a prison sentence. She re-presented at 20 weeks pregnant saying 'I know you f**kers were included when "J" [baby] was taken. I hated you but it was right. I want to do better this time, will you help?' She hugged various staff members and was reassessed urgently.
- A long-term male client of the clinic approached staff to tell us that his girlfriend, who was not a patient of the service, had become pregnant. He disclosed that she had both been abusing alcohol and taking heroin for some months and he was very concerned about the baby. She was offered an urgent appointment at the clinic where it was clear that she was both alcohol and opiate dependent. Her partner was known to have a past history of serious violence and was a polydrug user himself. The couple agreed to voluntary support from district social services which was arranged early in the pregnancy and a multi-disciplinary planning meeting was held to determine a comprehensive care plan involving all services. Flexible and easy

access to services is critically important and it was vital that a supportive, multi-agency care plan was put in place well before the birth of the baby.

- A local GP approached the specialist health visitor regarding a female patient who had been receiving methadone maintenance prescriptions and low dose diazepam for some years with no problems. He become concerned when she unexpectedly attacked him. He subsequently asked us for an urgent assessment. She was seen at the pregnancy clinic and transferred for further management within the Specialist Service Team. She has some mild, chronic depressive symptoms and the attack on her GP seemed to be related to benzodiazepine withdrawal. Her pregnancy was complicated by the fact that she had a history of previous caesarean sections, had quite severe abdominal adhesions and was very apprehensive regarding this pregnancy, which was unplanned. She was offered additional support, managed to reduce her diazepam markedly before the birth of her baby and stabilised well. The plan is to return her to primary care management soon. Her GP has accepted that her attack on him was out of character and her previously good relationship with him is likely to be restored.

INITIAL ASSESSMENT BY THE DRUG SERVICES

This is carried out jointly by an experienced doctor and the specialist health visitor who works within the service. We aim to assess comprehensively the nature and extent of the individual's drug problems and how drug use is impacting on their physical and mental health and their social functioning. It is the start of the process of a care plan and it gives the woman an opportunity to discuss her views of her problems, her coping strategies and support mechanisms, as well as her fears and anxieties regarding the pregnancy. The specialist health visitor is a relatively recent addition to the service. She has extensive child protection experience. We believe that health visitors have a less threatening reputation than a social worker, which is important at the initial meeting. Her role will be discussed later in this chapter.

The assessment covers in detail the following areas.

Illicit drug history

- Current drug use, route, amount and duration of use. Risk behaviours and the primary problem drug.
- Drugs taken in pregnancy and any changes since becoming pregnant.
- Detailed history of past drug use.

- Whether the woman is dependent on drugs.
- Tolerance, withdrawal symptoms, drug-seeking behaviours.
- Funding of her drug use.
- Whether she is on probation, and if there are any charges pending, fines outstanding or warrants for her arrest.

Treatment history

The following questions are asked about previous treatment:

- Is the woman already in treatment or known to other agencies?
- The length of her treatment and response to it.
- If prescribed methadone: the dose, form, compliance, and her attitude to this form of treatment and the reasons for its termination.
- If previously in treatment, why did she stop attending?
- The reasons for wanting specialist drug input during this pregnancy and the behaviours she wants to address and change.
- A history of her social relationships.

Sexual partner

Details regarding the woman's partner:

- Is he a significant person in her life?
- The quality of the relationship.
- Is he supportive?
- Is he aware of her drug use and is he a drug user and if so, is he in treatment?
- His attitude towards the woman and the pregnancy.

Significant family members and cohabitees:

- Their drug use and the level of support they give.
- Whether the woman has other children and whether they are living with her.
- The status of children, for example: whether under a care order; residency order; child protection.

Housing

- Do they have a home?
- Access to standard amenities: gas, water and electricity. Whether there are bills unpaid.
- The condition of the home and the number of bedrooms.

Register

* Does the family have a district social worker?

Full medical history

Documenting comprehensive details of the client's medical history is very important since some women make poor use of medical services and may have no general practitioner or access to primary care. Most are heavy cigarette smokers and have poor nutritional status and dental health. In addition there are other medical problems that may be relevant that could alter the obstetric management of the client, for example: asthma, anaemia, epilepsy, previous deep vein thrombosis (common in injecting drug users). Some women are already aware of their hepatitis and HIV status but screening for hepatitis B and C, and for HIV are offered by the maternity services at booking. An initial drug screen is performed using urinalysis in order to confirm illicit drug use and provide a baseline for subsequent changes.

THE CARE PLAN

At the end of the initial assessment, a workable care plan is negotiated with the client. The overwhelming majority of pregnant drug users seen in Liverpool are opiate dependent, with a high proportion also abusing crack cocaine, benzodiazepines or alcohol. We work within a broad harm minimisation model, which aims to help the individual to change their drug taking behaviour, take more responsibility for and control of their drug use, and move towards a long-term goal of abstinence with identified short-term goals, as described in Advisory Council on the Misuse of Drugs (ACMD) reports (ACMD, 1988, 1993).

Aims and objectives of the care plan

The overall aim is to minimise the impact of illicit drug use on the woman's ability to parent her child within the following hierarchy of harm reduction objectives:

* Cease to share injecting equipment.
* Reduce injecting, stabilise on oral methadone and reduce the use of all other illicit substances.
* Stabilise on oral methadone alone.
* Reduce dose of oral methadone.
* Total abstinence from all drugs.

Research suggests (Gossop, 1989) that abstinence is not achieved by most users in the short term and that drug dependence is often characterised by relapse to more chaotic behaviour patterns. In addition, many in our client group have other problems as well as drug use, such as poor family relationships, a history of being in care, poor educational attainment and little experience of employment. Many have limited coping strategies and have previously seen drug taking as a means of coping with a range of problems. This seems to contribute to the chronically low self-esteem seen within the group.

Prescribing methadone

For opiate-dependent drug users, there is overwhelming evidence for the role of methadone in assisting change. After assessment, most opiate-dependent pregnant women are offered oral methadone as part of their care plan, in conjunction with counselling, support and advice. Oral methadone without other input is known to be of less value as is just counselling without the use of methadone (Farrell et al., 1994). If methadone is to be prescribed, the dose needs to be determined based on the assessment and in Liverpool we aim to prescribe the lowest dose possible in pregnancy while recognising that some women will require higher doses to stabilise. We believe that this is preferable to continuing illicit drug use, although it is clear that with higher doses of methadone, the risk of neonatal withdrawal also increases, (Jarvis and Schnoll, 1994; Strauss et al., 1976).

All methadone is prescribed via community pharmacists. Initially most women are on daily pick-ups with weekly clinic reviews to assess their progress, and stability at the prescribed dose level. If a women is already on a methadone prescription and stable in her drug use, this level of stringent monitoring will not be required.

The dose levels required for stability vary greatly but in our experience they lie between 30 mg and 50 mg daily. Studies of methadone (Finnegan, 1991) in pregnant women show that there is considerable variation in plasma levels during pregnancy and that methadone levels may drop particularly in the last trimester of pregnancy, which then can require a slight increase in dose. We tend to adopt a regimen of multiple small doses, which seems to be acceptable to our client group. The woman divides her daily dose of methadone into two and takes it morning and evening. This seems to bring about greater stability at the end of pregnancy. Clearly some individuals may require a slight increase in dose but we are keen to try to keep the methadone dose as low as possible whilst keeping the woman comfortable as well.

The possible effects of methadone and other drugs on the foetus are always fully discussed at assessment. It is important that women are made aware of the risk of neonatal withdrawal and that some newborn babies will show severe withdrawal symptoms, even on lower doses of methadone. We emphasise that this is preferable to the foetus being exposed to intermittent withdrawal when the mother uses illicit heroin.

The use of street drugs

Women are encouraged and supported to make positive steps towards reducing their illicit drug use and this involves agreeing with the staff what lifestyle changes they will aim for between clinic visits. This occurs in the context of counselling sessions that cover relapse prevention strategies, coping with cravings, diversional tactics and the utilisation of other support mechanisms such as family, non-using friends and other professional sources of support.

Shared care

At the initial assessment we clarify with the client the details of her care plan including the identities of those who share in her care. In general, we share our care plan with the client's GP and (potential) health visitor, the hospital where she is to attend her antenatal care, and a district social worker, if one is already involved with the woman. If there are no current child protection concerns, we would discuss with the woman whether she wishes supportive input from members of the Drug and Alcohol Social Work Team.

It is important to address the issue of child protection and we explain in some detail that if there are child protection concerns during the pregnancy then we would have to involve the District Child Protection Team, even if this was not the wish of the client. Explaining very clearly what our expectations are of the woman, we reassure her that if we were to make a child protection referral we would discuss this fully with her and give a clear explanation as to the reasons. We also reassure her that the aim is to support her by agreeing a plan that will assist in coping with the child. In our experience, if information is given in a clear and logical way, then pregnant drug users understand. This produces less anxiety and helps to develop a more trusting relationship with staff.

Continuing care

The consultant, the specialist health visitor and an experienced drugs worker hold a weekly pregnancy clinic at the DDU. The local specialist midwife for drug misuse is also present to provide opportunistic antenatal care, and a member of the Drug and Alcohol Social Work Team is available to see clients if necessary. Part of the programme includes random urine screening to assist in the monitoring process. This is variable and depends on the stability of the client and our suspicions regarding illicit drug use that are not being openly discussed. However, all pregnant women will have several urine tests during the course of their pregnancy.

The clinic aims to be friendly and welcoming to the pregnant drug user. The counselling and support sessions vary in their content, depending on the agreed care plan and the progress made by individual women. The aim is to identify drug-related problems and look at ways to deal with them. These can be challenging sessions, particularly where women are continuing to use other illicit drugs and may present to the clinic clearly under the influence of a range of substances, are not complying with taking their medical treatment and do not appear to be taking the agreed steps to address and control their drug use. We recognise that we wish to continue in a positive relationship with women but that inadvertent collusion and manipulation can commonly occur when working with drug users.

We wish to continue in a positive relationship with the woman, but in adverse circumstances, collusion and manipulation can occur. For example, the woman may attempt to play down the extent of her drug use or the effects that it is having on her life and social stability. She may also ask workers not to share information on the outcomes of urine screening or details of clinic attendance with the district social workers. We believe that challenging attitudinal and behavioural issues associated with drug use within a trusting relationship should be a positive help to the woman and our experience is that women are often grateful for firm, decisive feedback around our assessment of their problems. This allows them to reflect on their attitudes and is a way of preventing collusive relationships which can arise when working with this group.

Although we aim to be a non-judgemental service, nonetheless we have duties and responsibilities as professionals. The women need to understand that professional judgements are made as part of our monitoring through the Pregnancy Support Group meetings.

It is important to allow the clients to vent their anger and frustration at times and be given an opportunity to work this through with our help. Where there are complex child protection issues the drug team wishes to continue to work with the woman and we need to be aware of the importance of maintaining an open and honest relationship so that a therapeutic relationship with the woman can be established and continue in the future. Women are seen regularly right up to delivery and we have excellent liaison with the local maternity services who inform staff when a women is in labour and when they are leaving the hospital post-delivery.

If a pregnant woman is known to be continuing to abuse drugs, such as alcohol, cocaine and benzodiazepines, this is shared with maternity services and enables them to be alerted to the risk of medical problems in the neonate. In our service, about a third continue with multiple drug use. This group is most likely to raise professional concerns about child protection, particularly if their partner is also a drug user.

Detoxification during pregnancy

Many drug-dependent women say they aim to become totally drug free during pregnancy and this should be considered as a feasible option. Some women see pregnancy as affording them the opportunity to make a fresh start and change how they view their drug use. Detoxification seems as likely to succeed in pregnant as in non-pregnant individuals when it is planned, the woman has high motivation to change and an appropriate level of social support and aftercare can be offered. If a woman manages to become and sustain a drug-free state in pregnancy then the foetus will also be drug free at birth. It is generally agreed in the literature that the mid-trimester is the safest time to attempt detoxification and this is our usual practice.

For opiate-dependent women, we consider a methadone detoxification the safest option during pregnancy. Detoxification using lofexidine has not been established as safe in pregnant women and we certainly would not consider any of the rapid detoxification methods while under sedation or anaesthesia, which are still controversial at the time of writing. Detoxification can be carried out either as an out-patient or as an in-patient.

It is essential that a thorough assessment is made to determine whether an individual woman is an appropriate candidate for this procedure and inevitably there is a high risk of relapse following detoxification. An assessment is made of the woman's motivation and reasons for wishing to detoxify and ensures that she is making an informed choice having considered all the options for her care during the pregnancy. Guilt about the baby, undue pressure which often comes from family members, and fears of the neonatal withdrawal syndrome may lead a woman to choose detoxification – with the consequent risk of the attempt failing. The assessment should ensure that the woman is fully prepared and motivated for detoxification.

We do not prescribe naltrexone, the opiate antagonist, following detoxification in pregnancy, as its safety is not established so this would not be an option in assisting relapse prevention.

Our detoxification regime for pregnant patients is that we reduce the methadone more slowly than for non-pregnant women and the majority of our patients choose an in-patient setting to undertake this. They receive the same package of care as non-pregnant clients in the in-patient setting and join in all usual therapeutic activities and diversional therapies whilst in-patients. We do not, however, offer alternative therapies such as reflexology, herbal remedies or acupuncture to pregnant clients, as their safety or appropriateness has not been established clinically.

When they are in the drug detoxification unit, the women are visited by their community midwife and attend all usual antenatal appointments. We have an arrangement with local maternity hospitals for emergency assessment if the woman or staff are concerned about the well-being of the foetus. Pregnant women are allowed to slow down the process of methadone reduction or stop reducing it if they feel unable to cope or if they change their mind about their ability to become abstinent during pregnancy.

If the pregnant woman is a polydrug abuser and is also benzodiazepine dependent, we attempt to detoxify her from benzodiazepines during pregnancy by using a slow reducing regime of diazepam. If this is not possible, we try to reduce her to the lowest possible dose of benzodiazepines. This is very important given the known effects of benzodiazepines on neonatal withdrawals (Sutton and Hinderliter, 1990).

On entering an in-patient detoxification programme, a pregnant woman is continued on her usual dose of methadone for the first 24 to 48 hours to ensure that she is comfortable before starting to reduce the dose. If she is on street heroin only, the first few days are spent in establishing an appropriate dose of oral methadone before reducing the dose. For women dependent on crack cocaine or other stimulants, no medication is given and they are offered psychological treatments and intensive support.

If during the detoxification process, vomiting, diarrhoea, cramps and insomnia are problematic, then symptomatic treatments may be offered after discussion with local maternity services to establish that any medications used are safe during pregnancy. An experienced pharmacist is of great assistance in these cases. In-patient care can also be used to stabilise a chaotic pregnant drug user on an appropriate dose of oral methadone or simply to reduce the higher level.

In Liverpool, only a small number of pregnant women opt for detoxification during pregnancy and they require intensive support and counselling afterwards. If they do relapse and resume heroin use, they are offered immediate assessment in order to initiate the resumption of oral methadone. From 1996 to 1998, only five pregnant drug users in Liverpool opted for detoxification during pregnancy and of these, only two actually became drug free.

SHARING ANTENATAL CARE: THE ROLE OF THE SPECIALIST HEALTH VISITOR

For some pregnant drug users, the pregnancy clinic at the Liverpool Drug Dependency Clinic may be the first contact with a health visitor. Whilst it is acknowledged that the health visitor may be less threatening than a social worker, it is most important that the client is made aware from the outset that should the specialist health visitor have any concerns of a child protection nature, she must refer to the District Social Services Department. This is not an automatic process but is based upon close monitoring of the client's illicit drug use and associated lifestyle. It includes a home assessment to ensure that the domestic environment would be suitable for a young baby to live in and an assessment of the likely impact of illicit drug use and the associated lifestyle on the woman's ability to parent adequately. Referrals are made accordingly.

The specialist health visitor may also refer to the Drug and Alcohol Social Work Team for assistance regarding housing problems, benefits and assessment for drug rehabilitation and works closely with colleagues in this team. Information gathered in the pregnancy clinic is shared with them and the Maternity Service Social Work Department through the distribution of the Pregnancy Support Group minutes. In addition, there are direct lines of communication between the specialist health visitor, district social worker, family health visitor and the general practitioner. Such a communication network is essential when monitoring chaotic drug use. The communication of concerns between professionals is deemed a priority.

The specialist health visitor has six specific dimensions to her role in the Liverpool Drug Dependency Clinic:

- To act as a resource, raise awareness and provide training in child protection and substance misuse to staff, in what is essentially an adult-centred service.
- To be the point of contact for other agencies and professionals and to offer specialist advice on the impact of drug use within the context of child protection issues.
- To provide health care advice and support to those clients with children where there are child protection concerns.
- To provide a specific service for pregnant drug users.
- To maintain a database of all child protection conferences held regarding children of the Liverpool Drug Dependency Clinic and attend conferences, reviews, planning meetings and professional meetings as required.
- To audit and evaluate the outcome of children who have been the subject of such conferences.

SHARING POSTNATAL CARE

The postnatal period can be stressful for a drug-misusing mother. She has all the stresses of any new mother and may be dealing with a baby with some residual withdrawal symptoms, who may be fractious and difficult to feed. This exacerbates feelings of guilt and if the woman has poor coping strategies can lead her back to more regular illicit drug use (see Klee and Jackson, 1998 and Chapter 11). Some degree of postnatal depression is common and since the rates of depression in opiate-dependent women are higher than in the general population (Farrell *et al.*, 1998), we feel that extra support and prompt treatment of postnatal depression is vital.

The specialist health visitor sees all women at least twice postnatally, either at the DDU or at home. She discusses a range of issues with them, including contraception, and offers additional support. She liaises with the family health visitor and may arrange a joint visit if there are more complex problems. Her task at this time is to pass clients on to other key workers at the DDU while maintaining uninterrupted continuation of the care plan. If key workers express concerns regarding childcare or possible child protection concerns, these are discussed both with the specialist health visitor and the worker's line manager and the care plan may be renegotiated or amended with involvement of other agencies including district social services, if child protection concerns emerge in the postnatal period. In addition, if clients become more chaotic, they will receive closer medical supervision and interventions.

The Drug Dependency Clinic may be the agency with most regular contact with clients, and the importance of good communication with the primary health care team and, in particular, the family health visitor cannot be overemphasised. This underpins the philosophy of working in open partnership with the client group and the need for adult drug services to work positively with other professionals involved with drug users and their children.

SUMMARY

This chapter aims to discuss the model of service delivery to pregnant drug users in Liverpool. Drug-misusing pregnant women have complex and differing needs and problems, and this chapter emphasises the importance of multi-agency and multi-disciplinary approaches to working collaboratively. It also describes in some detail the practicalities of this work. This approach does not lead to a large number of child protection conferences but it should be noted that when a conference has been held, all the children concerned have subsequently been placed on the Child Protection Register. This suggests that our multi-agency assessment process is effective whilst not being overly interventionist or utilising child protection procedures inappropriately. We know that drug-misusing pregnant women still feel marginalised and often exclude themselves from service provision available to the general population. Achieving a balance between child protection and support is a challenging problem for all professionals involved with this group but is, we believe, possible within this model.

We recognise that we must continue to strive to improve our service with more emphasis on assisting pregnant women with parenting skills. We are aware that very few of our clients attend the ParentCraft classes locally and we would hope to develop more structured ParentCraft facilities to meet their needs. These could be added to our routine pregnancy clinic services, if resources were available.

We do not maintain that this is the only possible model for working with pregnant drug users. Each local area should consider the most creative way to organise service provision to meet their own particular local needs and to mobilise most effectively the resources available locally. This model seems to be working well in Liverpool and, together with the strong will to improve and refine, there is a belief that the feelings of social exclusion and discrimination that affect many pregnant drug users will ultimately decline.

REFERENCES

ACMD (1988) *AIDS and Drug Misuse: part 1*. London: HMSO.
ACMD (1993) *AIDS and Drug Misuse Update*. Advisory Council on the Misuse of Drugs, London: HMSO, p. 10.
Farrell, M., House, S., Taylor, S. *et al.* (1998) Substance misuse and psychiatric comorbidity: an overview of the OPCS National Psychiatric Morbidity Survey. *Addictive Behaviours* 23, 909–918.
Farrell, M., Ward, J., Mattick, R. *et al.* (1994) Methadone maintenance treatment in opiate dependence – a review. *British Medical Journal* 309, 997–1001.
Finnegan, L.P. (1991) Treatment issues for opioid dependent women during the perinatal period. *Journal Psycho-Active Drugs* 23(2), 191–202.
Gossop, M. (1989) Introduction, in: M. Gossop (ed.) *Relapse and Addictive Behaviour*, London: Routledge, 1–8.
Jarvis, M.A.E. and Schnoll, S.H. (1994) Methadone treatment during pregnancy. *Journal of Psychoactive Drugs* 26, 155–161.
Klee, H. and Jackson, M. (1998) *Illicit Drug Use, Pregnancy and Early Motherhood: an analysis of the impediments to effective service delivery*. Final Report to the Department of Health Task Force to Review Services for Drug Misusers.
Strauss, M.E., Andresekon, J., Stryker, J.C. *et al.* (1976) Relationship of neo-natal withdrawal to maternal methadone dose. *American Journal Drug & Alcohol Abuse* 3, 339–345.
Sutton, L.R. and Hinderliter, S.A. (1990) Diazepam abuse in pregnant women on methadone maintenance: Implications for the neonate. *Clinical Pediatrics* 29, 108–111.

Chapter 16

The drug liaison midwife

Developing a model of maternity
services for drug-using women from
conception to creation

Faye Macrory

It is well documented in the literature that pregnant drug users are seen
to present a great problem to health care services. This is an area where
there is much misunderstanding, not infrequently based on unfounded myth
and stereotype. This chapter charts the conception and creation of a
specialised maternity service for drug-using women in the inner-city area
of Manchester.

THE BACKGROUND TO THE PROJECT

Initial action

In June 1993 a multi-agency steering group was formed in Manchester to
discuss the complex and wide-ranging issues associated with drug use,
pregnancy and childcare. The catalyst for this was partly in response to
media debate about a mother accused of manslaughter following the death
of her three-year-old child from ingesting methadone.

The steering group was based at the Zion Community Health and
Resource Centre in Hulme, a deprived area of the city of Manchester, that
was to undergo an impressive regeneration programme in the following
years. Members were from both the voluntary and statutory sectors, and
included myself (working then on the delivery unit at St Mary's Hospital),
other interested midwives, drug and social workers, probation officers,
health visitors and health promotion/HIV advisors.

The meetings were set up initially on an informal basis where workers
could share and exchange information, and discuss how to try to improve
different services to attract this particular client group. The overriding
question facing the group was 'what should we be doing?' Could we
support drug-using women and their families better? Where do we begin?

Assessing the problem

Among the various issues raised were concerns as to why many drug-
using women accessed antenatal care so infrequently, if at all. A realistic

assessment of potential parenting connected with a drug-using lifestyle was then usually not possible because of poor inter-agency communication and continuity of care in the antenatal period. Difficulties increased and crisis interventions frequently occurred when, for real or perceived reasons, some women persistently avoided contact with statutory services. This led to considerable time having to be devoted by the community midwives in trying to locate these clients, often unsuccessfully.

This scenario inevitably led to social services involvement following the delivery and the subsequent admission of the baby to the Special Care Baby Unit. Not surprisingly, conflict often occurred between service providers and service users. This admission policy was in direct contrast to other maternity centres such as Glasgow and Liverpool, where the babies of drug users are nursed on the ward with their mothers participating in their care.

At Manchester Metropolitan University, empirical research by Klee confirmed that drug-using women avoid statutory maternity services mainly because of their concern about possible negative attitudes of service providers, and their fears that their baby would be taken into care. Knowing that their baby would automatically be admitted to the Special Care Baby Unit appeared significantly to increase their anxiety. Drug-using women want to be treated in the same way as other women, and not be identified and labelled through their disclosed drug use. The research revealed that the relationships between the client and health professionals were consistently good in those clinics and hospitals in which a specific policy for drug users had been developed. Prior to 1995 there was no such policy in operation at St Mary's Hospital.

A model of good practice

The Zion Steering Group decided it would be of benefit to visit a model of good practice and chose the Women's Reproductive Health Service (WHRS) in Glasgow. Developed by Dr Mary Hepburn, it has provided a city-wide service since 1990, for women with severe social problems, which include drug use.

Hepburn (1993) (see also Chapter 17) suggests that there should be a pragmatic approach to appropriate individual management and that control of drug use with subsequent stabilisation of lifestyle should be the objective, with prescription of substitute therapy being only one of a range of measures that can help achieve this end. As pregnancy often provides motivation for a change in lifestyle, many women who use drugs want to stop doing so for the sake of their babies. The Glasgow model was a great inspiration and a decison was made to apply for funding that would support a specialist midwife who would liaise between clients and care providers.

Applying for funding

The bid for funding was supported by a retrospective audit of St Mary's services. Admissions to the Special Care Baby Unit were examined over a 15-month period between 1992 and 1993 (Macrory, 1994). Forty-three women were identified as using drugs in pregnancy, other than alcohol or tobacco. These included heroin, methadone, cocaine, cannabis, amphetamines and benzodiazepines, either alone or in combination. A previous audit over 1989–1998 had identified less than half this number. It is worth noting that the women all smoked cigarettes.

Of the 43 women, approximately 30 per cent were over 30 weeks' gestation at the time of booking in, and 20 per cent had presented for the first time in labour. It was unclear as to what contact with the drug services the women had, or what, if any, treatment they were receiving. It was also difficult to ascertain from the audit whether there were informed concerns among staff around child protection issues, since the general consensus appeared to be that all types and patterns of drug use are incompatible with parenting. Comments that were irrelevant to the pregnancy, but were based on the subjective views of staff members were made, while important and relevant information was absent. This appeared to derive from an emphasis on antenatal care that was heavily influenced by the label 'drug addict'.

The audit also indicated that pressure was being exerted by staff to persuade them to undergo HIV testing on the basis of assumptions about their supposed lifestyle. It was apparent that all grades of staff had very little awareness of the significance of the implications of HIV testing for the client. Furthermore, it seemed that many of them interpreted counselling as being synonymous with giving advice. Toxicological screening of urine specimens had also been carried out for the presence of drugs without informed consent being obtained from any of the women.

From the audit findings alone, it was apparent that extensive education was clearly necessary for all levels and grades of staff on complex aspects of drug use and HIV issues. The maternity care offered at that time appeared to be both insensitive and inappropriate to the needs of drug-using women. The dilemma lay in how best to provide a maternity service that would not stigmatise them, but would offer specialist care and support in a sensitive and non-judgemental way. It was clear to the Zion Steering Group that a lead midwife with the necessary expertise would be essential should a new improved service be created.

Access to clients

The work of Manchester Action on Street Health (MASH) is particularly relevant to this chapter. This is a street-based sexual health service for prostitutes and makes contact with large numbers of women, primarily

opiate users, but also those using a range of other drugs. MASH repre-
sents a particularly successful outreach model in terms of attracting
traditionally 'hard-to-reach' client groups. However, while many women
will fund their drug habit by working in this way not all drug users work
as prostitutes and some who do are not involved in either drugs or alcohol.
MASH staff engage in a whole range of conversations with the client,
and only when a particular level of rapport has been developed do they
initiate discussions that focus more specifically on sexual health, harm-
reduction and drugs issues. The trust established by this approach enables
staff to make more focused interventions at a later stage without having
alienated the clients (Crosby, 1994).

Within my previous role as a volunteer in this organisation I could only
give the women advice, and encourage them to approach mainstream maternity services. It became increasingly apparent that combining the roles of
practising midwife and trusted volunteer had great potential in promoting
the uptake of such services. The fear and suspicion about the medical and
social services among drug-using women convinced Weissman (1991) that
it is critical to put outreach activities into the hands of those who know the
women, and, most importantly, those who will not judge them. Other similar
projects have found that sensitivity is the key factor in overcoming the barriers. The best, perhaps the only, workable strategy, is to listen to the women
and to address the issues, problems, and concerns that *they* identify as the
most pressing in their lives rather than those that staff may identify for them.
The reality is that, while programmes might be organised around or funded
for a single specific issue such as substance misuse, antenatal care or HIV
prevention, the women they are attempting to serve cannot be categorised
so neatly. Most of this client group are afflicted by multiple problems and
in designing projects for these women, it must be remembered that neither
they nor their use of drugs exist in a vacuum.

BUILDING THE FRAMEWORK

The underlying philosophy

The Zion Steering Group wanted to build a framework that would create
a service reflecting the view that drug use and parenting are not automatically considered mutually exclusive. It would be a service where
women would be offered up-to-date, relevant and factual information in
a non-judgemental and sympathetic manner, *not* directive, subjective and
uninformed advice.

Clients would be partners in their own care and would be encouraged
to contribute to decisions relating to that care. Such empowerment should
be beneficial to physical and mental health and they could begin to move
down the ladder of drugs-related harm within a good therapeutic rela-

tionship, where trust prevails and a sense of positive self-worth is fostered. Thus, a foundation will be established on which to address other needs.

Such a model is explicitly rooted in the belief that health needs and social needs are inextricably linked and must be considered together in order to improve outcomes for this population in the long term. It was hoped that the service from the project would diminish the need for: consultant-led time; community midwifery input in trying to locate non-attendees; and ultimately infant care in a Special Care Baby Unit. The expertise offered would also give hospital staff the opportunity to access a liaison midwife as an additional resource when decisions were needed about procedures with members of this client group.

The proposed role for such a midwife within the Manchester area was to enable services to be offered in community and hospital settings, working in both voluntary and statutory sectors, including outreach sessions such as MASH. Referral would be accessible to drug-using women through any of these routes.

The role of education

One of the main aims of this innovative development was to set up a permanent specialised service. In this context the liaison midwife would have an expanded teaching role in a multi-disciplinary education programme for other health professionals involved in providing maternity care. Additional experience in HIV counselling and drug use issues was felt to be an important resource when implementing education programmes and policy change.

The importance of understanding the women's circumstances and views and providing support to the women in the course of any reduction or detoxification programmes they may undertake is vital for a service that the women will regard as user-friendly. Raising awareness of the potential effects of different drugs on the foetus and baby is also very important so that the women concerned are well informed. However, it is equally important that this information is communicated in a credible and non-alarmist way.

The aim of regular collaboration and sharing of information with the different agencies, both in the statutory and voluntary sectors, was to allow the proposed coalition ultimately to function as a single and integrated service while making maximum use of the treatment opportunity of every client contact. Ethical issues would be addressed within the relevant codes of professional conduct as and when they occurred. The liaison midwife would be responsible for the development, implementation and evaluation of individual programmes of care, ensuring that these objectives would be achieved by ongoing audit.

The anticipated impact of such a comprehensive education programme for service providers was that women who use drugs in pregnancy would feel comfortable in using mainstream maternity services, even if a liaison midwife was not always available. It was also hoped that the women would then feel more confident about addressing, with professional help, other difficulties in their lives. The knowledge and expertise contained within the team would enable specialised care to be offered in a manner that was appropriate to each woman and sensitive to her individual needs. Such a service would be cost effective, flexible and accessible, and provide women with continuity of care acceptable to them. At the same time it would supply hospital staff with reliable, ongoing support from the liaison midwife.

Fundraising

The proposals for a change from existing practice began to gain support among consultant paediatricians, consultant obstetricians and midwifery managers at St Mary's Hospital. Presenting the findings of the audit to relevant service providers proved to be a vital and useful tool in persuading them of the need for a change in this direction.

Although this model of care prevention was attracting increasing attention (Macrory and Crosby, 1995) bids for funding to support the post of drug liaison midwife were initially unsuccessful. Ultimately, funding was agreed that would share costs between Salford Mental Health Services NHS Trust and Central Manchester Health Care Trust. The job description included reference to voluntary work, which was important since this would now be subject to the UK Code of Professional Conduct and mean that access routes to maternity services through outreach agencies such as MASH would be formally and legally recognised. The post became finally official on 1 August 1995 amid great celebrations among all those who had been involved for so long in its conception and creation.

THE ROLE OF THE DRUG LIAISON MIDWIFE

Responsibilities

Jointly employed by Central Manchester Healthcare Trust and the Mental Health Services of Salford NHS Trust, I am now responsible for leading the development of good policy and practice in caring for the pregnant drug user in the Manchester Drug Services at St Mary's Hospital, other maternity services in Manchester, and in Primary Health Care Teams.

This includes giving advice about preconceptual problems, contraception, sexual problems and sexually transmitted diseases, and referral for the termination of a pregnancy. Other problems can include domestic violence, rape and sexual assault, associated legal problems, and relationships in general.

Each drug worker has a responsibility to notify the drug liaison midwife of any pregnant client, whether or not she wants a consultation, and irrespective of which hospital she will be attending. Such referrals come from a wide variety of sources, including the voluntary sector and include cases of self-referral. With a city-wide responsibility for Manchester Drug Service this role facilitates access to the other maternity services in the city.

Outcomes

Since its inception the model of care has enhanced communication and good practice between the drug and the maternity services in the city. Among other improvements, it has led to the cessation of the standard procedure of removing the babies of drug-using women to the Special Care Baby Unit in the hospitals. In addition, antenatal care and advice is given to women admitted to the drug detoxification unit at the regional psychiatric hospital.

Although not an aspect of the model that will apply in all locations, a weekly sessional basis with MASH enables women who are working as street prostitutes to be given antenatal care and access to maternity services and other support agencies. Such contacts can offer opportunities to reduce the number of crisis interventions that occur among hard to reach groups. Commonly these arise when an unknown, unbooked drug user who is already in labour presents to maternity services.

The work of a drug liaison midwife has relevance to the training of health professionals. A significant contribution can be made at both local and national levels while information levels are low and demand is high. Training on a city-wide basis has commenced in Manchester. The topics covered by the author include pregnancy, childbirth and childcare issues associated with women with drug-related problems. HIV and hepatitis tests are offered to all pregnant women and training will be informed by work with HIV-positive women through referral or special clinics.

Since the implementation of this service the number of clients has been steadily rising. In the first year 152 women were notified from a wide variety of statutory and voluntary sources. In the second year this increased to 177, and 57 babies were delivered in that year at St Mary's Hospital. There has been a substantial increase in the number of women disclosing excessive alcohol use and closer collaboration has been established with the Community Alcohol Team.

An information leaflet for clients, *Pregnant and Using?*, and a booklet for parents about the signs and symptoms of neonatal drug withdrawal have been produced. A guide for professionals, 'Pregnancy, Drug Use and Care of the Newborn', was completed in March 1997 and has since been used by many other maternity services when implementing their own change in practice.

ANTENATALLY: THROUGH BIRTH AND BEYOND

Achievements and boundaries

The hope is that an environment has been created where women can feel free to disclose at any stage their substance use/misuse without fear of being judged and criticised. Our service can demonstrate that when women are aware that the reason for asking questions is to offer support, rather than to marginalise them further, increasing numbers will disclose information and seek reassurance and advice.

Boundaries have been set for the service. For example, women with problematic drug use are not admitted to the ward for detoxification or stabilisation. It is considered by our service not to be the most appropriate place to address the many complex issues associated with a drug problem. Pregnant women get priority into assessment at the in-patient unit at the regional psychiatric hospital, but this requires a detailed and individualised assessment prior to admission. However, with no other option available, for some women admission to an antenatal ward *may* be beneficial in the short term, but only with very close involvement and supervision by the drug team or key worker.

For many women, illicit drug use is a chronic relapsing condition, and clients presenting for drug treatment will almost invariably have been using drugs for several years. The prescribed and non-prescribed drugs used can include methadone, heroin, crack cocaine, benzodiazepines, amphetamines, cannabis, alcohol and tobacco. Some women combine several of the above. Some will comply with their prescribed treatment for their dependence while others will not (see Chapter 6).

Medication

The treatment of drug misuse in a maternity unit should be a planned exercise. The service has set up the parameters that govern methadone administration. As a general rule, should methadone be requested by a client and staff are unable to confirm the dose level/frequency with the prescriber, 5 to 10 ml doses at four-hourly intervals may be given if the client is showing symptoms of withdrawal. We recommend that no medication should be given if the woman appears drowsy or intoxicated. Confirmation must be obtained from the drug service, the GP or dispensing chemist, and specialist advice sought as soon as possible. Benzodiazepines should not be prescribed at all, unless verified. A urine sample for drug screening should be taken prior to commencing prescribing under these circumstances, as this will aid the assessment of those new into treatment.

During labour, standard analgesia is indicated since a daily dose of methadone will not provide pain relief. If we remind ourselves that pain is an individual subjective experience, the requirements of opiate-dependent women should be no different than other women, provided they have their normal level maintained (Siney *et al.*, 1995).

Infant care

After delivery, the mother and baby are transferred to the ward together, unless medical reasons dictate otherwise. Should babies require treatment, they usually return to the Special Care Baby Unit, but as ward staff gain more experience they are now increasingly treated on the ward. As most *major* symptoms of withdrawal will show, in the main, between 24 and 72 hours, a stay of 72 hours in the hospital is recommended (Shaw and McIvor, 1994). Babies are observed on the ward by the mother and the staff, using a modified score chart. The staff are encouraged to view the babies' condition holistically, using the chart as a guide, rather than as a prescriptive tool. The amount and type of drug used is not a reliable indicator as to how the baby may react.

Good liaison with the community midwifery service and the health visitor ensures extra support once discharged home. Staff now recognise that should a woman wish to go home before the recommended 72 hours, it is usually because of other childcare issues, not because they are irresponsible and uncaring. Where this previously led to conflict, greater communication between staff and clients has led to the development of mutual respect and understanding and a more harmonious resolution to such problems.

Without the threat of automatic admission of the baby to the Special Care Baby Unit the women have the chance realistically to address their drug use during pregnancy, rather than try desperately and unsuccessfully to be drug free by the birth. Anxiety from anticipating that their babies would be separated from them, and fear of confidentiality being compromised by such an action, has been shown seriously to disrupt a previously stable treatment programme (Klee and Jackson, 1998). The focus is now on giving parents support and encouragement to help them cope with what is often an irritable and unsettled baby. There is good liaison with social services although their involvement is no longer automatic, and each woman's particular need is assessed on an individual basis. Many already have ongoing and long-term involvement, but not necessarily because of child protection issues. Drug use is not now considered incompatible with good parenting, but it is acknowledged that a drug-oriented lifestyle may have damaging effects (SCODA, 1989).

Breast feeding should be encouraged even if the mother is continuing to take drugs. Very small amounts of the drugs being taken will pass across in the breast milk, matching exactly the combination of drugs the baby received *in utero*. This will help reduce the withdrawals and diminish the need for treatment (Hepburn, 1997). Our service has found that those women who wish to breast feed are, in general, those more motivated to deal with their drug use.

It has been encouraging to observe that such changes in practice have led to a dramatic reduction in the use of pharmacological treatments.

CONCLUSION

It was recognised at the outset of the project that there might be diffi-culties in attempting to provide a specialist service that did not appear to stigmatise the client. Although drug-using women certainly need indi-vidualised services, projects may run several risks in concentrating the delivery of help to women during this time of their life. The intensive nature of care in the antenatal period for all women can simply rein-force the already strong societal message that women's sole value is in producing offspring, and that the only attention they will get is in their role as potential mothers (see Chapter 3). For women whose sense of self and self-esteem is already precarious, the feeling that they are only valued when pregnant can leave them feeling used and even more vulnerable once the baby comes home and they are left to cope on their own.

Ongoing and accessible support is vital for the staff who work with this client group since their pregnancies cannot be supported in a way that takes no account of the more complex problems that are often part of the client's lifestyle. If a user-friendly service for staff and clients alike is available, the potential for strain among those involved in the plan of care is reduced. Ideally a seamless service between the drug and maternity services will develop that has benefit for clients and health professionals alike. A client group's particular needs will not be met until all those involved are regarded as important contributors, and are informed and supported in their delivery of care. The past mistakes that have led to client alienation can be avoided through such action. What is needed now is a period of improvement that establishes a way of working together that is free from prejudice, conflict and confrontation.

REFERENCES

Crosby, S. (1994) *Working with Prostitutes: reducing risks, expanding services.* Presented to the 5th International Conference on the Reduction of Drug Related Harm, Toronto.

Hepburn, M. (1993) Drug misuse in pregnancy. *Current Obstetrics and Gynaecology* 3, 54–58.

Hepburn, M. (1997) Caring for the pregnant drug user, in: B. Beaumont (ed.) *Care of Drug Users in General Practice: a harm minimisation approach*. London: Radcliffe Medical Press.

Klee, H. and Jackson, M. (1998) *Illicit Drug Use, Pregnancy and Early Motherhood*. The Manchester Metropolitan University, UK: SRHSA.

Macrory, F. (1994) *Maternal Drug Use and Pregnancy*. Audit 1992–1993. St Mary's Hospital for Women and Children. Unpublished. Available from the author.

Macrory, F. and Crosby, S. (1995) *Drug Use, Pregnancy and Care of the Newborn: a guide for professionals*. Unpublished. Available from the author.

Shaw, N.J. and McIvor, L. (1994) Neonatal Abstinence Syndrome after maternal methadone treatment. *Archives of Disease in Childhood* 71, 203–220.

Siney, C., Kidd, M., Walkinshaw, S., Morrison, C. and Manasse, P. (1995) Opiate dependence in pregnancy. *British Journal of Midwifery* 3(2), 69–73.

Standing Conference on Drug Abuse (SCODA) (1989). *Drug Using Parents and their Children: the second report of the National Local Authority Forum on Drug Abuse in conjunction with SCODA*. London: Association of Metropolitan Authorities.

Weissmann, G. (1991) *Working With Pregnant Women at High Risk for HIV Infection: outreach and intervention*. Rockville, Maryland: National Institute on Drug Abuse.

Chapter 17

Providing care for pregnant women who use drugs
The Glasgow Women's Reproductive Health Service

Mary Hepburn

Drug use occurs throughout the social spectrum but is not a uniform phenomenon. Problem drug use, especially injecting drug use, that involves significant addiction and that causes major medical and social problems is closely associated with socio-economic deprivation (British Medical Association, 1997) which itself causes significant medical and social problems. As a result, the drug use that concerns obstetric services should be recognised as being one of a range of problems associated with deprivation that consequently cannot be managed effectively in isolation. Drug use can adversely affect pregnancy outcome (Chasnoff, 1991; Finnegan, 1982) either directly or as a consequence of its medical complications. Pregnant drug-using women should therefore be recognised as having potentially high-risk pregnancies, and, while much of their maternity care can be delivered by midwives, their management should be obstetrically led. Moreover since both the health and social problems associated with deprivation and with drug use can adversely affect pregnancy outcome, joint health and social management is essential. While deprivation and problem drug use are both associated with poorer health, including poorer pregnancy outcomes, they are also associated with ineffective service use, with pregnant drug-using women tending to attend late and irregularly for antenatal care. The challenge for service providers therefore is to provide maternity care which is appropriate to the women's needs and which the women will want to use.

THE GLASGOW WOMEN'S REPRODUCTIVE HEALTH SERVICE

Service design

The Glasgow Women's Reproductive Health Service (WRHS) is a city-wide service for women with social problems, including drug use, who require additional support. It was established to provide care for those women reluctant or unable to attend standard services, or for whom such services were inappropriate, or did not meet their needs (Hepburn, 1997a). From a single clinic opened in the mid-1980s it expanded to provide a city-wide service in 1990. Based in the Glasgow Royal Maternity Hospital, medically led out-patient care is delivered through a network of community-based multi-disciplinary clinics, each providing a full range of reproductive health care.

Each clinic is staffed by an obstetrician, a midwife and a health visitor, all experienced in providing information and counselling about HIV, hepatitis B and C, and other blood-borne infections. Additional personnel provide help with social problems including information and advice about housing and benefits and help with drug problems. There are local variations, and other professionals participate as available and appropriate, while others contribute on an ad hoc basis. The service is immediately accessible by any route, medical or non-medical, including self-referral; women who attend the service can obtain not only a full range of reproductive health care, but also help with both medical and social problems within a single setting.

Service delivery

Care of pregnant women involves lengthy episodes of care, and since drug-using women have potentially high-risk pregnancies, specialist maternity services should play a lead role; the WRHS therefore provides care for pregnant drug-using women within its own health care-based clinics to which other agencies contribute. While it is obviously sometimes appropriate and necessary to provide some maternity care within addiction services, this should not be the only or even the main setting for delivery of specialised maternity care. Maternity service-based care for pregnant drug-using women is the ideal since it recognises that pregnant drug-using women are pregnant women who have a drug problem and therefore require specialist maternity care rather than drug users who happen to be pregnant. It is therefore less stigmatising and as an additional advantage the broader remit of the WRHS allows women not yet willing or able to admit their drug use to receive appropriate care. Reproductive health care for *non*-pregnant drug-using women does not require lengthy periods of contact and since the WRHS is only one of a number of relevant services, it provides care for non-pregnant women not only in WRHS clinics but also within services co-ordinated by other agencies.

Prevalence and patterns of drug use

As discussed earlier, the service is not exclusively for drug users but drug use is recognised as one of a range of social problems and is managed in this context. Since the service was first established in 1986, the number of drug-using pregnant women attending has steadily risen to the current level of more than 150. A similar number of non-pregnant drug-using women attend. In Glasgow, heroin is the drug of first choice followed by, and often in association with, benzodiazepines, especially temazepam. Both are commonly injected. There is a moderate amount of problem amphetamine use, both oral and injected, while cocaine use, although on the increase, is used recreationally and rarely injected. The majority of drug-using women who attend also use cannabis, and use of tobacco is almost universal. However, we have found that regular consumption of alcohol by drug-using women is extremely uncommon, although some women attempt to stop using drugs by switching to alcohol or use them concurrently.

EFFECTS OF DRUG USE ON PREGNANCY

General effects

Drug use in pregnancy is associated with higher rates of perinatal mortality and morbidity and can affect pregnancy in a number of ways. Women are often concerned that the drugs they use may cause developmental anomalies in the foetus but there is no good evidence of teratogenesis by any of the drugs that are commonly used illicitly. While drug use can affect placental function and hence foetal growth, minor drug withdrawals due to erratic use of opiates can also increase the risk of preterm labour. Consequently there is an increased incidence of low birth weight due either to poor growth or early delivery. This together with other effects of placental compromise, contribute to higher rates of perinatal mortality and morbidity (British Medical Association, 1997). These increases are multifactorial in origin with a major contribution from underlying social circumstances and medical and/or social problems caused by drug use. The effects are exacerbated by erratic drug use and can therefore be minimised through stabilising drug use and/or by use of drugs with a longer half-life.

Neonatal withdrawal symptoms

Opiate/opioid use can cause withdrawal effects before or after birth. Before birth these can include passage of meconium or bowel contents, which, if aspirated, cause lung damage. After birth they include symptoms of varying severity ranging from mild irritability and poor feeding to convulsions. Typically babies are difficult to settle (with a characteristic high pitched cry) and require a high level of nursing. They are hungry but feed ineffectively, and may suffer excessive weight loss. They may have diarrhoea and if they have aspirated bowel contents either before or during delivery, may have breathing problems which can be severe and sometimes life threatening. They may have difficulty in controlling their body temperature.

Neonatal withdrawal symptoms can include a range of other problems, with convulsions an extreme but uncommon manifestation. Benzodiazepines also cause withdrawal symptoms which may be similar to those due to opiates. If both drugs are used simultaneously withdrawals may be particularly severe.

The severity of neonatal withdrawal symptoms is influenced by other health problems in the baby but paradoxically, prematurity may be associated with reduced severity due to the immaturity of the baby's neurological system. The level and pattern of maternal drug use is also important. While in general the degree of severity is dose dependent, the influence of other factors makes it impossible to predict accurately from the level of maternal use, the likelihood or likely severity of withdrawals in an individual baby. However, the risk will be minimised by reducing drug doses as far as possible. Since polydrug use often causes more severe withdrawals, reduction should not be at the expense of stability and the appearance of unexpectedly severe withdrawal symptoms should raise the suspicion of polydrug use, or 'topping up' on prescribed drugs.

Cocaine use is associated with a number of specific problems due to its powerful action in causing blood vessels to constrict. This can cause separation of the placenta and consequently death of the baby in the uterus (Chasnoff et al., 1985). It can also interfere with blood supply to the foetus preventing normal development of parts of the foetus including limbs or bowel. It has also been reported to cause withdrawal symptoms in the baby after birth, but any such problems are a consequence of antenatal complications rather than true withdrawals. Reports of bad pregnancy outcomes may be unduly alarmist since there is evidence of a bias towards publication of such data rather than data showing no adverse effects (Koren et al., 1989). The more severe problems may be restricted to chaotic use and/or injecting.

MANAGEMENT OF PROBLEM DRUG USE IN PREGNANCY: GENERAL PRINCIPLES

Management of opiate/opioid use

There is a lack of consensus over the management of illicit drug use in general. The arguments largely centre on harm reduction through prescription of substitute medication versus detoxification with a view to abstinence. These options are often viewed as absolute and mutually exclusive. The arguments over management in pregnancy follow similar lines. In favour of substitution therapy is that it promotes stability of lifestyle and facilitates regular contact with services while removing the need to obtain drugs illegally or money to procure drugs (Farrell et al., 1994). Additionally, for opiate/opioid use, substitution with methadone with its long half-life reduces fluctuations in levels of drug in the body with beneficial effects on the pregnancy. The WRHS provides substitute prescribing of methadone on an in-patient and/or out-patient basis for pregnant opiate/opioid-using women.

While the role of substitution therapy for opiate users is acknowledged, antenatal detoxification from opiates is still widely perceived as risky with 'cold turkey' detoxification considered unacceptably hazardous to the foetus. Various regimes are advocated, usually with very slow rates of reduction and often restricted to the mid-trimester. However, this has not been the experience of the WRHS (Hepburn, 1997b). Opiate/opioid-using women attending the WRHS have the option of antenatal detoxification at any stage of pregnancy, at any speed and as often as required. Although not unacceptably hazardous to the foetus, opiate detoxification should always be carried out under close obstetric supervision; rapid detoxification is often unsuccessful on an out-patient basis and in this situation the maternity ward will usually be the most appropriate setting.

Given that the severity of neonatal withdrawal symptoms can be influenced by the maternal drug dose, there is no dose above which withdrawal symptoms are inevitable or below which their avoidance can be guaranteed. While withdrawal symptoms will be minimised by keeping maternal drug use as low as possible, overzealous attempts to reduce drug use, including unrealistic attempts to achieve abstinence, may jeopardise stability. Equally, while it has undoubted benefits, methadone is not without disadvantages and as an opioid has actions in common with the drugs it replaces. Very high doses of methadone will have adverse effects on the pregnancy and will exacerbate neonatal withdrawal symptoms. Methadone remains the substitute opioid of choice because of its long duration of action, its documented medical and social benefits, and the absence of evidence to date of superiority of alternative drugs, but its benefits must be weighed against its disadvantages. Detoxification should be suspended at any stage if failure seems likely. On the other hand, total elimination of illicit drug use may not be feasible and increasing the dose of methadone to very high levels in pursuit of this goal may be counterproductive.

It is therefore important to remember that the aims of prescribing for pregnant and non-pregnant drug-using women are not identical and during pregnancy the aim should simply be to reduce overall drug use to the lowest level compatible with acceptable stability. For any individual woman this level may not be constant during pregnancy. Maintenance and detoxification should therefore be interchangeable with the dose of methadone increased, decreased, or kept constant as deemed appropriate by ongoing assessment. It is often suggested that methadone doses will need to rise in later pregnancy but this has not been the experience of the WRHS. Indeed, the converse usually proves true and women often achieve the greatest reductions in dosage in the third trimester being motivated by a desire to reduce neonatal withdrawal symptoms. Pregnancy provides motivation for short-term reductions in methadone dosage to levels which may not be sustainable in the long term. There should be recognition of the possible temporary nature of this reduction and consequently the likely need to increase methadone doses after delivery.

Management of other types of drug use

The argument for substitution therapy for other types of drug use is less clear. Amongst heavy chaotic-injecting amphetamine users substitute prescribing may improve stability of lifestyle and be helpful in promoting contact with services. However, amphetamines per se have no major impact on pregnancy outcome and there is no good evidence of benefit from prescribing. There is no evidence of any kind of benefit from maintenance prescription of substitute benzodiazepines, and, in view of their harmful effects, both medically and socially on mother and baby, they should not be prescribed to pregnant women. There is no effective substitute for cocaine. Within the WRHS, maintenance substitution therapy is therefore limited to prescription of methadone.

For those drugs for which substitution therapy is not appropriate, ante-natal detoxification is the only option and there is no evidence that this is unsafe for the foetus. Benzodiazepine withdrawal, however, carries a risk of maternal convulsions; consequently, in the maternal interests, the WRHS offers in-patient detoxification covered by a reducing benzodiazepine regime with diazepam the drug of choice because of its relatively long half-life. There is continuing debate about the timescale advisable for benzodiazepine withdrawal in general, with a relatively slow speed usually advocated in the interests of long-term success. However, this is not the priority in pregnancy, when the damaging effects make rapid reduction more important. Experience in the WRHS has demonstrated that a detoxification period as short as a week is adequate to prevent convulsions regardless of the dose of benzodiazepines used. This allows safe detoxification under supervision without out-patient prescription of benzodiazepines and without a prolonged in-patient stay. Relapse can be managed in the same way and does not indicate that the original detoxification constituted inappropriate management.

Administration of substitution therapy

Appropriate management of problem drug use involves participation by maternity, primary care, addiction and social services and requires close collaboration between them. Few maternity services will have the volume of experience required to undertake substitute prescribing; this will therefore usually be provided by addiction services based on either a primary care or psychiatric model. Nevertheless, maternity services should always be involved in decisions about substitution therapy, particularly changes in therapy, and should monitor the effect on the pregnancy of such therapy. Moreover, if reduction in prescribed drugs is planned at a speed that requires in-patient care this should ideally be carried out in a maternity hospital and certainly under maternity supervision. Circumstances in Glasgow, however, are unusual in that the WRHS was developed before an effective prescribing service was established and consequently undertook prescription of methadone for pregnant women. Because of its city-wide remit and the high level of problem drug use locally the WRHS gained considerable experience and continues to provide substitute prescribing in most cases. This has the advantage of allowing speedy response when changes need to be made and flexibility when co-ordinating in-patient and out-patient care.

Regardless of the source of substitution therapy during pregnancy it is essential to ensure that the woman will have access to prescribing services after delivery. This is important even if the woman plans to be drug free by delivery since the need for future medication, while hopefully unnecessary, cannot be ruled out.

OBSTETRIC MANAGEMENT

Antenatal care

When a drug-using woman presents for antenatal care it is important to obtain information about her pattern of drug use – which drugs, how much, how often, by what route, for how long, at what cost and how financed – and then to agree a strategy for dealing with her problem. It is also important to take a social history including information about a partner (if any), sources of support (including professional agencies, especially drugs and social services, with which she may be involved), previous children and their care arrangements, current housing, sources of income and legal problems, including outstanding prosecutions. It is essential, as in the care of all pregnant women, to establish the circumstances of the pregnancy – whether it was planned, intended and/or wanted, whether her partner is the baby's father and the nature of the woman's relationship with the baby's father (particularly relevant if she has been financing her drug use by prostitution).

Drug-using women are often reported to attend late for antenatal care making it difficult to establish gestation accurately. Late presentation is often attributed to ignorance of the pregnancy due to the amenorrhoea that frequently accompanies drug use. This has not been the experience of the WRHS. In the presence of amenorrhoea women have overdiagnosed rather than underdiagnosed pregnancy and the average booking gestation of 14 weeks is comparable to the hospital average (Hepburn and Elliott, 1997).

Content of care

The woman should be given factual information about the effects of drug use on pregnancy but reassured that major damage to the foetus is very unlikely and that subsequent adverse effects will be limited by control of her drug use. Liaison with paediatric services is important and antenatal visits to the labour ward and the special care nursery are helpful. In the absence of significant risk of teratogenesis, a detailed scan to screen for foetal anomaly is not especially indicated for drug-using women but can be reassuring. Regular weighing while ineffective as a measure of foetal well-being is a useful indicator of stability of drug use. Serial scans in the third trimester to assess foetal growth and well-being are necessary if there is evidence of problems.

While cervical smears are not routinely carried out during pregnancy women attending the WRHS, who may not attend at other times, are encouraged to have this done if due. Screening for genital tract infection can be carried out at the same time and is especially relevant for women financing drug use by prostitution. All women attending the WRHS are given information about, and the offer of, screening for hepatitis B, hepatitis C and HIV infections. Women are also screened for immunity to hepatitis B. Those with no evidence of prior exposure are offered a course of hepatitis B vaccine during pregnancy.

Taking blood for routine investigations may be difficult if there is significant damage to veins from drug injecting. However, under no circumstances is it ever appropriate to invite women to take their own blood. When carried out by health care professionals this is a therapeutic intervention but for drug-using women injecting is part of a problem they are trying to give up. The two situations should never be confused.

Drug-using women should be screened for drug-related health problems which may affect their pregnancy or its management. A history of endocarditis may indicate damage to the heart valves and the need for antibiotic cover during labour or any surgical procedure. A history of deep vein thrombosis is usually related to drug injection and merits prophylactic anticoagulant therapy. However, such women should also be screened for susceptibility to thrombosis. Constipation is common among drug-using women due to poor diet and also to use of opiate or opioid drugs. Dietary advice is therefore indicated. Poor diet, together with poor hygiene, contributes to dental problems often exacerbated by drinking methadone syrup. Pregnancy provides an opportunity to deal with carious teeth, which in the presence of damaged heart valves are a focus of infection that should be removed. In this situation extraction should be carried out under antibiotic cover.

It may be difficult to persuade drug-using women to attend antenatal classes. ParentCraft instruction, which addresses their specific needs, may be more appropriately delivered on a one-to-one basis.

Intrapartum and postpartum care

Midwives in the WRHS provide continuity in in-patient and out-patient care both antenatally and postnatally but do not undertake intrapartum care, which is provided by standard labour ward staff. WRHS staff can, however, maintain contact during labour. Formal evaluation of the service confirms that the women are happy with this arrangement and do not feel it is important for them to be delivered by a midwife personally known to them (Hepburn and Elliott, 1997).

Drug use is associated with an increased risk of preterm labour but even those who do not deliver early rarely go beyond term, and usually labour quickly. Therefore while women on methadone or related drugs may in theory need increased doses of opiate analgesics in labour, this has not proved to be the case for women attending the WRHS. Equally, while there is a low threshold for epidural anaesthesia, drug-using women do not choose this more often than other women. Thus the problems which might be anticipated on theoretical grounds often prove irrelevant in practice.

After delivery, mothers and babies go together to the maternity ward. Neonatal withdrawal symptoms do not invariably lead to admission to the nursery nor are they considered an automatic indication for medication. Babies of drug-using women like all other babies are therefore managed as medically indicated.

In the absence of absolute contraindications and provided their drug use is stable, drug-using women are encouraged to breast feed to minimise neo-natal withdrawal symptoms. Maternal HIV infection is a contraindication because of the increased risk of vertical transmission. The evidence suggests that hepatitis C is not transmitted by breast feeding but there is no absolute proof of this. However, the enormous benefits of breast feeding for these particularly vulnerable babies outweighs any tiny theoretical risk. Maternal hepatitis B infection is not a contraindication to breast feeding. Stability of drug use cannot be rigidly defined by a particular level of use and should be individually assessed. However, the successful establishment of breast feeding is in itself adequate evidence of acceptable stability. Women should be aware that breast feeding must not be suddenly discontinued.

SOCIAL MANAGEMENT

During pregnancy

Close collaboration between medical and social services is essential, and drug-using women should be encouraged to accept early input from social services. This should be supportive and aimed at prevention rather than crisis intervention. In the WRHS, weekly liaison meetings are held in asso-ciation with each of the clinics. These meetings are attended by the clinic staff and chaired by a senior social worker from a local team. The social work department's policy is one of early allocation. At the liaison meetings information is shared with the women's knowledge and consent. Their problems are discussed and plans made to provide appropriate support. Other professionals involved with the women can attend to share information on an ad hoc basis. Multi-disciplinary planning meetings for individual women are held at 32 weeks' gestation and again postnatally.

The woman's stability of lifestyle should be assessed throughout pregnancy with support provided as necessary to ensure she will be able to care for her child. It is inappropriate to wait until after delivery and then only take action if problems arise. It is particularly inappropriate to base this assessment on the presence or absence of neonatal withdrawal symptoms. The mother's level of drug use cannot give an accurate prediction of the baby's condition. It is equally impossible to use the baby's condition as a measure of the severity of the mother's drug use.

After delivery

While the remit of the WRHS allows antenatal admission on social grounds it also allows a longer postnatal stay to continue support and instruction in the necessary childcare skills, as well as assessment of parenting abilities. The early involvement of social services enables rapid preventative action that can reduce the risk of crises which might delay the woman's postnatal discharge home with her baby or jeopardise her chances of retaining care of her child. This approach has been the joint policy of health and social services in Glasgow since the mid-1980s and is also the nationally recognised model of good practice (LGDF & SCODA, 1997).

After the woman's return home with her baby, maternity services have a limited role. However, since the WRHS provides a full range of reproductive health care, including contraceptive care, it often has an ongoing though less intense relationship with women for whom it has provided maternity care. Although it no longer prescribes substitute medication, the service can nevertheless continue to collaborate with the main partners in primary care, addiction and social services. In Glasgow community drug prescribing services are primary care based, so there is considerable overlap between the three services, which enhances effective collaboration.

SUMMARY

The Glasgow Women's Reproductive Health Service provides city-wide community-based multi-disciplinary care for women with social problems and it is in this context that pregnant drug-using women are managed. They are therefore regarded as pregnant women who have social problems including drug use. The service adopts a social model of health with close collaboration between all relevant agencies both medical and non-medical. Early social support is provided with a philosophy of prevention rather than crisis intervention to help women to have healthy babies for whom they can be effective parents. The aim of the service is to provide women with appropriate care which meets their needs and which they will be willing and able to use to help them achieve these outcomes. That the service is acceptable to the women is demonstrated by a high rate of self-referral and has been confirmed by formal evaluation (Hepburn and Elliott, 1997).

REFERENCES

British Medical Association (1997) *The Misuse of Drugs*. Amsterdam: Harwood Academic Publishers.
Chasnoff, I.J. (1991) Chemical dependency and pregnancy. *Clinics in Perinatology* 18, 1–191.
Chasnoff, I.J., Burns, W.J., Schnoll, S.H. and Burns, K.A. (1985) Cocaine use in pregnancy. *New England Journal of Medicine* 313, 666–669.
Farrell, M., Ward, J. and Mattick, R. *et al.* (1994) Methadone maintenance treatment in opiate dependence: a review. *British Medical Journal* 309, 997–1001.
Finnegan, L.P. (1982) Outcome of children born to women dependent on narcotics, in: B. Stimmel (ed.) *The Effects of Maternal Alcohol and Drug Abuse on the New Born*, 55–102. New York: Haworth Press.
Hepburn, M. (1997a) Horses for courses: developing services for women with special needs. *British Journal of Midwifery* 5(8), 482–484.
Hepburn, M. (1997b) Drugs of addiction, in: F. Cockburn (ed.) *Advances in Perinatal Medicine*, 120–124. Carnforth: Parthenon Publishing Group.
Hepburn, M. and Elliott, L. (1997) A community obstetric service for women with special needs. *British Journal of Midwifery* 5(8), 485–488.
Koren, G., Graham, K., Shear, H. and Einarson, T. (1989) Bias against the null hypothesis: the reproductive hazards of cocaine. *The Lancet*, 16 December 1440–1442.
Local Government Drugs Forum (LGDF) and Standing Conference on Drug Abuse (SCODA) (1997) *Drug Using Parents: policy guidelines for inter-agency working*. London: LGA Publications.

Part V

Implications for policy

The data produced by our research on pregnant drug users highlighted aspects of the delivery of care that generated anxiety, fear, deception, confusion and antagonism among the women who took part. They are the barriers to productive relationships between health and social service providers and their drug-using clients.

These barriers are the subjects of the first chapter in this part, and some ideas are offered that may be useful in overcoming them. This analysis focuses on issues with implications for service delivery and the uptake of services by drug-using mothers. We hope that other implications, perhaps more apparent to practitioners, will be identified in our data and actively pursued in order to improve the service.

The second chapter returns to the problems of child welfare that are associated with drug dependence and poses the question of whether it is possible to ensure that children are safeguarded while cultivating bonds with drug-using parents. Attitudes towards child protection, and the dilemmas faced by social welfare workers are explored in the US literature, and recent models of family interventions examined to assess their wider relevance to other cultures.

The final chapter looks at policy and practice development in the UK in the context of global trends in service delivery to pregnant drug users. The concept of 'shared care' is the cornerstone of UK government policy on drugs and is a reflection of trends elsewhere in advocating multi-agency teams. Some of the problems associated with achieving full professional liaison between agencies are described here. Two examples of care provision are outlined that are not necessarily independent procedurally, the drugs liaison midwife and the multi-agency service.

Chapter 18

Overcoming the barriers

Hilary Klee

Although it is several years since the deficiencies in services for drug-using women were identified in Europe, they remain poor. Expert meetings, reports, recommendations for improvements and a slow but steady growth in support among professional and research communities (see Chapter 20) have not led to much improvement. The 'cause' seems to have languished in a state of virtual reality in which the main players are missing and only their representatives take the stage. Deterred by what they see as insurmountable barriers, the women themselves do not appear. It seems that these barriers are not imaginary; they are revealed as soon as safe concealment has to be abandoned and the women are obliged to invite scrutiny by health professionals.

Pregnancy and early motherhood for many drug-using women is a time of anxiety and stress in which uncertainty and fear are common emotions. The failure of services to acknowledge this and neutralise those fears that originate in the services themselves perpetuates these responses. It is interesting that a recent national survey of mothers (Birth in Britain Today: Survey 2001) has revealed general dissatisfaction about aspects of antenatal care and hospital confinement. Only drug-using women, however, are likely to face active hostility and lack of understanding and support. Whether through ignorance or prejudice these deficiencies can have serious consequences for the more vulnerable among them. Explicit attribution of blame for withdrawal symptoms in the child and its subsequent removal can threaten the bonding process that is the root of mother–child attachment. Problematic childcare is added to the constellation of their anxieties. If an early relapse follows, the opportunity for an escape from the drug-oriented lifestyle for them and their children slips away.

The recurring themes that run through the chapters in this book emanate from negative attitudes and discriminatory procedures revealed by this research that are incompatible with good practice. An ideal service would be run by staff who are universally well informed, insightful, consistent, sympathetic, supportive and work well together. There are a number of barriers to be overcome before such a goal is reached. The main barriers are revisited in this chapter with recommendations on how they may be approached.

NEGATIVE DISCRIMINATION: BEING JUDGED

I do feel sympathy for them when they've had a terrible time at the hospital . . . I've been there myself when one person has been dealt with in not a very nice manner by the doctor . . . I've thought 'I'm glad I'm not in your shoes.' Really, there was no need for that to occur.

The drug-using woman fails to conform to societal ideals of a 'good' mother, or even a 'good enough' mother. She may be attributed a particularly unpleasant set of characteristics associated with specific versions of the general stereotype: devious manipulator; aggressive troublemaker; weak-willed helpless victim; unwashed self-neglecting junkie; sex worker; and, of course, someone who puts her own self-gratification before the care of her children. The stereotype precedes her during pregnancy into encounters with those who are charged with her care. She may believe that they will expect her to conform to the ideal. If she is sensible she will be compliant. If she is resentful, she will be additionally labelled as a troublemaker, and this will conveniently reinforce the stereotype.

No service can be effective if its clients will not willingly co-operate. For some time many of those who treat drug users have settled for compliance, which is a poor substitute for active co-operation since the behavioural change in following the rules or wishes of those with power will not be underpinned by the attitudinal change that is necessary to sustain it in the long term. Compliance is skin deep and closely allied to the use of deception, as we have witnessed in this and other studies of drug users in treatment (Klee and Wright, 1999).

The data from this study, although based on a limited sample of professionals, suggest a growing awareness of the specific needs of drug-using women. However, it is evident from the women's accounts that the impact of those that lack understanding and sensitivity has strong and long-lasting effects. Maternity staff can acquire a reputation as judgemental and insensitive autocrats, and social workers are seen as nosy, interfering and positively dangerous. Such summary evaluations spread easily through drug-using networks. When both carer and client have rigid stereotypes of the other, effective communication becomes impossible. It is an unpleasant experience for both the woman and those who are responsible for her care.

Recommendation

Greater familiarity with the social precursors of drug use among women and their current lifestyle will help to soften the stereotype. Education and training, particularly if this includes some input from drug-using mothers, may go some way to broaden the views of medical staff. However, progress is likely to be impeded by problematic interactions in which the women's fears result in a level of defensiveness that is difficult to transcend, and it is at this point that specialist help is needed.

EXPOSURE OF DRUG USE

I think it's lack of thought rather than people intentionally breaking confidentiality. They discuss things without thinking who else is within earshot.

Unnecessary exposure is another fear that leads women to protect themselves through concealment and deception. The most dangerous environment for a new mother is the Special Care Baby Unit. If the staff are put under pressure to lie to relatives, alienation is almost inevitable. It puts into question the appropriateness of the child's presence there unless there is serious risk to health. More generally, unless there is an agreed definition among professionals about what can be shared and with whom that is made known to her in advance, she will not be able with any certainty to identify disclosures that are 'safe'. Without knowledge of the rules she fears entrapment. The need for agreement on confidentiality is particularly acute for her since such details may lead to the breakdown of personal relationships and interventions that can result in the removal of her child. Exposure of the women's drug use was mostly unintentional and those procedures that risked a breach of confidentiality may be less typical in the future. However, such lapses quickly become part of the folklore of drug-using networks that has a long life, and they seem to have a disproportionate effect on the image that services present.

Recommendation

It should be of concern that the exercise of confidentiality seemed idiosyncratic and open to various interpretations in this study. There were differences of opinion between different categories of service providers that undermined the process of 'working together'. It appeared to be largely resolved in those services with a high degree of liaison between professional groups, or a multi-disciplinary team with formal procedures and regular meetings. These are emerging in urban areas in the UK but there are still regions where such developments have very low priority and need to be put further up the agenda.

PROFESSIONAL INCONSISTENCY ON DRUG MANAGEMENT

The lack of credibility of service providers also contributed to the negative image of some services. Much of this concerned the effects of methadone on the foetus. Not only did drug workers disagree with maternity staff on the best way to manage the administration of methadone during pregnancy, they also disagreed among themselves:

> There was conflicting advice at the antenatal stage between the drug team and the hospital . . . the antenatal service was not preparing the women, not giving them reliable information on what they could expect postnatally both for them and their baby. It caused a lot of problems.

The outcome of this disagreement was manifest in the women's independent action on the amount of methadone they used. It was also hidden since they were dependent on the agency staff for their supply, and did not wish to risk their disapproval or the possibility that a temporary change to their prescription would become permanent. A way of improving the credibility of health professionals is needed – the woman's psychological well-being depends in part on a belief that she and her child are in safe hands.

Recommendation

It seems that the discovery of a reliable method of relating drug consumption during pregnancy to neonatal withdrawal is unlikely in the near future. The use of illicit drugs of uncertain quality and polydrug use is common in early pregnancy and it is difficult to see a solution to this problem other than communicating more compelling prevention messages about the need for birth control until a pregnancy is planned. However, although the probability of NAS may remain uncertain, the advice about methadone consumption should be consistent across professional groups. This may then limit independent action by the woman and remove the sense of total responsibility for the child's state that some women have.

PROFESSIONAL CREDIBILITY AND PATIENT CONFIDENCE

A user-friendly service does not necessarily mean an improved service. The lack of knowledge about drug use among maternity staff also affects the quality of their care. Respondents were surprised when medical staff admitted to knowing little about drugs and their effects. It was evident that some staff, possibly aware of the danger to their credibility of such an admission, volunteered an opinion anyway. Similarly, there were drug workers who lacked information concerning midwifery services and procedures.

The home environment

It is critical that health service personnel should have good insights into the nature of the problems faced by their patients in the home. Apart from counteracting stereotypic profiles, they sensitise staff to signs of dysfunction and risks to the health of mother and child. If support is deficient or missing in the home environment there need to be procedures ready to supplement or replace them.

A case in point is the powerful influence of partners. The majority of the respondents were living with a drug-using partner and although there were agreements between them to reduce drugs, apparently with the best of intentions, few partners persisted in their efforts after the first few weeks. This is a disappointing outcome since most women made serious efforts to modify their use. Those who reduced their drug use and maintained the reduction were those with supportive partners and mothers.

Services can play a major role in providing support where family support is missing but health professionals may not be alerted to the need, particularly if the woman is fearful of admitting that she is having difficulty in coping. If there are attempts at concealment by the patient, then family dysfunction may go unnoticed until it reaches crisis proportions.

Recommendations

If both the mother and her partner are in treatment there is an opportunity for drug workers to work with both of them as a unit. Accurate evaluation of the level of coping simply on the basis of the mother's self-report is difficult. After the birth of the child the health visitor is best placed to acquire information (*Working Together*, 1999). In this study there were several that took action at this time and provided support. Multi-disciplinary interventions based on family units have been the subject of considerable research in the US (for example, Kumpfer, 1994; Kumpfer, 1998; Kumpfer *et al.*, 1989) and this is an approach that could be investigated elsewhere.

Drug workers identified a need for information about antenatal and hospital procedures. This would facilitate better communication with midwifery services. In addition, their understanding of drug dependence was restricted mostly to heroin; they needed information about stimulants in general and amphetamine in particular. These deficits should be easily remedied with brief, but regularly updated, training courses, and also seminars on these topics that are open to all professional groups involved in the care of drug-using women.

Understanding drug dependence and relapse

The relationship between dependence on drugs and health and social problems is also an important part of the information that should be made available to maternity and social welfare staff. Ideally such general knowledge should be enhanced by specific information about a patient's level of dependence. It is particularly important to include information about relapse and the circumstances that precipitate a return to street drug use. An environmental cue will act as a trigger, for example the presence of another drug user, drug administration paraphernalia, a place associated with past drug use, or even talking about drugs. The range of cues is as extensive as the number of variables habitually present when drugs are taken. There are multiple risk factors but few protective factors. The study consistently supported the notion that a new infant is a powerful motivating force towards abstinence. Apart from the attachment behaviour that is initiated by signs of distress – the baby's presence is a distraction and its demands require active engagement with an adult carer. The common complaint of drug users trying to stay off drugs is that the structure of day-to-day life disappears and there is nothing to replace the drug-focused activities: buying the drugs, administering them and getting the money to buy more. With a new baby the day is easily filled and in a positive way for most mothers of healthy babies.

Recommendation

The baby's influence has to be powerful to compete with drug cues but this remains the most likely life event that will empower a woman to abstain. Other changes are needed to support her, however. Research has consistently shown that the domestic and social context has to be radically changed. While strong environmental cues are present only limited success can be anticipated and relocation is often sought. Drug and social workers are well aware of this but are limited by the level of resources available for aftercare. This would be a wise form of investment that would reap dividends if it reduced the incidence of relapse and avoided removal of the child with its damaging emotional costs to mother and child and high financial costs to the state.

FEAR OF SOCIAL WORK INTERVENTION

The overwhelming concern of the women was to avoid the child being taken into care. Their fears centred on social workers but there was more agreement between drug workers and social workers than would have been anticipated from the differences between them in terms of their respective professional interests. Most acknowledged that parenting behaviour among drug users fell into the same range as non-users:

I suppose if I'm being totally objective I don't think they make any worse or any better parents than most other people. They've got the same potential for abusing their children physically, emotionally or whatever.

(Drug worker)

There are some drug users and it's not a particular problem . . . but in other cases the drug use is part of the problem. If they're chaotic and intoxicated they're not capable of caring.

(Social worker)

Once the child is born, the key professionals in the mother's life in the early months are the health visitor, a drug worker if she is in treatment and possibly a social worker. An admission that she is not coping may invite an intervention. There are reasons why she may find childcare difficult and there are likely to be problems in relating to the child, particularly if it is ill or disturbed.

Social workers were aware of these factors and were making efforts to promote an image that was less threatening to drug-using women. However, there were barriers to productive relationships between them: the mother's uncontrolled drug use; poor bonding and care of the baby; poor parenting skills; and her fear of social services.

Using drugs: restoring stability

Uncontrolled drug use by the mother or a family member is hazardous for a child and it requires a sensitive approach by a health professional or social worker to maintain constructive contact with the mother that improves the prospect of adequate care. It was evident from this research that there were some social workers who were very skilled in reassuring the mother that there were ways of surviving this phase that would not result in the removal of her child (Klee and Jackson, 1998). The women who had lost earlier children through care orders and had a known history had been chastened by the experience and were determined not to allow it to happen again. However, their experiences did not always mean that their child rearing practices were improved, the guilt in some cases producing overanxious, sometimes overprotective, interactions that could lead to different problems (Klee *et al.*, 1998). Again this might be remediated by a watchful health visitor or social worker. Such monitoring over an extended period of time is needed and adequate resources should be available for the professionals concerned.

Bonding

For the women the problems began immediately the baby was born if it was removed for observation into a Special Care Baby Unit. Current UK guidelines (LGDF/SCODA, 1997) indicate that this should be avoided as long as there is no risk to the child. However, not only is there variation in professional estimates of risk, it seems that there are practical considerations of human resource management in hospitals. In practice the decision seems to be made increasingly on the basis of a number of factors in addition to the state of health of the infant. It is recognised that the potential for adequate childcare is badly affected by early and prolonged disruption to the bonding process. This may persist if the child continues to be sick.

Recommendation

There was little real preparation for the task of nursing a baby with NAS. It is possible that advance information about such a depressing prospect for a woman, who may already be in a state of anxiety, was considered unwise by maternity staff. Recourse to drugs was an option that offered her the easiest solution if there was no other form of support. Guidance in coping with such infants and subsequent reassurance is needed. For these respondents health visitors fulfilled this role well but inevitably the positive aspects of mothering disappeared at this time. Reviving them requires more intensive counselling interventions that will lessen the strain on the mother and afford some relief from her sense of guilt and heavy responsibility.

Parenting

The parenting skills of many respondents were perceived by them to be inadequate to cope with an infant suffering withdrawal. There was praise for health visitors, and their role in helping the mother was critical to the mother's perception of her abilities. Apart from this there seemed to be few ways of acquiring information or developing skills in childcare that were attractive to the women, which are, perhaps, more important for these mothers than many others. It may be that help was available to the respondents in difficulties but was not pursued. In particular, the women's accounts of protecting the child from the drug-oriented environment showed at times a poor understanding of a child's capacity to notice drug-related activities or adult conversations. This may be remediable with educational interventions or family therapy but such a strategy faces problems if it is not invited by the mother. In the US, courts in some states are empowered to order compliance with parenting programmes (Reid *et al.*, 1999) but European developments, which are somewhat more liberal, are some way behind these initiatives on family dysfunction. Meanwhile, the mother's fear of the consequences of admitting problems to health professionals remains strong and will be difficult to remove.

Recommendation

Initial advice and subsequent guidance is vital over the first few weeks or months. Other interventions seemed less useful. The mixed classes in parenting that are currently available in some areas are unlikely to be popular with this group since exposure will remain a concern for them and they could be demoralised by contact with women who do not face similar problems and who are more successful.

Avoiding the attention of social services

The reticence of mothers in seeking information and advice was noted by different groups of professionals in this research. It seems to be due mainly to their fear of exposure or engaging in dialogue over which they have no control. This is particularly apparent in their attitude to social workers whose reputation for removing the children of drug-using parents still persisted.

The potential value of social work is seriously undermined at present if the observations made of this sample are characteristic of the situation elsewhere. The women did not want to seek help, believing that they put themselves at risk by doing so. Given their key role in family support, the service needs, and in some areas probably already deserves, a better image. From the woman's point of view what is missing is a way of making an accurate assessment of the risk in approaching them. Information about the aims of social workers in preserving the family, offering guidance rather than judgement and so forth, does not appear to be generally filtering through to them. This will be the case particularly for those women who are not receiving drug treatment.

Recommendation

It seems that there is still a need to quell the fears of mothers. They apparently do not believe social work statements about the constructive approach now adopted towards family support (see Chapter 13). Until this is established in the minds of drug-using women it will be difficult to convince them that the stories they hear on their network are not examples of unwarranted interference. There is a need for a more radical approach to working with parents, preferably one that is seen to encompass all vulnerable families and not visibly single out drug users as an especially difficult case. It should be proactive and empowering in publicly acknowledging the real bonds that can exist between drug-using mothers and their children.

WORKING TOGETHER: PROFESSIONAL CONSISTENCY

Attitude change and resistance to compromise

Increasing professional awareness of the factors underlying the women's behaviour cannot be guaranteed to change attitudes and produce greater tolerance. The pressure to agree on common policy appeared to be an irritant to some staff. Drug workers were 'adult centred' – a term used by them and implying a contrast with 'child-centred' care. The health of the woman was the major focus, although the requirement to safeguard the interests of children was admitted in interview. There were differences between agencies and drug workers within agencies in how far they pursued an assessment of such issues with the client. This was due to a concern to ensure that the service should be regarded as user-friendly by women and a conviction that no aspect of treatment should drive women away or deter others from presenting. This was a pragmatic approach that gave high priority to the danger of driving drug-related problems underground, which made them inaccessible to interventions and hence risk greater damage to the client and her family.

> I would be the last person in the world to see a child hurt or injured or at risk, but at the end of the day I think people have to accept that this service is not about protecting the child. Our responsibility is not children . . . there are agencies out there whose responsibility is children. I think that once we start crossing that line all we do is frighten people off, and that won't protect children at all because the parents won't come here.
>
> (Drug worker)

Because of their efforts and experiences with drug users, drug workers believed they knew the capacities and limitations of their client group and felt these were not appreciated by other professional groups.

Among obstetricians, nurses and midwives there was a combination of sympathy for the mother and of substantial concern for the child. The maternity staff were likely to endorse conventional social expectations, which was very rare in drug workers. If the mother was seen to be trying to meet those demands, hospital staff were more likely to be sympathetic. Those in paediatric departments and Special Care Baby Units were least likely to excuse the mother's drug use during pregnancy and most likely to apply negative stereotypes indiscriminately. This was also true of some of the social workers specialising in child protection.

Sharing information

In addition to the issues that relate to face-to-face interactions with drug-using pregnant women, the deficiencies in communication between professional groups generated problems for them if they assumed their details were known or were uncertain whether they had been passed on:

> I think the problem with all of these agencies is the fact that everyone is under a different umbrella . . . they feel that everything that they have is confidential and I think they forget that we've got a confidentiality clause as well and that presents a problem.
>
> (Community midwife, on getting information from drug agencies)

> I think it just needs someone to sit down and . . . well . . . it needs someone to bang their heads together in some ways . . . there's no reason why your information shouldn't be available to us. It's daft really. It's not being used in a punitive way, all being well, so there's no reason not to share it between professional people who need to know. Obviously you don't want everyone knowing about it, but professional people do need to know about these things.
>
> (Paediatrician)

We found a high proportion of professionals who were in disagreement about the procedures governing the sharing of information and the relative importance of infant and maternal health and welfare. In some cases this seemed to be a way of protecting traditional professional views and practices and did not allow for flexibility in dealing with other professional groups.

Nonetheless, on childcare issues there was general recognition and agreement that child safety overrides confidentiality, and that there is an obligation to notify child protection teams of problems. Drug workers seemed to be the targets of most criticism from other groups. The inclusion of certain professional groups in the 'need to know' category was not consistent in any professional group and there was no mention of discussions aimed at resolving the problems. Confidentiality was the cornerstone of the difficulties observed in inter-agency co-operation and co-ordination and is an issue that must have high priority when developing models of care.

There were many complaints about the lack of communication of critical information. For example, a health visitor complained that she was not supplied with advance information about new mothers with problems but was expected to pick up the case and proceed on the basis of case notes alone. Poor communication was sometimes blamed on inadequate resourcing in the form of staff shortages on antenatal and postnatal wards, and among drugs and social workers. Some peripatetic workers were described as 'elusive' and problems had been dealt with by the time contact was made with them. Lines of communication in most regions where liaison was not formally developed were deficient in some way and gave rise to exasperation and resentment. It seems that working together is adversely affected by several factors and will not improve until they are addressed and resolved at procedural levels:

* Disparities in definitions of confidentiality.
* Differences in attitudes towards drug use and priorities between professional groups.
* A restricted focus on one aspect of the client at the expense of others; for example, the health of the foetus, drug dependence, the capacity to care for the child.

Recommendation

The exhortation for professionals to work together is not enough to ensure their engagement in this process. In the field of services for pregnant drug users there are notable successes, but failures too. It can be argued that radical change requires time for participants to adapt. However, there seems to have been no independent research in the UK that focuses specifically on the impediments to full collaboration that inhibit the development of multi-disciplinary teams, or research on the critical predictors of success. Given that working together or 'shared care' (DoH, 1999: 10–15) is allocated the status of a universal principle in 'tackling drugs' (UK Government Cm 2846, 1995), this should now be considered. There are many versions of shared care protocols currently in operation in the UK (Gerada and Tighe, 1999) and profiling and evaluating them would accelerate progress towards a consistently high quality service.

SUMMARY AND CONCLUSIONS

Services designed for non-drug users are based on a model of motherhood that sets standards that are unattainable by the majority of pregnant drug users. This is now changing as their numbers increase, but the education and training of staff lags behind. The first point that needs to be addressed is education and training for medical staff across a broad range of areas that includes not only social and medical aspects of drug use but also training in interpersonal skills that can defuse hostile situations and deal with defensiveness. The second point is consistency. There is a need to agree to a policy that cuts across professional boundaries and resolving issues of confidentiality should be given high priority. Consistency in advice given to mothers is important despite the differences in opinion within and between groups. Guidelines have been constructed on the best available data and it is in the interests of the women that they feel secure in following them.

These measures should result in an increasingly skilled workforce that delivers high quality support for the mother. Support is critical for a drug-using woman throughout pregnancy, childbirth and into early motherhood while she is in danger of relapse. When informal support in the home is lacking this should be detected and professional help offered that will complement any existing support. There should be provision for aftercare facilities that will be sustained until family support is sufficient to achieve continued stability in drug use and an acceptable level of childcare is reached. The aim is efficient multi-disciplinary services that can intervene at any stage and co-operation between professional groups is essential.

REFERENCES

Birth in Britain Today: Survey 2001. An online survey.

DoH (1999) *Drug Misuse and Dependence: guidelines on clinical management.* London: Department of Health: The Stationery Office.

Gerada, C. and Tighe, J. (1999) A review of shared care protocols for the treatment of problem drug use in England, Scotland and Wales. *The British Journal of General Practice* 439, 125–126.

Klee, H. and Jackson, M. (1998) *Illicit Drug Use, Pregnancy and Early Motherhood.* The Manchester Metropolitan University, Manchester, UK: SRHSA Blue Book Series.

Klee, H. and Wright, S. (1999) *Amphetamine Use and Treatment: a study of individual and policy impediments to effective service delivery – Part 2 Treatment and its outcomes.* The Manchester Metropolitan University, Manchester, UK: SRHSA Blue Book Series.

Klee, H., Wright, S. and Rothwell, J. (1998) *Drug Using Parents and Their Children: risk and protective factors.* The Manchester Metropolitan University, Manchester, UK: SRHSA Blue Book Series.

Kumpfer, K.L. (1994) *Strengthening America's Families: promising parenting and family strategies for delinquency prevention: users' guide.* Office of Juvenile Justice and Delinquency Prevention, Silver Spring, MD: Aspen Systems.

Kumpfer, K.L. (1998) Links between prevention and treatment for drug-abusing women and their children, in: C.L. Wetherington and A.B. Roman (eds) *Drug Addiction Research and the Health of Women.* National Institute on Drug Abuse, Washington DC: Government Printing Office.

Kumpfer, K.L., DeMarsh, J. and Child, W. (1989) *The Strengthening Families Program.* Salt Lake City, UT: Department of Health Education, University of Utah.

LGDF/SCODA (1997) *Drug Using Parents and their Children.* London: Local Government Drugs Forum and the Standing Conference on Drug Abuse.

Reid, J., Macchetto, P. and Foster, S. (1999) *No Safe Haven.* National Center on Addiction and Substance Abuse (CASA), New York: Columbia University.

UK Government Cm 2846 (1995) *Tackling Drugs Together: a strategy for England 1995–1998.* London: HMSO.

Working Together to Safeguard Children (1999) Department of Health, Home Office, Department for Education and Employment, London: The Stationery Office. www.doh.gov.uk/pub/doh/safeguard/pdf

Chapter 19

Dilemmas of child welfare and drug dependence

Hilary Klee

There can be no denying that while a woman uses certain drugs, there are risks to the foetus during pregnancy, and different, possibly even more damaging, risks later from within the home. A harm reduction approach tries to set limits on these risks rather than attempt to remove them; for example, by controlling drug use rather than advocating abstinence. This is not seen as good enough by critics of this philosophy because using drugs is seen as a choice and there is an 'innocent child' that will be hurt. The combination of these two words tends to induce a variety of emotional reactions that in the context of drug use may initiate protective action on behalf of the child and restraining, often punitive, action against the mother. The common answer to this is to point out that reality dictates a more pragmatic approach, one that avoids repressive and moralising actions, since these only alienate drug users and may interfere with treatment and control outcomes. The critical task for services is to safeguard the child and yet cultivate the bond with a drug-using mother. Accepting that there are significant risks to the child, what is the best way of minimising them?

RECONCILING THE IRRECONCILABLE

The immediate, though facile, answer is to get the woman off drugs as soon as possible. Although relapse is regarded as commonplace, the period of pregnancy and early motherhood is still regarded by both women drug users and drug workers as one of the best chances a woman will have to change. The early months after returning home are particularly critical since a return to illicit drugs is likely to invite action by social services and the removal of her child. Most women in this study eventually returned to their earlier patterns of drug use. Many women increased their methadone but regretted the need. They were both seen as failures.

A number of stressors were identified that started at the point of aware-ness of a woman's pregnancy and continued into motherhood without remitting. At the end of the study there were very few 'happy endings' among our respondents, but for some there was hope of a better future. However, although the data have offered insights that could lead to improvement in the welfare of drug-using women and their children, they provide no real solution to the root problem of reducing her drug dependence that so directly affects the potential for damage to her child. The most compelling data on this from the study is the negative influence of the partner's drug use and the drug orientation of the home environment. Similar observations have been made from research on amphetamine users in treatment (Klee and Wright, 1999).

That this unique 'window of opportunity' did not result in abstinence and a new life suggests that it has assumed an undeserved reputation. Nonetheless, the study revealed that motivation was high at this time and this can still be used to support other interventions, most notably family therapy. However, it would be best if other procedures could be found that predate the time when motivation has been worn thin by anxiety and relapse is imminent.

REDUCING THE RISK

A starting point of an intervention that aims to reduce the number of children at risk is to attract more women into treatment, a goal now adopted internationally (see Chapter 20). Once in contact with health professionals, health issues can be addressed that include their fertility. The results of this study suggest that a strongly proactive birth control programme is needed in treatment agencies. The majority (72 per cent) of these respondents had not planned their pregnancy and the impact of the news was severe. Forty per cent considered abortion, which suggests that there were many others not enrolled into the study that chose to terminate their pregnancy. Those who considered abortion were more likely later to have problems with their partner and with the baby, and return to street drugs early.

Drug workers usually warn their clients not to make assumptions about their fertility but this is not working; respondents had either not retained the information, did not believe it or were unable to use reliably the recommended contraceptive measures. The aim should be to make every baby planned and expect a proportion of drug users to want a family. Male clients should be included as targets for all kinds of information about conception and contraception since they may be important channels of communication for their partners.

A reduction in unplanned pregnancies would make a significant contribution to reducing the strain on health and social welfare services. For those that remain there is a need for more powerful interventions. Given the influential role of partners, one option would be to attempt to draw on any resources within the family to help the mother maintain control of her drugs and set up an environment free of drug-related risks. Partners varied in their own control but this study and previous data (Klee and Wright, 1999) have consistently shown the benefits of a supportive partner who can not only control his own use but will co-operate in making joint plans for a combined effort that will protect the child. Unfortunately such partners are rare and it is for this reason that help should be provided.

SOCIAL WORK DILEMMAS

The US experience of child protection and its relationship with drug use is extensive and research on family interventions is well developed. Despite the differences in the nature and patterns of drug use and family structures, an examination of US data may offer a basis for interventions that could be used in other cultures with suitable modification.

A search of the US research literature on child protection and drug use produced a number of features in common with the UK. One is the extreme nature of attitudes towards drug-using parents, not only by the public but also among professionals. There are health and social welfare professionals that base their judgements on the child's perspective and recognise parental needs only insofar as they contribute to the health and safety of the child. A vivid example is the account of research among a large number of social welfare workers by Reid and her colleagues (1999). In their report for the National Center on Addiction and Substance Abuse (CASA) they came to the conclusion that parental substance abuse was the major factor in the vast majority of child welfare cases brought before the US courts. The graphic language used in some parts of the report does not encourage a balanced and objective response in the reader:

> The human costs are incalculable: broken families; children who are malnourished; babies who are neglected, beaten, and sometimes killed by alcohol and crack-addicted parents; eight year olds sent out to steal or buy drugs for addicted parents; sick children wallowing in unsanitary conditions; child victims of sodomy, rape and incest; children in such agony and despair that they themselves resort to drugs and alcohol for relief. For some it may be possible to cauterise the bleeding but the scars of drug and alcohol-spawned parental abuse and neglect are likely to be permanent.
>
> (Reid et al., 1999)

Uncharitably, the writing could be characterised as a tub-thumping crescendo of rhetoric ending in the ultimate defamation of the perpetrators of these evils that might have resulted in earlier days in a public lynching. Public opinion is moulded by such imaginings and they have lasting effects that are manifest in powerful stereotypes that disable those who are stereotyped in their capacity to break free and achieve rehabilitation. The fierce emotions stirred by the unimaginably cruel treatment of children by drug-using parents are quick to rise and slow to respond to reasoned attempts at alternative interpretations of the alleged dynamics of their parenting.

If this is an accurate reflection of the majority view, then attempts at a moderate and realistic approach to prevention and remedial interventions will face considerable resistance. However, the undercurrent of despair that the situation is out of control in the US is palpable. Drugs policy, the demographic profiles and the patterns of drug consumption are all very different from those in Europe, but there is now a growing concern in the UK at the increasing number of children born into drug-using families. Preventative interventions are needed now and action should be taken early. Health and social services are already hard pressed and should case loads increase it would be wise to be armed with workable procedures if damage to mothers and their children is to be avoided in the coming years.

The focus of the CASA report was the overwhelming tide of child protection cases associated with substance misuse that has gathered momentum in the US: 'Parental alcohol and drug abuse and addiction have thrown the nation's system of child welfare beyond crisis and calamity into chaos.' A major concern among social welfare workers is the need for urgent action for the sake of the child. This is set in a context of lengthy delay caused by the slow progress towards rehabilitation made by the parent, and results in the dilemma of whether or not to remove the child. This is worsened by the unsatisfactory nature of many of the fostering options that are available. Social welfare workers in the US feel they need to act but complain about the inadequacies of their work, which may resonate among their UK counterparts, for example: timely access to other services, the absence of strategies to motivate parents to control their use, and the lack of efforts to prevent or prepare for relapse.

While the situation in the US may not translate easily to the European culture, these concerns are likely to be shared by most professionals with a primary role in child welfare. The report goes on to examine a number of interventions that are designed to limit the impact of parental drug use on the child. Some focus on increasing caseworker skills through training, or supplementing them with imported expertise in the form of drug/alcohol counsellors, mostly recovered addicts. In some states the whole area of child protection was being outsourced to private consultancy.

Many thorny dilemmas and procedural problems were identified in the CASA report that were similar to those noted among the professionals in this study; for example, how to safeguard the child while dealing sympathetically with the parent, how to deal with repeated relapse, the increased load on staff, and issues of inter-agency confidentiality. There was also confusion about professional role boundaries and difficulties in retraining staff.

Many problems were similar between US and UK data, and so too were the solutions. A number of recommendations were made in the report for comprehensive and co-ordinated services that would ideally include general health care, social welfare, parenting skills, literacy and job training for drug-using clients, and substance abuse training for all professionals working with them. It was suggested that the need to integrate services across agency lines was essential even if this required a change in their organisational culture and practice. The report ends with an observation that in dealing with child safety, service provision should start with prevention by anticipating need, treating drug dependence in pregnancy and then extending home-based support.

THE ADVANTAGES OF FAMILY THERAPY

Acknowledging the primary role of the family in preventing drug misuse and the need to increase understanding of that role, a programme of work on family prevention intervention research was launched by the National Institute on Drug Abuse (NIDA). Protective factors and risk factors are identified and the aim is to strengthen the former and reduce the latter. In addition to the health and social benefits to the parents the intergenerational transmission of drug misuse to their children is addressed.

An advantage of an approach to drug misuse control based on working with the family is that influential social dynamics can be observed through home visits. By contrast, the disadvantage of a drug treatment intervention that deals with only one member of a family, which is the traditional approach in the UK, is to be unaware of factors that may be critically important in the life of that person. These include the way he or she interacts with family members and children. Additionally, family interventions can address dysfunctional behaviours that may or may not be associated with drug use, for example mental health problems that arise through damaging social relationships and social isolation. If care is provided that is not visibly labelled with a reference to drugs, this avoids the associated stigma. As a result it will be more attractive to parents who are acutely sensitive to interpersonal and environmental cues that suggest they are being stereotyped. The same principle applies to treatment for dependence that includes as options the alternative therapies used by many people in society at large, such as stress management, social skill learning and acupuncture. These 'camouflage' techniques are useful in establishing contact with hidden populations.

Acquiring skills

The emphasis on skill building is a critical aspect of many family intervention programmes and allows for practice and feedback during interactive sessions. According to Etz and her colleagues (Etz *et al.*, 1998), although parental drug use poses serious risks for the children, protective monitoring of children can be taught. The sessions are flexible in allowing the focus to be on the parents and child separately or together. There are diverse family-based interventions but as yet few have been evaluated. In their development there has been increased emphasis on creating prevention programmes for subgroups, largely defined in terms of racial and cultural differences. Kumpfer (1998) outlines their key elements which comprise: the targeting and selection of high-risk groups known for their specific risk profiles and resource based factors; working with smaller groups with longer or more intensive contact; high staff–client ratios; and greater expense. Although they require considerable resources, it is claimed that they are more likely to have positive effects on parenting. The 'Strengthening Families Programme' developed by Kumpfer is now being tested and is produced as a video training package (NIDA, 1994).

Another type of programme with similar aims but a very different approach is 'Focus on Families' (Catalano *et al.*, 1997; Catalano *et al.*, 1999). The aims of this study trial were to reduce parental use of drugs by teaching parents how to cope with underlying problems that are associated with their dependence and also how to manage family problems. An intensive course of four months of twice weekly treatment sessions was followed up with weekly home visits for nine months. A control group was used to measure progress. After two years the improvement in parenting persisted but the difference in illicit drug use was no longer significantly different from the controls. The high incidence of relapse led to the conclusion that aftercare would be needed while parents had any association with the drug scene.

RELEVANCE TO THE UK

The results of many years of research effort in the US are still to be evaluated. Although it is too early to identify those practices that may have relevance to UK populations, the studies have already revealed correspondences with observations here. Combined, they demonstrate the complexity of problems that are a part of working with families irrespective of culture and the need to overcome certain barriers. There are some aspects that are particularly worth noting:

1   Identifying protective factors within a family is a positive feature that facilitates a proactive approach built on strengths. This is in contrast to the more reactive and critical mode that focuses on the presence of risk. Overt recognition of such strengths helps to attenuate the defensiveness in parents caused by implied faults that so often makes communication difficult.

2   The nature of the intervention changes in various ways with the size and composition of the unit. Are educative messages delivered or are they discussed? Are disclosures expected? Group dynamics in a family group are quite different from those where participants are not related. Free-flowing confrontations between family members may be informative and ultimately useful but they are difficult to manage and require trained personnel to run them.

3   The availability of resources raises issues concerning the medium of communication. Working with families encompasses more than offering skill building in parenting: it implies a broader coverage of issues that are specific to a particular family whereas parenting education offers a narrower and more formal focus that is less likely to take account of idiosyncratic features of the recipients. The latter is less demanding of resources and easier to implement.

4   The research to support such interventions has yet to be done. Parents should be used as informants in developing the syllabus for the training of professionals and also for parenting education aimed at drug users. With a core syllabus of child development, educators could then incorporate the known protective strategies used by parents and involve parents in critical evaluation of these strategies. When interacting with disadvantaged and/or socially isolated people, dialogue empowers whereas didactic delivery is likely to alienate, especially if the information comes from a source with low credibility.

5   Various factors deter drug users from attending treatment (Wright *et al.*, 1999); and they will also deter parents or parents-to-be from attending other events outside the home. For example, the location of the intervention is important, whether held in drug agencies or health centres that are regularly visited or in more unfamiliar places. There are associated concerns about the distance to travel, particularly with a child. The time of day and the lack of crèche facilities prevent attendance by many mothers. Parents may anticipate that the intervention will have little relevance and hence be of little value. Some respondents in this study attended general classes in parenting and felt alienated.

6   Most international guidelines emphasise easy access to treatment. In the UK a woman's pregnancy ensures immediate access. Women presenting at this time, if not very late in pregnancy, can benefit from educational interventions on childcare at a time when they are maximally motivated to become abstinent or reduce their dependence. Support should be at its highest at this stage and also into the early months postpartum in order to avoid relapse and subsequent deterioration.

Many culturally sensitive interventions are possible, and having several options available is advisable.

CONCLUSION: AVOIDING FAMILY BREAK-UP

It is in the specific design and implementation of multi-disciplinary systems of 'shared care' that good intentions will be tested for their effectiveness in providing an acceptable service that will attract women, gain their trust and co-operation rather than compliance, produce outcomes that lead to improved health for them and their children, and result in fewer children removed from them. Although it is likely that underlying negative attitudes to drug-using mothers will continue to exert a powerful effect for some time, the view that adequate parenting is possible with good control, professional support and education, would become more widespread if a range of family-based options was available. The research on which this book is based has shown that the majority of mothers and many of their partners wanted to be good parents. It should be possible for professionals to work with such motivation and empower them to reach the stage that allows them to seek help without fear, something that non-drug users can do without a thought. Part of the empowerment lies in making it known that their potential for good parenting is recognised by health and social workers. Brief parenting education sessions may help but are unlikely to be sufficient, and support should be available for extended periods. It is hard to say from these data the forms that such support should take for drug-using families in the UK. Some of the components of the US systems could be taken on; others would be inappropriate in view of the UK orientation towards harm reduction, less punitive legislation and free access to treatment.

Many drug-using women have a history of childhood deprivation and abuse. The legacy of this may be a dysfunctional adulthood and an effect on their children that perpetuates that dysfunction. Breaking the pattern is hard, but important for later generations. It is essential that support is available for them to change to a more rewarding lifestyle with their children that can ensure the safety of those children. When there are so many opportunities for great joy and fulfilment in family life, it is sad that so much fear, ignorance and prejudice pervades their lives. This can only be remedied effectively with non-judgemental and well-informed policy and practice. At present such a Utopian state is a far cry from the experiences of drug-using mothers.

REFERENCES

Catalano, R.F., Gainey, R.R., Fleming, C.B., Haggerty, K.P. and Johnson, N.O. (1999) An experimental intervention with families of substance abusers: One year follow-up of the Focus on Families project. *Addiction* 94 (2), 241–254.

Catalano, R.F., Haggerty, K.P., Gainey, R.R. and Hoppe, M.J. (1997) Reducing parental risk factors for children's substance misuse: preliminary outcomes with opiate-addicted parents. *Substance Use and Misuse* 32, 622–721.

Etz, K.E., Robertson, E.B. and Ashery, R.S. (1998) Risk and protective factors in the family context, in: C.L. Wetherington and A.B. Roman (eds) *Drug Addiction Research and the Health of Women*. National Institute on Drug Abuse (NIDA), Rockville, MD: US Department of Health and Human Services.

Klee, H. and Wright, S. (1999) Amphetamine use and treatment: a study of the impediments to effective service delivery. The Manchester Metropolitan University, Manchester, UK: SRHSA Blue Book Series.

Kumpfer, K.L. (1998) Links between prevention and treatment for drug-abusing women and their children, in: C.L. Wetherington and A.B. Roman (eds) *Drug Addiction Research and the Health of Women*. National Institute on Drug Abuse, Washington DC: Government Printing Office.

NIDA (1994) *Coming Together on Prevention*. (Video). National Institute on Drug Abuse. Produced for the National Clearinghouse for Alcohol and Drug Information Videotape Resource Program, Washington DC.

Reid, J., Macchetto, P. and Foster, S. (1999) *No Safe Haven*. National Center on Addiction and Substance Abuse (CASA). New York: Columbia University.

Wright, S., Klee, H. and Reid, P. (1999) Attitudes of amphetamine users towards treatment services. *Drugs: Education, Prevention and Policy* 6(1), 71–86.

Chapter 20

Drugs policy and practice development in the United Kingdom

Hilary Klee

The primary aim of this chapter is to summarise the models of care for drug-using pregnant women under development in the UK. It is useful, however, to set these in a wider context. There are many aspects of them that have their roots in developments that have been occurring at an international level over the past decade. The global concordance in the principles that should inform policy and practice is impressive. It is also heartening, since the opportunities for productive exchange of information should be high. The key elements in the search for appropriate and humane services in the US, Australia and Europe are described before going on to describe in more detail the paths that have been taken in the UK to translate these principles into practice.

The fundamental issues concerning services for women drug users were addressed early in the 1990s by the United Nations in their position paper on *Women and Drug Abuse* (UNDCP, 1994). This revealed that there had been only 'limited prevention, treatment and rehabilitation efforts for women' worldwide at a time when female drug use was increasing. There were serious deficiencies in services for women: 'Most treatment programmes are based on the needs of men who, in contrast with women, often can count on somebody else to care for their children and who do not have the same feelings of gender-based shame and guilt', and such programmes 'do not consider the special needs of women'. The paper recommended (*inter alia*) that action should be taken to:

- improve women's access to drug services;
- develop outreach services for women drug users and their families;
- improve family counselling sources in out-patient and family practices;
- promote counselling services for drug users and their partners;
- strengthen social reintegration programmes for former drug users with an emphasis on parenting and job skills training;
- promote training and gender sensitisation for health and social service professionals.

The international community of policy makers, researchers and practitioners seems to have responded as far as resources allow in developing models of care. It is interesting that they share so many common features, though the operationalisation of the model may reflect the overall political, cultural and perhaps moral orientation of the country concerned. Almost without exception they espouse the idea of comprehensive care undertaken by different categories of professional groups working together.

INTERNATIONAL SERVICE GUIDELINES AND RECOMMENDATIONS

The United States of America

Concepts of service development for drug-using mothers in the North American literature are strongly influenced by the woman's role within the family as mother. Although there has been a general decline in federal funding for treatment services for women since the late 1970s (Gerstein and Harwood, 1990) the exception is research on pregnant drug users that has been encouraged by the National Institute on Drug Abuse (NIDA). Studies that were initiated in the early 1990s have now reached the stage of dissemination of findings and the development of models of care (Kumpfer, 1998).

As early as 1993 and in parallel with the research initiative, Treatment Improvement Protocols (TIP, 1993) were provided that emphasised 'comprehensive services' and a 'continuum of care' in which the support service is available over an extended period of time. In addition, programmes should be accessible, confidential, collaborative, co-ordinated, culturally sensitive, and have a supportive orientation. Two years later, thirty different programmes for drug-using parents across the US were described that indicate considerable diversity (TIP, 1995). The list of components of the services largely correspond to those in Europe and Australia, namely:

- health care: family planning, obstetrics, check-ups for children, counselling;
- treatment for drug dependence;
- other services: housing, legal, vocational, child welfare, home management including nutrition;
- psychosocial: stress management, counselling, interpersonal skills, mental health, domestic violence counselling;
- parental education and training in child growth and needs; child-rearing practices, counselling for couples and family therapy.

Australia

The contribution made by Australian research to our knowledge of drug use and ways of measuring and treating dependence has been outstanding over the past decade. Although progressive work in the area of women, pregnancy and drugs has been under way for some time in major cities (see, for example, Copeland, 1997, 1998; Copeland and Hall, 1992; Copeland et al., 1993; Wan and Sunjic, 1998) only fairly recently have government advisors, clinicians and health services increased their demands for commonwealth funding to develop collaborative guidelines.

The guidelines on services for pregnant drug users for New South Wales (NSW Health, 1999) state that an aim of treatment for opioid-dependent women is 'to provide comprehensive antenatal and postnatal care'. Advice is given on achieving stabilisation on methadone in pregnancy and decisions to change dose levels. Antenatal care should be managed if possible in collaboration with obstetric services that specialise in managing drug dependency during pregnancy.

The Sydney-based Drugs and Pregnancy Service (DAPS) conducted retrospective research that covered a 54-month period and reported on obstetric outcomes for mothers and birth outcomes for their drug-exposed infants. Among the recommendations arising from the research were:

• service providers should be encouraged to obtain a thorough drug use history on first contact;
• trained carers should provide counselling on drug use during pregnancy and be able to offer appropriate interventions to women at risk;
• the initiation of education and prevention programmes;
• a flexible antenatal appointments system that sustains contact with the women;
• a comprehensive postpartum home visit schedule;
• evaluation of services to identify barriers to access and uptake.

Europe

The changes in the UK are a part of a broader strategy that has been heavily influenced by a number of European initiatives. The need to address the issue of women's use of drugs and the implications for health and welfare services was taken up by the Council of Europe in a series of expert meetings and symposia on Women and Drugs, and Pregnancy and Drug Misuse held by the Pompidou Group[1] over several years (Klee, 1998; Pompidou, 1993, 1995, 1997, 1998). Among the key points from the recommendations on pregnancy and drug misuse were that:

• low-threshold harm reduction services should be provided;
• pregnant drug users should receive counselling and treatment;

- the family, or the mother and her child should get support in order to stay together;
- abortion should be available as an option;
- substitute opioid medication should be available for detoxification or maintenance purposes;
- substitution therapy should continue after delivery in all cases where relapse is expected.

Principles of shared care were espoused in the recommendations for services: 'In order to ensure best care for pregnant drug users and their children there is a need for a multidisciplinary approach.' The service should include:

- medical care;
- close co-ordination between professionals delivering that care;
- social care: housing and financial support; outreach activities;
- psychological care: single and group therapies;
- social welfare;
- educational provision: parenting and basics in child education;
- nutritional care;
- opportunities for partners of pregnant drug-dependent women to participate.

A consultancy document brought together the conclusions of the Pompidou Group meetings along with a survey of women's drug services in the European Union and a literature survey (Hedrich, 2000). This identified the main priorities as first making services attractive to women, and then making sure they are aware of them. The desirable characteristics of the service would be an appropriate location and service ambience (with childcare facilities, flexible opening hours and an option of a women-only environment); a drop-in facility for preliminary informal uncommitted contact; and a service run by trained personnel. Best practice would require a comprehensive range of services that are delivered by a multi-professional team in which health and welfare personnel are aware of the background, lifestyle and other contextual features of their clients.

THE UNITED KINGDOM

The global developments in addressing the needs of women drug users are mirrored in the UK. Policy on prevention and treatment for drug misuse has been undergoing radical change since the mid-1990s. The principle of 'shared care' was adopted at that time as part of the national UK government initiative on drug misuse (UK Government Cm 2846, 1995) and co-ordination between government agencies at a central level was matched at local levels with the development of Drug Action Teams comprising representatives from police, probation, prison and health services and also the private sector. This was followed up by the appointment of an Anti-Drugs Co-ordinator to develop and implement a ten-year strategy that continued with the theme of partnership at every level. In 1998 (UK Government Cm 3945, 1998: 22–23) the links between the health problems of drug users and public health concerns about mental health and social exclusion were acknowledged and a commitment made to provide an 'integrated, effective and efficient response' to people with drugs problems; 'develop collaborative, coherent, accessible and cost-effective service provision'; and support drug misusers in changing their lifestyles by 'linking up where appropriate with accommodation, education and employment services'.

SERVICES FOR DRUG-USING PARENTS: THE UK GUIDELINES FOR INTER-AGENCY WORKING

Models of 'shared care' in the delivery of drugs and midwifery services are gradually being developed across the UK to replace, by a painstaking process of trial and error, the previous, less formalised arrangements between professional groups. There are a number of local working models but as yet no defined principles or protocols of good practice. In the past, disparate groups of health and social welfare professionals (GPs, nurses, drug agencies, social workers) governed by their own well-established norms, values, rules and regulations, were not required to co-ordinate with others. Attempts to change procedures have exposed the many problems in assembling a team in which roles and responsibilities are defined and agreed, and the mechanisms determined, that will produce a smooth running, co-ordinated service.

The theme of inter-agency working was the focus of guidelines on drug-using parents published by the Local Government Drugs Forum (LGDF) and the Standing Conference on Drug Abuse (SCODA) in 1997. At that time the recommendations were that all drug-using parents in treatment should be routinely asked about their parenting and childcare practices and where serious problems are detected to carry out a joint assessment by child and adult agencies. It was advisable to work in partnership with parents and note contextual aspects of their lives that would affect their parenting, such as poor health, unemployment, housing and poverty. Drug workers discovering evidence of risk that could lead to significant harm to the child were to contact social services. Social service personnel should examine ways of 'providing packages of care to meet the needs of the child and to support the family' (LGDF/SCODA, 1997: 23).

Two years later, in identifying the challenges presented by multi-agency work, the revised UK Guidelines on Clinical Management of Drug Misuse and Dependence (DoH, 1999 Annex 5) revisited the same theme, that is, the need for comprehensive care: 'involving obstetricians, paediatricians, midwives, drug services, general practice and social service representatives'. Informed in part by the outcomes of the pregnancy research presented here, they included the need for drug services to attract women and to address problems of confidentiality. The role of the partner was identified as 'an important aspect of enabling the pregnant woman to achieve progress at the earliest possible stage' and aftercare was important 'which may need to include parenting advice and skills training, [and] is essential after dis-charge if the ideal outcome of maintaining mother and child together is to be achieved'.

Another document produced by three government departments with shared responsibility for childcare and education (*Working Together to Safeguard Children*, 1999) aimed 'to set out how all agencies and professionals should work together to promote children's welfare and protect them from abuse and neglect'. As befitting a document with a designated readership of all services that are in contact with children and families, it is both detailed and comprehensive. The national framework it provides allows for local variations in setting up systems of communication and corporate responsibility across a range of agencies. The short section devoted to Drug and Alcohol Misuse (2.24) echoes the social service directive to refrain from making assumptions about the effects on a child of parental drug use. In general, services are asked to work *with* families, promoting a positive but realistic image to encourage parents to seek help. Among the recommendations are many that are supported by this research:

- A key role for health visitors.
- A role for midwives and nurses in identifying potential problems during pregnancy and childbirth.
- Children and families should have access to an advice and advocacy service.
- That issues of sharing information and confidentiality should be addressed and priorities and rules be determined.
- Training needs should be identified and resources made available.
- The strengths of families should be used through Family Group Conferences in which the membership is defined by the family. This would operate as the primary planning group for dealing with difficult problems.

In terms of inter-agency collaboration the document goes beyond the development of structures and procedures to advise that services 'should create an ethos which values working collaboratively with other professionals and promote partnerships with children and families that recognise families' strengths in responding to the needs of children'.

MODELS OF CARE: THE DRUG LIAISON MIDWIFE

> She's the one that's going to be directly involved with them so it's all passed over to her now . . . which is quite a relief really to have somebody that's specially involved.
>
> (Antenatal midwife)

> It's excellent. There's one person to deal with it, we know how to get hold of her. If there's a problem she comes in, speaks to them and sorts it out.
>
> (Postnatal midwife)

As a model of care that has rapidly gained in popularity, the drugs liaison midwife mediates between the main players in services for drug-using pregnant women: the client, maternity services, drug agencies and social services. The midwife may be operating in the context of a community-based maternity service or a drug agency. In these early days of development there has been no research that shows the extent and nature of local variations. The essential ingredient seems to be personal involvement with all pregnant women in the area who are known to be using drugs. The initiatives tend to come from midwives with a special interest in this client group. They monitor the client's progress and are a major resource for the woman during her pregnancy and hospital confinement. When midwives are part of a multi-disciplinary group they are a resource for the members of that group and also for antenatal and hospital staff, since they are involved directly with clients. The job may involve providing in-service training as well as information to other professionals on demand.

Although access to a specialist like the drugs liaison midwife may be important for both the women and the service providers, such a facility should contribute to a partnership between them, not replace it. There were signs that this could happen since many midwifery, hospital and drug staff were obviously very pleased to have someone to relieve them of the responsibility of decision making. It was unlikely that the severance of all individual communications between agencies was the intent but one drug worker welcomed it:

> I hardly ever speak to the hospital . . . it's all done through the two midwives here.

The development of formal, local policies is hard work for drugs liaison midwives and there could be teething problems in the early days:

> We've got policies now and we can sort out some individual care plans, we know where to refer to and the facilities are there to refer people. Before, it was a hit and miss affair but now I think it's improving.

There are both advantages and disadvantages to this model. Different levels of formality in the exchange of information and decision making are possible, which may be an advantage in allowing for flexibility and greater relevance to local conditions, but there may be disadvantages if informal systems of communication are exploited. For example, if most of the mediation is between the midwife and various agencies, there may be little incentive to initiate a forum for direct communication between them and the success of the enterprise may depend heavily on the individual's energy and personality. Under these circumstances there may be considerable work overload.

This is the more precarious option if continuity of working practices is important, since personal style may play a major role and a successor or replacement may prefer alternative procedures. If the drugs liaison midwife acts as advocate and counsellor in a one-to-one relationship with the pregnant drug user, an exclusive relationship is likely to develop that may inhibit the development of relationships with other carers. Ultimately this may not be in the woman's best interests.

MODELS OF CARE: MULTI-AGENCY COLLABORATION

A structured multi-agency model is an alternative that can operate without liaison midwives. The Glasgow model described in Chapter 17 has no need for specific liaison roles. In models such as this, which operate out of a hospital or clinic maternity service, low threshold access that includes self-referral is important. Some clients will not be in contact with drug services and their drug use may not be known to their GP. The Glasgow service has an advantage in that although located within the hospital itself, it has satellite clinics elsewhere. The existence of a number of points of entry into the services is important to women with children. They can face arduous and expensive journeys to centralised locations if they cannot find a childminder.

In Glasgow the mother's care is the responsibility of all midwives in the team and an exclusive relationship with one midwife is discouraged. Junior midwives in the hospital rotate in and out of the team so that their experience can be applied elsewhere. The Pregnancy Support Group in Liverpool includes among its core members a midwife who liaises with the hospital, a health visitor and a social worker working in tandem with obstetric, paediatric and drugs services in a way that facilitates sharing of relevant information. Here, too, self-referral is possible. The principal difference is that the team is based in a large drug agency. This has significant implications for the way that the woman's use of methadone is handled. The lead is taken by the agency and her treatment continues to be determined by the prescribing physician and her key worker during her pregnancy. Through the liaison midwife the hospital staff are kept informed. This is in contrast to the Glasgow model, which is hospital based and obstetrically led. The woman's methadone treatment is handled by the obstetrician, the argument being that this is a medical matter that affects both mother and the foetus. There is likely to be variation in other aspects of care, if one looks at the fine detail, which depends on local conditions, existing provision and available resources. For example, hospital confinement may be in a general labour ward rather than a specialist ward catering for women with drug problems, or more generally in the case of Glasgow, for social problems, that make standard care options inappropriate. It seems that in all models there will be health visitors and social service representation and possibly the involvement of local doctors but there could be an array of other professional groups serving more specific needs like housing or legal advice.

Hepburn was well ahead of her time in putting shared care principles into practice in Glasgow's midwifery services in the mid-1980s. The models that are now emerging elsewhere in the UK (see, for example, Lawrence, 2000; Speed and Janikiewicz, 2000) are diverse in operational terms though similar in their objectives.

The advantage of multi-agency care, in the form of a team throughout pregnancy, is that the assessment of the woman's needs and planning for her return home can be a standard feature of her care, and decisions are informed by issues associated with child welfare as well as the woman's health. One particular benefit is that stigmatisation through exposure is less likely although at present this is not guaranteed. Whatever the base of care, whether in hospital or drug clinic, there may be a tendency to focus primarily on medical issues and health, avoiding the complexities of social influences that affect many aspects of her life: housing, finances and informal support. Nonetheless these models offer opportunities to address these issues. Involvement of social workers from the start also allows prediction or early diagnosis of parenting and child safety problems that can reduce the risk of crises later.

An advantage to a multi-disciplinary model with a formal structure and procedures is that decisions concerning client care are agreed at regular intervals by several agencies that all know what is happening. They are less reliant on informal communication channels. Another advantage is that their procedures can be evaluated more easily and such a model can be replicated elsewhere if thought to be appropriate. However, as with the liaison midwife the sharing of managerial responsibilities may not be well balanced across the group and not well supported with appropriate administrative help. In this period of innovation and growth, the pioneers succeed in the fight for resources helped by their own dedication and charisma. Their own survival and that of the model they have constructed depends subsequently on clearly recorded protocols, good administration and willing co-operation between team members.

MODELS OF CARE: ADVOCACY

The data suggested that drug-using pregnant women need support in their uptake of services, particularly if they lack a partner and family. A drug liaison midwife or a drug worker cannot be expected to help navigate through all the complexities of maternity and childcare services, social security, housing departments and so on. This requires different forms of experience, extensive knowledge and time. It also requires other skills if the woman needs to present her case to the authorities. Under these circumstances it may be better to have a mentor or advocate, whose role is to advise and guide the woman in dealing with such problems. This research revealed that some social workers, drug workers and drugs liaison midwives were taking on this role, though it was a strain on them at times. The development of a post of advocate for pregnant women in difficulties would not only facilitate appropriate responses to a wider range of problems, but could be located in antenatal services and hence be accessible to those women who do not disclose their use of drugs and are not known to drug services.

THE CASE CONFERENCE

For drug-using mothers in the UK perhaps their greatest fear is the possibility of a case conference being called to determine the adequacy of the arrangements for care of the infant. The service providers reported that case conferences were not automatic simply because the mother was a drug user. This was a view that was generally supported. There were a number of reasons for setting up a conference; for example, if there was some doubt about the capacity of the mother to meet the needs of the child, or if there was no existing input from a health visitor or social worker, or nothing was known of the mother's history of childcare.

Case conferences were attended by hospital maternity staff, SCBU staff, social workers and drug workers. Parents, or in some cases, grandparents, were invited to attend and usually did. They sometimes also involved police officers, probation, and, if there were older children, head teachers and school nurses. GPs were invited but apparently seldom attended. The factors that were taken into account in deciding on the fate of the child included parenting skills, past history, home environment, the partner's drug use and support, criminal offences and the stability of drug taking.

However, drug workers were more likely to feel that there was too much emphasis on the woman's drug use. They tended to complain that it was difficult to communicate with non-specialists and felt a lone voice in challenging the stereotypes that emerged in discussions. There were also different views concerning the presence of the parents. Most believed that this had the positive effect of increasing honesty and openness, of involving parents in the decisions and also ensuring that they were aware of the reasons for those decisions. However, some community midwives felt inhibited by the presence of parents since their role in continuing home care meant that future interactions might be difficult.

The participants tended to have mixed views on the advisability of set guidelines for the conducting of case conferences. It was apparent that these varied across the region and were not always known to staff. The disadvantage of guidelines to some of them was that they could become too prescriptive. All respondents were agreed that each case should be decided on individual merit.

THE FUTURE OF SERVICES FOR DRUG-USING PREGNANT WOMEN

The dominant theme for the future is about accelerating progress towards midwifery and child protection services that are based on the principle of shared care. It has been observed that greater liaison helps to improve attitudes and tolerance among staff more than in those services with no such protocol. Effective collaboration has also been shown to reduce fear of social workers among the women. It is generally recognised that services with inter-agency teams are in the best position to reduce or remove their fears.

A lack of communication between professionals, and in some cases visible antagonism, not only diminishes the faith that clients have in their carers but also leads some professionals to question the integrity of other workers. In an environment where co-operation is now being encouraged between mainstream maternity services, social services and specialist drug agencies, such mistrust is unhelpful. Ultimately it is drug-using women and their children who lose out when professionals are reluctant to communicate. Although the potential value of 'shared care' is not challenged and the problems of professional territorialism are well known, reluctance to engage in full collaboration could result in the most important partner in this network, the pregnant drug user herself, being left confused and uncertain while the struggle goes on.

REFERENCES

Copeland, J. (1997) A qualitative study of the perceptions of treatment services and 12-step programs among women who self-managed change in addictive behaviours. *Journal of Substance Abuse Treatment* 14(2), 183–190.

Copeland, J. (1998) A qualitative study of self-managed change in substance dependence among women. *Contemporary Drug Problems* 25(2), 321–345.

Copeland, J. and Hall, W. (1992) A comparison of women seeking drug and alcohol treatment in a specialist women's and two traditional mixed-sex treatment services. *British Journal of Addiction* 87, 1293–1302.

Copeland, J., Hall, W., Didcott, P. and Biggs, V. (1993) A comparison of a specialist women's alcohol and other drug treatment services with two traditional mixed-sex services: client characteristics and treatment outcome. *Drug and Alcohol Dependence* 32, 81–92.

DoH (1999) *Drug Misuse and Dependence: guidelines on clinical management.* London: Department of Health: The Stationery Office.

Gerstein, D. and Harwood, H. (1990) *Treating Drug Problems Volume 1: A Study of the evolution, effectiveness and financing of public and private drug treatment systems.* Washington DC: National Academic Press.

Hedrich, D. (2000) *Problem Drug Use by Women: focus on community-based interventions.* Strasbourg: Pompidou Group, Council of Europe Publishing.

Klee, H. (1998) *Health Care Delivery to Pregnant Drug Users.* Presentation to the Pompidou Group Symposium: Pregnancy and Drug Misuse 1997 Proceedings, Strasbourg.

Kumpfer, K.L. (1998) Links between prevention and treatment for drug-abusing women and their children, in: C.L. Wetherington and A.B. Roman (eds) Drug Addiction Research and the Health of Women. National Institute on Drug Abuse, Washington DC: Government Printing Office.

Lawrence, S. (2000) Models of primary care for substance misusers: St Martins Practice, Chapeltown, Leeds – secondary provision in a primary care setting. *Drugs: Education, Prevention and Policy* 7, 279–291.

LGDF/SCODA (1997) *Drug-using Parents: policy guidelines for inter-agency working.* London: Local Government Drugs Forum and the Standing Conference on Drug Abuse.

NSW Health (1999) *New South Wales Methadone Maintenance Treatment: clinical practice guidelines.* Publication Number DTS 980181. Sydney: NSW Health Department.

Pompidou Group (1993) *Symposium on Women and Drugs: proceedings.* Strasbourg: Council of Europe Publishing.

Pompidou Group (1995) *Women and Drugs: proceedings of the seminar held in Prague, 1993.* Strasbourg: Council of Europe Publishing.

Pompidou Group (1997) *Symposium on Women and Drugs – focus on prevention 1995 proceedings.* Strasbourg: Council of Europe Publishing.

Pompidou Group (1998) *Symposium on Pregnancy and Drug Misuse 1997 Proceedings.* Strasbourg: Council of Europe Publishing.

Speed, S. and Janikiewicz, S.M.J. (2000) Providing care for drug users on Wirral: a case study analysis of a primary health care/general practice-led drug service. *Drugs: Education, Prevention and Policy* 7, 256–277.

TIP (1993) *Pregnant, Substance-Using Women: Treatment Improvement Protocol (TIP) Series no. 2*. Rockville, MD: Department of Health and Human Services, Center for Substance Abuse Treatment.

TIP (1995) *Improving Treatment for Drug Exposed Infants*: *Treatment Improvement Protocol (TIP) Series no. 5,* Publication No. 95–3057. Rockville, MD: Department of Health and Human Services, Center for Substance Abuse Treatment.

UK Government Cm 2846 (1995) *Tackling Drugs Together: a strategy for England 1995–1998*. London: HMSO.

UK Government Cm 3945 (1998) *Tackling Drugs to Build a Better Britain: the government's 10-year strategy for tackling drug misuse*. London: HMSO.

UNDCP (1994) *Women and Drug Abuse: a position paper*. Vienna: United Nations Drugs Control Programme.

Wan, L. and Sunjic, S. (1998) *Report on Perinatal Use of Drugs of Dependence and Birth Outcomes*. Sydney: SW Sydney Area Health Authority, Drugs and Pregnancy Service.

Working Together to Safeguard Children (1999) Department of Health, Home Office, Department for Education and Employment, London: The Stationery Office. www.doh.gov.uk/pub/doh/safeguard.pdf

Notes

1 Women, family and drugs

1   Established in 1974 the National Institute on Drug Abuse is part of the United States National Institutes of Health, Department of Health and Human Services and claims to have supported over 85 per cent of the world's research on the health aspects of drug misuse and addiction. A part of its mission is to disseminate widely and rapidly research information to policy makers and practitioners. It has a large and user-friendly web site with a search facility: http://www.nida.nih.gov/NIDA

13 Child protection: social workers' views

1   Every local authority in the UK has responsibility for the establishment and effective functioning of an Area Child Protection Committee (ACPC). ACPCs include members from each of the main agencies responsible for working together to safeguard children, who can contribute to developing and maintaining strong and effective inter-agency child protection protocols, and ensure that local child protection services are adequately resourced. It is the multi-agency forum which acts as a focal point for co-operation to safeguard children.

20 Drugs policy and practice development in the United Kingdom

1   The Pompidou group is a multi-disciplinary, intergovernmental body comprising thirty-one member states in Europe. Set up in 1971 by the French President at that time, it was incorporated into the Council of Europe in 1980. Its aims are to 'stimulate the exchange of knowledge and experience between policy makers, professional groups and researchers on drug-related issues, policies and programmes'. For information: http://www.pompidou.coe.int

Index

abortion 49, 50–1, 186, 277
abstinence: desirability 276; motivation
54–5, 150; partners 94–5; pregnancy
78, 80–6, 88, 230–1; structure of day
268; success 167, 191–2; *see also*
detoxification; relapse
abuse: drug users' own childhood 5,
177; sexual 19; use of word 199; *see
also* child protection
adolescents, drug use 10
adoption, unborn child 51
advocacy 75, 294
aggression, amphetamines 153–4
AIDS *see* HIV
alcohol: foetal alcohol syndrome 218;
US child welfare 278–9; use in
pregnancy 245, 252
alternative therapies 234, 280
ambivalence, motherhood 38–9, 146–7
amphetamines: anorectics 7; case
studies 183–90; coping with stress
185; effect on pregnancy outcomes
255; increasing energy 53; injecting
186; irritability 153–4; mental health
188; OTC 6; parents' assessment of
harm 148–9, 155; preferences 18;
pregnancy 80–1, 120; reduction 184;
relapse 166
antenatal care 63–76; care plan 230–5;
clinics 226–8; collaboration 75–6,
232; confidentiality 74; doctors'
attitudes 105–7; Glasgow 250–60;
information 69–70, 71–3; initial
assessment 228–30; judgemental
attitudes 65–7, 241; late presentation
67, 106; Liverpool 224–36;
Manchester 239–48; non-attendance
63–8, 106, 226–7, 239–40, 245;

procedures 257; specialist health
visitors 235–6; users' evaluation
73–5; *see also* drug liaison midwives;
midwives
Area Child Protection Committees
(ACPCs), UK 208, 298
'at risk' register 179, 181, 187, 203–4
audit, Manchester maternity services
241
Australia, policy and practice 287

babies *see* foetal; infants
barriers, professionals and drug users
63–75, 105–7, 263–75
benefits, welfare state reforms 200–2
benzodiazepines: detoxification 235,
255; hospital 246; Neonatal
Abstinence Syndrome 217–18,
220–1, 253; pregnancy 80; prescribed
6, 20; substitute prescription 255
biphasic withdrawal 220–1
blame, by professionals 68, 135, 263
bonding process: disruption 134, 140,
142, 143, 263; importance 146–7,
150, 269–70
boredom 192
breast feeding 71–2, 120–1, 247–8, 258

camouflage techniques 280
cannabis use 133, 153–4, 166, 192
caring concepts 36–7
CASA *see* National Center on
Addiction and Substance Abuse
case studies 177–94, 227–8
CDT *see* Community Drug Teams
changing lifestyle 54–5, 149–50, 276–7
child abuse, drug users' own history
177

child protection 195–209, 276–83; Area
    Child Protection Committee 298;
    case conferences 236, 294–5; case
    study 187–8; drug workers' views
    272; guidelines 290, 295; ideology
    196–200; Liverpool Pregnancy
    Support Group 232, 235–7;
    minimising risks 276, 277–8; parents'
    fears 58–9, 110, 114, 169, 195–6,
    271; public enquiries 196–8;
    recommendations 208–9; registration
    179, 181, 187, 203–4; sharing
    information 233, 273; social workers'
    views 114, 202–7
childcare: service access 23, 26, 282,
    288, 292; working mothers 37–8
children: accidentally consuming drugs
    109, 160, 239; awareness of drugs
    159, 161, 270; disease transmission
    4; environment risks 148, 156–61;
    giving up custody voluntarily 173,
    180; long term effects 8, 161–2;
    maternal influence 39–40, 152–4;
    neglect 5, 8–9, 113, 154–5; positive
    influence 95–6, 185, 191, 268; public
    enquiries 196–7; relationship with
    mother 109, 153–4, 159, 185, 188–9;
    risks 109, 148, 156–61; role
    modelling 157–8; single-parent
    families 7–8; standards of care
    179–80, 185, 190; supporting mother
    158–9; taking drugs 148
Children Act (1989) 201
cigarettes 65, 80, 170, 252
'Cinderella syndrome' 159
clinics see antenatal care; drug
    treatment services
cocaine 186, 190–3, 214–15, 217, 235,
    253
colic 146
collaboration see inter-agency working;
    liaison; multi-disciplinary approach;
    shared care
collusion, Liverpool Drug Dependency
    Unit 233
communication: between agencies
    272–4, 291–2, 295; breakdown 264;
    Liverpool Drug Dependency Unit
    236; multi-disciplinary meetings 226,
    258–9
Community Drug Teams (CDT) 115,
    117
compliance 70, 264

concealment: from children 156–8, 159,
    161; from families 100, 132, 139,
    171, 265; from hospital 64–5, 129
conception, drug effects 79
confidentiality: antenatal care 74; child
    protection issues 204, 273; drug
    workers 110; hospitals 247; inter-
    agency co-operation 272–4; Liverpool
    Drug Dependency Unit 233; post
    natal wards 131–2; professional
    collaboration 115, 116–17; Special
    Care Baby Units 138–40, 265
confinement 127–44
contraception 236, 244, 259, 277
cot death, worries 151
counselling: blood-borne diseases 251;
    couples 25; HIV 251; illicit drug use
    232–3; maternity services 243;
    Neonatal Abstinence Syndrome 231
crime, funding drugs 181, 186–8
crisis intervention 240, 245
'culture of dependency', welfare state
    reforms 200–2

delivery see labour
dental care 257
depression: after birth 147, 178, 184–5,
    236; improving 182; new mothers
    47–8; prozac 6, 184–5; relationship
    with partner 168; risks 152–3
detoxification 83–4, 88, 188, 233–5,
    246, 254–5; see also abstinence
diazepam see benzodiazepines
discrimination by professionals 66–7,
    135, 196, 241, 263–5
diseases see hepatitis; HIV
doctors: attitudes 105–7, 109, 113,
    272–3; discharging babies 142;
    prescribing drugs 6–7
Drug Action Teams 289
Drug Dependency Unit, Liverpool
    225–37
drug liaison midwives 115–16, 138,
    143, 239–48, 291–2, 294
drug management in pregnancy 52–5,
    68, 78–91, 253–6, 266; see also
    methadone
drug screening tests 232, 233, 241, 246
drug treatment services: attracting
    women 277; barriers 21;
    collaboration 75–6, 115–18, 138,
    142, 143; family therapy 280–1;
    gender differences 20–7; outcomes

23; pregnancy 224–38, 244–5,
250–60; social context 25
drug workers: advocacy 75, 294;
attitude to hospitals 117; attitudes to
women 108, 109–11; breast feeding
71–2; child protection views 272;
counselling 279; methadone use
88–90; sharing information 272–4;
social workers relationship 115, 117;
supporting women 75, 172; treating
couples 267

economic exclusion 7–8, 199, 201, 250
ecstasy 186
education see training
environmental risks 82, 156–61, 187,
235, 268
erratic drug use 179–81, 188–9, 252
Europe 5, 287–8, 298

families: division of labour 33;
dysfunction 7–11, 101, 267; family
therapy 280–1; single-parent 7–8,
40–1; support 21, 56–7, 179, 180,
183–4
fathers 33, 40; see also partners;
stepfathers
fear, of professionals 58–9, 110, 114,
169, 195–6, 271
female workers, drug treatment services
24
fertility 79, 277
financing drug habit 181, 186–8, 190,
206
Finnegan neonatal abstinence score 214,
216
fluoxetine see Prozac
foetal alcohol syndrome 218
foetal drug effects 4, 78, 133, 252, 253,
257
friends 86, 171–2, 192
funding, specialist maternity services
241, 244

gender differences, drug use and
services 15–20
Glasgow Women's Reproductive Health
Service 240, 250–60, 292
good intentions 162, 166
'good mother' concept 34–5, 61, 108,
185–6, 264
good practice 239–60, 263, 281–2,
291–4

government guidelines 286–91
grandmothers see mothers (of drug
users)
guilt 35, 38–9, 49, 68, 101, 147

health professionals: attitudes 65–71,
105–22, 137–8, 241, 272–3; drug
knowledge and training 119–22; drug
users policy 240; guidance 245;
inconsistent advice 71–2, 84–5,
88–91, 110, 266
health visitors 172–4, 204–5, 225, 228,
235–6, 270
hepatitis 4, 245, 257, 258
Hepburn, Mary 240, 293
heroin use: attitudes 188–9; case
studies 188–9, 190–3; effects on
family 152–3; infant health 137,
141; Neonatal Abstinence
Syndrome 214–15; in pregnancy
79–80
HIV: antenatal testing 52, 66, 241, 245,
257; breast feeding 258; drug
injection 3; hospital precautions
65–6, 139; risks to children 161;
transmission 4
home environment 82, 156–61, 187,
235, 268
hospitals: confidentiality 131–2,
138–40; confinement 127–44; early
discharge 113, 128–9, 141–2, 247;
in-patient detoxification 234–5, 246,
254, 256; infant care 216–21, 247–8;
inter-agency collaboration 115–17;
length of stay 141–3; limited
resources 140, 144–5; medication
130–1, 246–7; mothers' attitudes
127–8; see also Special Care Baby
Units
housekeeping 58–9, 154–5
housing 187, 235–6

inconsistent advice 71–2, 84–5, 88–91,
110, 266
inebriation, risks 154, 156
infants: crying 135, 136–7, 145–6,
165; effects on mother 145–7;
health 133–41; hospital care 140–1,
247–8; observation on ward 247;
perinatal mortality 252; withdrawal
see Neonatal Abstinence
Syndrome
infections see hepatitis; HIV

information: antenatal care 69–70, 71–3; inconsistent 71–2, 84–5, 88–91; leaflets 245

injecting drugs: pregnancy 80, 97, 186, 230; relapse 166; relationship with partner 168; risks to children 156–7, 161; sexual partnerships 20; stigma 67; vein problems 257

inter-agency working: child protection 194–5, 202, 205–9; communication 191–2, 272–4, 295; guidelines 289–90; maternity services/drug services 75–6, 115–18, 138, 243, 259, 290–1

international perspective 285–8

irritability, amphetamines 153–4

judgemental attitudes 66–7, 135, 198–9, 241, 264–5

labour 129–30, 246–7, 252, 258

lefexidrine 234

legislation 4

LGDF see Local Government Drugs Forum

liaison see collaboration; communication; drug liaison midwives; inter-agency working

Liverpool: Neonatal Abstinence Syndrome care 213–21; Pregnancy Support Group 224–38, 292–3

Local Government Drugs Forum (LGDF), UK 289

lone mothers 7–8, 40–1, 54

low birth weight 215, 252

Manchester specialist maternity services 239–48

maternity services: drug specialists 224–38, 239–48, 250–60; see also antenatal care; hospitals

meconium aspiration 252

menstrual abnormalities 78

mental health problems 79, 152–6

mental health services 20, 244

methadone use: abstinence 83–6, 88–90, 233–5; advantages 254; after birth 166, 170, 178–9, 191; antenatal care 66, 68; case history 177–83; conflicting advice 71–2, 84–5, 88–91, 110, 266; detoxification 234–5; dosage 214, 231, 266; effect on foetus 110–11; gender differences 23;

half-life 254; hospitals 130–1, 246; independent dosage change 86–7, 266; infant withdrawal 137, 141; pregnancy 82–91, 191, 231, 253–4; reduction 82–7, 134, 137, 152, 234–5, 254–5; stabilizing drug levels 89, 254; tolerance 181

methylphenidate 7

midwives: attitudes 65, 67–8, 111–13; breast feeding 71; drug liaison 115–16, 138, 143, 239–48, 291–2, 294; experience of drug users 292; giving information 72–3; labour wards 129–30; methadone use 85, 88–9, 110–11; post-natal wards 128, 130–2, 135, 140; specialist 225

miscarriage 85, 110

models: maternity services 224–38, 239–48, 250–60, 291–4; motherhood 60–1

morphine 134, 141

motherhood 32–42, 125–210; ambivalence 38–9, 146–7; blaming culture 39–41; 'good mothers' 34–5; models 60–1, 151; natural instincts 32–4; positive aspects 149–50; responsibilities 36–7; social construction 37–8, 145; working mothers 35

mothers (of drug users): concealing drug use 100, 131–2, 139, 171; getting custody of children 170–1; influence 60–1; lack of support 151; relationship breakdown 101–2, 185; support 50, 56, 99–102, 170, 183–4, 191–3

motivation: help-seeking behaviour 22; methadone reduction 254–5

multi-disciplinary approach 224–38, 265, 274, 288; see also inter-agency working; shared care

naltrexone 234

NAS see Neonatal Abstinence Syndrome

National Center on Addiction and Substance Abuse (CASA) 278–9

National Institute on Drug Abuse (NIDA), US 280, 298

neglect, children and home 5, 8–9, 113, 154–5

Neonatal Abstinence Syndrome (NAS) 133–7, 213–21; after discharge 113,

147, 217–18; assessment 216–17, 218, 219, 247; before birth 252; benzodiazepines 235; breast feeding 71–2, 247–8; diagnosis 134, 135; effects on mother 165, 178; Finnegan scoring 214, 216; guidance for parents 245, 270–1; Liverpool Pregnancy Support Group 231; long term effects 134, 160; mothers' uncertainty 68, 84, 135; precautions 134, 142; prediction 84, 133, 136–7, 214–15; relapse 165; symptoms 216, 252–3; time course 217–18; treatment 121, 140–1, 218–21
Neonatal Intensive Care Units *see* Special Care Baby Units
neonatal opiate withdrawal *see* Neonatal Abstinence Syndrome
NHS and Community Care Act (1990) 201

opiate use *see* heroin use; methadone use
outreach activities 242
over the counter (OTC) drugs 6–7
over-protectiveness 269

pacdiatricians, attitudes 109, 113, 272–3
pain relief, labour 246–7
parent–child relationship 109, 153–4, 159, 185, 188–9
ParentCraft instruction 237, 257, 259, 271
parenting capacity: drug users' views 52–3, 55–6, 150; lack of information 270–1; practitioners' views 108–9, 204–5, 206–7, 208, 241, 247; recognition 283; skills training 161, 237, 257, 259; social workers support 269; studies 162
partners: approaching services 227; attitude to pregnancy 49–50; bad influences 188–9; couple counselling 25; drug use reduction 82, 94–7, 168–70; evaluation of couple 267; gender differences 19–20, 21; ignorance of mothers' drug use 139; mothers' relapsing 168–70; in prison 95, 99, 179–81; separation 98–9, 180–2, 185, 187–8; supplying drugs 96; support 94–9, 167–8, 178–9, 182, 191–2, 277–8
perinatal mortality 252

physical environment 160–1, 187, 268
physiology 18–19
placenta 78, 252
political/economic factors in drug use 200–2
polydrug use 214–15, 217–18, 220–1, 235, 253
Pompidou Group 287–8, 298
postnatal wards: confidentiality 131–2; diagnosing Neonatal Abstinence Syndrome 216; medication 130–1; treating babies 140–1
poverty 9, 200–1, 206; *see also* economic exclusion
pregnancy: continuing 49–51; early months 78, 79–82; emotional preparation 47–61; late recognition 52, 78, 79, 183; optimism 55–6; partner's attitude 49, 50; planning 49, 277; testing 226; *see also* antenatal care
Pregnancy Support Group (PSG), Liverpool 224–38, 292–3
prcmature birth 133, 151, 165, 215, 251, 252, 253
prostitution 4, 241–2, 257
Prozac 6, 184–5
PSG *see* Pregnancy Support Group

recreational drug use 186
referrals, specialist maternity services 226, 227, 243, 245, 251, 292–3
rehabilitation 190–3
relapse 54–5, 165–75, 255, 268, 276–7, 279
relocation, importance 187, 268
reproductive health care, non-pregnant drug users 244, 251, 259
role modelling, children 157–8

SCBU *see* Special Care Baby Units
SCODA *see* Standing Conference on Drug Abuse
self-esteem 24, 145, 150, 248
self-referral, specialist maternity services 226, 227, 245, 251, 259, 292–3
sexual abuse 19
sexual behaviour 4, 18, 25
shared-care 232, 236–7, 274, 288, 289–90, 295
siblings, drug users 101, 183–4
single-parent families 7–8, 40–1, 54

skill building 280–1
smoking *see* cannabis; cigarettes
social attitudes 3–6, 39–41, 198
social environment 19–20, 25, 156–60, 168–72, 268
social exclusion 7–8, 199, 201, 250
social services: assessing families 151; attitudes of mothers 57–9; 'culture of dependency' 201; disagreement between professionals 207–9; Glasgow 258–9; guidelines 289; ideology 196–202; Liverpool 224–5, 232; moral character judgements 198–9; recommendations 208–9; society's expectations 198; support versus child protection 199–200, 202, 207–8
social workers: advocacy 294; attitudes to mothers 4–5, 10–11, 108, 113–15, 278; case studies 180, 181–2, 189; changing perspectives 196–202, 207–9; child protection views 202–7; early involvement 293; fear of 58–9, 110, 114, 169, 195–6, 271; positive relationship 172–4; professional collaboration 115–18; proscribed roles 201
Special Care Baby Units (SCBU): automatic admission policy 137, 143–4, 240, 241, 245; bonding 134, 140, 143, 269–70; confidentiality 138–40, 265; disadvantages 121; fear of 68, 240, 247; length of stay 135; misuse 143–4; mothers' attitudes 134, 137, 139–40; staff attitudes 137–8; visiting 136, 140, 142–3
Specialist Drug Service, Liverpool 224–38
specialist maternity services: Glasgow 240, 250–60; Liverpool 224–38; Manchester 239–48
Standing Conference on Drug Abuse (SCODA), UK 289
stepfathers 187
stereotypes 33, 39–41, 264, 279, 295
stigmatisation 5–6, 21, 40–1
still birth 252
street drugs: effect on family 162; infant health 137; new mothers 147–8; pregnancy 78, 79–82, 88, 89, 95, 97–8; relapse 166–7
stress: hospital confinement 127–8; increased need for drugs 53–4;

motherhood 36; new baby 47, 145–6, 148, 166
substitution therapy: non-opiate users 255; *see also* methadone use
suicide attempts 19
support: early months 172–5; from children 158–9; from families 21, 56–7, 179, 180, 183–4; from friends 86, 171–2, 192; from mothers (of drug users) 50, 56, 99–102, 170, 183–4, 191–3; from partners 94–9, 167–8, 178–9, 182, 191–2, 277–8; from professional 55, 57–9, 75, 88–91, 172–4; needs 56–7, 93–103

'telescoping' drug-using careers 18–19
temazepam *see* benzodiazepines
teratogenesis, drug use 252, 257
termination (abortion) 49, 50–1, 186, 277
tobacco 65, 80, 170, 252
training: child protection issues 208, 236; drug use issues 119–22, 236, 245, 267, 279, 280; health professionals 243–4, 264–5; HIV issues 243, 245; needs 115, 241; parenting skills 161, 237, 257, 259; pregnancy issues 245; skill building for drug users 280–1
travel issues 23, 26, 282, 288, 292
Treatment Improvement Protocols (TIP), US 286
trust: between agencies 295; of health professionals 114, 116, 122, 242–3
'turkey' *see* Neonatal Abstinence Syndrome; withdrawal

ultrasound scans 257
unemployment 8, 9, 200–1
United Kingdom, policy and practice 9, 285, 288–95
United Nations, *Women and Drug Abuse* paper 283
United States of America; attitudes to drug-using mothers 278; child protection 278–80; National Institute on Drug Abuse 298; policy and practice 286; public opinion 4–5
urine tests 232, 233, 241, 246

violence: effects on women 5, 19, 25; from partners 181, 182, 188, 227; towards health professionals 228
viruses *see* hepatitis; HIV

welfare *see* social services
welfare state reforms 200–2
withdrawal: benzodiazepines 255; 'cold turkey' detoxification 254; depression 152–3; opiate users 53–4; *see also* Neonatal Abstinence Syndrome
women-only groups 24
Women's Reproductive Health Service (WRHS), Glasgow 240, 250–60, 292
working mothers 35, 37–8

working together *see* inter-agency working; liaison; multi-disciplinary approach; shared-care
Working Together guidelines (1991) 202
WRHS *see* Women's Reproductive Health Service

Zion Community Health and Resource Centre, Manchester, steering group 239–42